Clinical Utility of Applying PGx and Deprescribing-Based Decision Support in Polypharmacy: Future Perspectives

Clinical Utility of Applying PGx and Deprescribing-Based Decision Support in Polypharmacy: Future Perspectives

Editors

Charlotte Vermehren
Niels Westergaard

MDPI • Basel • Beijing • Wuhan • Barcelona • Belgrade • Manchester • Tokyo • Cluj • Tianjin

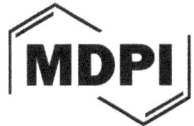

Editors
Charlotte Vermehren
University of Copenhagen
Department of Drug Design
and Pharmacology
Copenhagen
Denmark

Niels Westergaard
Centre for Nursing
University College Absalon
Roskilde
Denmark

Editorial Office
MDPI
St. Alban-Anlage 66
4052 Basel, Switzerland

This is a reprint of articles from the Special Issue published online in the open access journal *Pharmaceuticals* (ISSN 1424-8247) (available at: www.mdpi.com/journal/pharmaceuticals/special_issues/polypharmacy_perspectives).

For citation purposes, cite each article independently as indicated on the article page online and as indicated below:

LastName, A.A.; LastName, B.B.; LastName, C.C. Article Title. *Journal Name* **Year**, *Volume Number*, Page Range.

ISBN 978-3-0365-5162-3 (Hbk)
ISBN 978-3-0365-5161-6 (PDF)

© 2022 by the authors. Articles in this book are Open Access and distributed under the Creative Commons Attribution (CC BY) license, which allows users to download, copy and build upon published articles, as long as the author and publisher are properly credited, which ensures maximum dissemination and a wider impact of our publications.

The book as a whole is distributed by MDPI under the terms and conditions of the Creative Commons license CC BY-NC-ND.

Contents

About the Editors vii

Preface to "Clinical Utility of Applying PGx and Deprescribing-Based Decision Support in
Polypharmacy: Future Perspectives" ix

Carlotta Lunghi, Caterina Trevisan, Michele Fusaroli, Valentina Giunchi, Emanuel Raschi
and Elisa Sangiorgi et al.
Strategies and Tools for Supporting the Appropriateness of Drug Use in Older People
Reprinted from: *Pharmaceuticals* **2022**, *15*, 977, doi:10.3390/ph15080977 1

Robin Brünn, Dorothea Lemke, Jale Basten, Petra Kellermann-Mühlhoff, Juliane
Köberlein-Neu and Christiane Muth et al.
Use of an Electronic Medication Management Support System in Patients with Polypharmacy
in General Practice: A Quantitative Process Evaluation of the AdAM Trial
Reprinted from: *Pharmaceuticals* **2022**, *15*, 759, doi:10.3390/ph15060759 17

Armando Silva-Almodóvar and Milap C. Nahata
Clinical Utility of Medication-Based Risk Scores to Reduce Polypharmacy and Potentially
Avoidable Healthcare Utilization
Reprinted from: *Pharmaceuticals* **2022**, *15*, 681, doi:10.3390/ph15060681 37

Dagmar Abelone Dalin, Sara Frandsen, Gitte Krogh Madsen and Charlotte Vermehren
Exploration of Symptom Scale as an Outcome for Deprescribing: A Medication Review Study
in Nursing Homes
Reprinted from: *Pharmaceuticals* **2022**, *15*, 505, doi:10.3390/ph15050505 47

Tanja Stenholdt Andersen, Mia Nimb Gemmer, Hayley Rose Constance Sejberg, Lillian
Mørch Jørgensen, Thomas Kallemose and Ove Andersen et al.
Medicines Reconciliation in the Emergency Department: Important Prescribing Discrepancies
between the Shared Medication Record and Patients' Actual Use of Medication
Reprinted from: *Pharmaceuticals* **2022**, *15*, 142, doi:10.3390/ph15020142 61

Katja S. Just, Catharina Scholl, Miriam Boehme, Kathrin Kastenmüller, Johannes M. Just and
Markus Bleckwenn et al.
Individualized versus Standardized Risk Assessment in Patients at High Risk for Adverse Drug
Reactions (The IDrug Randomized Controlled Trial)–Never Change a Running System?
Reprinted from: *Pharmaceuticals* **2021**, *14*, 1056, doi:10.3390/ph14101056 75

Anne Byriel Walls, Anne Kathrine Bengaard, Esben Iversen, Camilla Ngoc Nguyen, Thomas
Kallemose and Helle Gybel Juul-Larsen et al.
Utility of suPAR and NGAL for AKI Risk Stratification and Early Optimization of Renal Risk
Medications among Older Patients in the Emergency Department
Reprinted from: *Pharmaceuticals* **2021**, *14*, 843, doi:10.3390/ph14090843 89

Akshaya Srikanth Bhagavathula, Mohammed Assen Seid, Aynishet Adane, Eyob
Alemayehu Gebreyohannes, Jovana Brkic and Daniela Fialová
Prevalence and Determinants of Multimorbidity, Polypharmacy, and Potentially Inappropriate
Medication Use in the Older Outpatients: Findings from EuroAgeism H2020 ESR7 Project
in Ethiopia
Reprinted from: *Pharmaceuticals* **2021**, *14*, 844, doi:10.3390/ph14090844 105

Liv S. Thiele, Kazi Ishtiak-Ahmed, Janne P. Thirstrup, Esben Agerbo, Carin A. T. C. Lunenburg and Daniel J. Müller et al.
Clinical Impact of Functional CYP2C19 and CYP2D6 Gene Variants on Treatment with Antidepressants in Young People with Depression: A Danish Cohort Study
Reprinted from: *Pharmaceuticals* **2022**, *15*, 870, doi:10.3390/ph15070870 . . . . **117**

Niels Westergaard, Lise Tarnow and Charlotte Vermehren
Comparison of Multidrug Use in the General Population and among Persons with Diabetes in Denmark for Drugs Having Pharmacogenomics (PGx) Based Dosing Guidelines
Reprinted from: *Pharmaceuticals* **2021**, *14*, 899, doi:10.3390/ph14090899 . . . . **133**

Diane Merino, Arnaud Fernandez, Alexandre O. Gérard, Nouha Ben Othman, Fanny Rocher and Florence Askenazy et al.
Adverse Drug Reactions of Olanzapine, Clozapine and Loxapine in Children and Youth: A Systematic Pharmacogenetic Review
Reprinted from: *Pharmaceuticals* **2022**, *15*, 749, doi:10.3390/ph15060749 . . . . **147**

Henok D. Habtemariam and Henk-Jan Guchelaar
The Potential Application of Extracellular Vesicles from Liquid Biopsies for Determination of Pharmacogene Expression
Reprinted from: *Pharmaceuticals* **2022**, *15*, 252, doi:10.3390/ph15020252 . . . . **175**

Jens Borggaard Larsen and Steffen Jørgensen
Simple and Robust Detection of *CYP2D6* Gene Deletions and Duplications Using *CYP2D8P* as Reference
Reprinted from: *Pharmaceuticals* **2022**, *15*, 166, doi:10.3390/ph15020166 . . . . **187**

Lisanne E. N. Manson, Wilbert B. van den Hout and Henk-Jan Guchelaar
Genotyping for HLA Risk Alleles to Prevent Drug Hypersensitivity Reactions: Impact Analysis
Reprinted from: *Pharmaceuticals* **2021**, *15*, 4, doi:10.3390/ph15010004 . . . . **201**

About the Editors

Charlotte Vermehren

Charlotte Vermehren has many years of experience within pharmaceutical research, development and use of medicines from both the pharmaceutical industry, biotech, the Danish healthcare system, and academia. For the past 10 years, Charlotte has had an intensive focus on rational pharmacotherapy and polypharmacy. She has published approximately 50 scientific papers and holds a PhD in pharmacology from the University of Copenhagen.

Niels Westergaard

Niels Westergaard has more than 25 years of experience from both academia and the pharmaceutical industry within pharmaceutical disciplines, which has provided him with a deep insight into the value chain from early drug discovery to development and marketing of new drugs. He has published more than 60 peer reviewed papers and holds a PhD and DSc –degree from the University of Copenhagen.

Preface to "Clinical Utility of Applying PGx and Deprescribing-Based Decision Support in Polypharmacy: Future Perspectives"

According to the World Health Organization (WHO), polypharmacy is one of the global key challenges for medication today. Polypharmacy is a necessary and important aspect of drug treatment; however, it becomes a challenge when the medication risks outweigh the benefits for an individual patient. Drug–drug interactions and the introduction of prescribing cascades are common features of polypharmacy, which can lead to ineffectiveness and increased risk of adverse drug reactions (ADR). Genes encoding CYP450 isozymes and other drug-related biomarkers have attracted considerable attention as targets for pharmacogenetic (PGx) testing due to their impact on drug metabolism and response. This Special Issue is devoted to explore the status and initiatives taken to improve medication and to reduce ADR in polypharmacy patients. The collection of articles spans many expert areas and disciplines dealing with drug–drug interactions and consequences thereof in therapeutic management, including PK- and PD-profiling; the application of PGx-based guidance and/or decision tools for drug–gene and drug–drug gene interactions; medication reviews; development and application of deprescribing tools; and drivers and barriers to overcome for successful implementation in the healthcare system. We hope by this Special Issue to stimulate to further actions and initiatives to be taken for the benefit of polypharmacy patients. We thank the authors of the individual articles for their creativity and ingenuity and for paving the way forward in developing new tools and approaches to the understanding of polypharmacy.

Charlotte Vermehren and Niels Westergaard
Editors

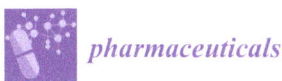

Review

Strategies and Tools for Supporting the Appropriateness of Drug Use in Older People

Carlotta Lunghi [1,2,3,†], Caterina Trevisan [4,†], Michele Fusaroli [1], Valentina Giunchi [1], Emanuel Raschi [1], Elisa Sangiorgi [5], Marco Domenicali [1,2], Stefano Volpato [4], Fabrizio De Ponti [1,2] and Elisabetta Poluzzi [1,2,*]

1 Department of Medical and Surgical Sciences, University of Bologna, 40126 Bologna, Italy
2 Centre of Studies and Research on Older Adults, University of Bologna, 40126 Bologna, Italy
3 Department of Health Sciences, Université du Québec à Rimouski, Lévis, QC G5L 3A1, Canada
4 Department of Medical Sciences, University of Ferrara, 44121 Ferrara, Italy
5 Pharmacy Service, Local Health Authority of Ferrara, 44121 Ferrara, Italy
* Correspondence: elisabetta.poluzzi@unibo.it
† These authors contributed equally to this work.

Abstract: Through this structured review of the published literature, we aimed to provide an up-to-date description of strategies (human-related) and tools (mainly from the digital field) facilitating the appropriateness of drug use in older adults. The evidence of each strategy and tool's effectiveness and sustainability largely derives from local and heterogeneous experiences, with contrasting results. As a general framework, three main steps should be considered in implementing measures to improve appropriateness: prescription, acceptance by the patient, and continuous monitoring of adherence and risk-benefit profile. Each step needs efforts from specific actors (physicians, patients, caregivers, healthcare professionals) and dedicated supporting tools. Moreover, how to support the appropriateness also strictly depends on the particular setting of care (hospital, ambulatory or primary care, nursing home, long-term care) and available economic resources. Therefore, it is urgent assigning to each approach proposed in the literature the following characteristics: level of effectiveness, strength of evidence, setting of implementation, needed resources, and issues for its sustainability.

Keywords: older adults; appropriateness; medication adherence; digital health; adverse drug reactions; polypharmacy

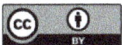

1. Introduction

With the ageing of the population, an increasing proportion of individuals are affected by more than one chronic condition, namely multimorbidity [1]. The treatment of different comorbidities often leads to the use of several medications. Thus, it is not unusual that an increasing proportion of older individuals is exposed to multiple medications, known as polypharmacy. Despite the lack of consensus on polypharmacy definition, researchers more often use this term to indicate the use of five (or ten) medications [2]. A global prevalence of polypharmacy of 32.1% was estimated in Europe when a definition of 5 or more medications was used [3]. Nevertheless, the prevalence of polypharmacy varies not only according to its definition or the type of assessment used but also the country, the setting and patients' age group. Current self-reported prevalence rates in older adults aged 70 years and above from seven European centres ranged from 16.4% (in Geneva) to 60.8% (in Coimbra) [4]. Another study reported prevalence estimates from 26.3% to 39.9%, depending on the country [3]. Different estimates are also reported for Italy: 49% of Italian patients older than 65 received polypharmacy (at least 5 concomitant medications) and 11.3% excessive polypharmacy (at least 10 medications)[5], with a higher prevalence in Southern Italy [6,7].

The aging population and the availability of new medications for chronic conditions can explain the rise in polypharmacy in many developed countries. On the other hand, it is not negligible the impact of the pharmaceutical industry and pharmaceutical sales representatives on the prescribing patterns of physicians. A recent systematic review found that the interaction with the pharmaceutical industry (through its sales representatives) is likely to affect physicians' prescribing behaviours and contribute to the irrational prescribing of different medications [8]. In this context, the concept of pharmaceuticalization has been introduced to emphasize the importance of pharmaceuticals and the pharmaceutical industry in modern life [9]. Pharmaceuticalization can also explain the rising pharmaceutical choices of purchasing and using medications bypassing physicians, through over-the-counter drugs, herbal medicines, supplements or even internet-purchased medications without prescriptions (i.e., opioids or drugs for erectile dysfunction) [10]. Medication-related problems have been exacerbated by the Covid-19 pandemic. Indeed, during the pandemic, physicians and other healthcare professionals were in short supply, and medication reviews and other "non-essential" services were delayed or suspended to reduce the spread of the disease [11,12]. The pandemic has also increased the use and misuse of some medications, such as antidepressants, benzodiazepines, or antipsychotics [13], and increased self-medication behaviours [14].

Despite the variability of polypharmacy estimates and the reasons underlying its rising, it is consistently reported that polypharmacy is associated with increased risk for drug-drug or drug-disease interactions, adverse effects, potentially inappropriate medications (PIMs), geriatric syndrome, falls, and mortality [15,16]. There is generally little guidance in treating multimorbidity in older adults. In Italy, Onder et al. have recently developed specific guidelines for managing individuals exposed to multimorbidity and polypharmacy [17]. These guidelines underline the importance of an individualized and multidisciplinary approach and identifying individuals at higher risk for adverse outcomes of polypharmacy, despite there being no evidence that the number of medications (polypharmacy), rather than inappropriate polypharmacy, is directly responsible for these adverse outcomes. Adverse drug reactions (ADR) are very frequent in geriatric patients: a meta-analysis estimates that ADRs are responsible for 8.7% (95% CI = 7.6–9.8%) of hospital admissions [18]. Non-steroidal anti-inflammatory drugs (NSAIDs) were among the most common classes related to hospital admissions, which ranged from 2.5% to 33.3% in the studies [19]. Other medications implicated in ADRs included beta-blockers (1.8–66.7%), antibiotics (1.1–22.2%), oral anticoagulants (3.3 to 55.6%), digoxin (1.6–18.8%), angiotensin-converting enzyme inhibitors (5.5–23.4%), oral antidiabetics (4.5–22.2%), and opioids (1.5–18.8%). Risk factors for ADR-related hospitalizations included the number of medications (in all the studies analyzing this variable), the number of comorbidities, female sex, age, and inappropriate medications. Therefore, reducing the number of prescriptions in older adults might improve health and reduce hospitalization and mortality [20,21]. In this context, interventions, strategies, and tools to minimize the iatrogenic risks for multimorbid older patients by reducing the number of drugs they take are strongly recommended.

In this paper, we aimed to give an up-to-date description of the strategies and tools supporting the appropriateness of drug use in older adults.

2. Diagnosis And Medical Prescription In Older Adults

The care pathways of older patients may substantially differ from those of their younger counterparts with the same disease, especially considering treatment options and choices. This is because the focus of geriatric medicine does not lie on the disease but on the whole individual. The main goal is not just the treatment of a pathologic condition but the maintenance as much as possible of self-sufficiency, social participation, and quality of life. Therefore, as recommended by the Italian guidelines for managing people with multimorbidity and polypharmacy, physicians should consider these patients' health trajectories, needs, and preferences and set realistic therapeutic targets [17,22]. After diagnosis, the medical prescription process is primarily driven by the need to avoid the disease's clinical manifestations and complications, including its interactions with coexistent conditions and pharmacologic therapies. This means that physicians should adjust the clinical recommendations reported in the guidelines for single diseases to each patient's characteristics. A further crucial point concerns the need for a frequent re-evaluation of the ongoing treatment appropriateness. Indeed, since older individuals frequently have unstable health trajectories, single therapies' risk/benefit ratios may vary with the changes in clinical conditions. Close follow-up assessments may also allow physicians to question the current patients' needs and treatment goals and consider the introduction, maintenance, or discontinuation of different treatments [17]. Hospitalization is a delicate moment in the management of drug therapy in older adults. Mucalo et al. describe that nearly one-third of patients have a potentially inappropriate prescription at discharge [23]. In geriatric units, performing a medication review may reduce the number of potentially inappropriate prescriptions (PIPs) and the risk of iatrogenic events [24]. The experience of a German university hospital showed that the number of PIP observed six months after discharge was significantly reduced in patients with at least one in-hospital therapeutic reconciliation. Nevertheless, no difference was found between reconciliation during hospitalization or at discharge [25].

3. Medication Adherence

Once the most appropriate therapeutic approach for the patient is defined, physicians should dedicate adequate efforts and time to inform and share the care plan with the patient, their caregivers (e.g., family members or non-healthcare professionals taking care of an older individual who is sick or not able to take care of themselves), and other healthcare professionals who play a role in their care process. Effective physician-patient interaction is a cornerstone to increasing the patient's comprehension of medical recommendations [26] and facilitating the acceptance of the prescribed therapies. In this regard, extensive literature has evidenced that deep communication between physician and patient on diagnosis and prescriptions with shared decision-making improves adherence to the medical recommendations and short- and medium-term clinical outcomes [27–29]. Previous reports found that around half of the patients discharged from the emergency department would not be able to understand written medical recommendations completely [30–33]. In addition to patients' and caregivers' awareness of the need, role and possible adverse effects of the prescribed recommendations, acceptance may be influenced by other aspects after initiation of the treatment. Among these are the drugs' beneficial effects on disease control and quality of life, the tolerability of the prescribed therapy [34], and the ease of administration in terms of drug formulations and dosage forms [35].

When dealing with older patients, maintaining a high level of adherence to the medical recommendations is still a challenge, especially among those coping with multimorbidity. In this population, previous reports estimated that the prevalence of medication adherence is only around 50% [36]. A crucial moment in the patient's care pathway is represented by the transition between secondary and primary care. Indeed, after hospital discharge, patients and caregivers may experience difficulties following new or modified medical recommendations. In a study comparing treatments prescribed at hospital discharge and those actually taken at home after 48 h in a sample of individuals aged 70 years or older, researchers found discordances in 56% [37].

A crucial enabling factor of medication adherence is interpersonal trust between physician and patient, which is a vital aspect of the patient-physician relationship, particularly for older patients [38,39]. According to Thom et al., low trust in physicians is associated with poorer adherence to medical recommendations, lower satisfaction with care, and diminished symptoms' improvement [40]. Moreover, trusting their physician leads patients to disclose their health-related behaviours, even those they believe are shameful [38]. Qualitative data suggest that patients' trust in general practitioners is crucial to establishing positive beliefs and becoming willing to deprescribe medications after a medication review [41]. Trust in physicians and the pharmaceutical industry seems to have been worsened by the recent Covid-19 pandemic because of the rapid growth in contradictory information on the internet, social media and traditional media [42].

Poor medication adherence is a prevalent problem in older age because geriatric patients have a complex set of risk factors, including the presence of multiple chronic diseases that co-exist with cognitive and functional deficits. It is essential to make older patients or their caregivers able to report possible use of over-the-counter medications, adverse events, and difficulties in following prescription recommendations. Identifying people with potential risk factors for non-adherence would be a key step for prescribers and healthcare providers in order to focus efforts on supporting adherence to medications. For instance, previous reports have observed that the use of over-the-counter medications was influenced by sociodemographic factors (e.g., educational and socioeconomic levels), individual aspects (e.g., health literacy, disease experience), and policies in the local healthcare system [43].

The consequences of non-adherence to medical recommendations can occur in the short- and longer-term. Indeed, poor medication adherence has been associated with scarcer disease control, higher hospitalization needs, lower quality of life and shorter survival [44–47]. In light of the relevance and impact of this factor, several intervention studies have evaluated the best strategies to improve medication adherence in adult and older patients in different settings of care. These concerned educational, pharmacist-led, nurse-led, or reminder/simplification approaches [25,48,49] (see below). However, an integrated multidisciplinary approach with these strategies combined may provide the best solution to promote adherence to medical recommendations in older patients and to positively influence clinically relevant outcomes.

4. Strategies Supporting The Appropriateness Of Medication Use
4.1. Prescriber'S Tools
4.1.1. Lists And Indexes

An appropriate prescription refers to the proper medication treatment for the patient's needs at the correct dose and the required duration. Many well-validated tools for evaluating the appropriateness of medications for older adults exist. A recent systematic review identified all the published tools to guide clinicians in optimizing drug treatment in older adults [50]. The most known are those based on lists of medications that should not be used (or that should be initiated) in older individuals, such as the Beers [51] or the Screening Tool to Alert to Right Treatment (START)/Screening Tool of Older Persons' Prescriptions (STOPP) criteria [52]. These widely used criteria are based on expert consensus processes (i.e., Delphi) and are revised periodically based on new evidence. Many other consensus-based lists of medications have been developed. The majority are based on consensus-based lists of medications to be avoided in older adults (and, sometimes, necessary drugs) [53–58]. The medication appropriateness index (MAI) [59] is based on a list of structured questions (i.e., on the presence of an approved and/or evidence-based indication, an effective dosage, and the lack of duplication), without addressing specific drugs. It is often used during the medication review process. The Fit fOR The Aged (FORTA) list [60] has classified all the medications used to treat chronic diseases in older adults into four classes according to the evidence on the efficacy and safety, and the appropriateness for the age group.

Although many of these lists repose on similar evidence to build classes of medications to avoid in older adults, differences exist, and the prevalence of PIMs may vary widely depending on the tool used. A recent study comparing the European Union Eu(7)-PIM list and Beers and STOPP criteria showed poor concordance among these tools in identifying inpatients exposed to PIMs [61]. Moreover, the applicability in different settings and countries of these tools has been studied only for a few tools, such as Beers and START/STOPP criteria. Many other country-specific criteria have been proposed in recent years to improve applicability to the specific healthcare system, especially because of the absence of specific medications in the country-specific market. Examples in Europe are the REview of potentially inappropriate MEDIcation pr[e]scribing in Seniors (REMEDI[e]S) in France [62], the PRISCUS list in Germany [54], and the NORGEP-NH criteria in Norway [63]. The Eu(7)-PIM list has been developed through a consensus of experts from 7 different European countries (Denmark, Estonia, Finland, France, Netherlands, Spain, and Sweden) with the aim of clinical applicability in Europe. Nevertheless, the applicability of these criteria to all European countries is still limited, especially for the Eastern and Central European Countries [64]. It is, therefore, necessary to define all the better strategies to improve the appropriateness of drug use in older adults according to the specific country but also to the specific care setting. Differences from a regulatory, legal and cultural point of view have to be acknowledged to implement the use of these tools in routine clinical practice.

4.1.2. Medication Review In Team

Although physicians have the main role and responsibility in prescribing medicines, optimization of drug use in older adults needs support from other healthcare professionals, especially for chronic therapies. The medication review process can be split into different steps, and trained nurses and clinical pharmacists may be active in some of these, with well-defined roles (Figure 1). At the discharge from the hospital, as well as after second or primary care access, when patients have to be aware of why, when, how much and how long to use prescribed medicines, both can support physicians in verifying patient and caregiver awareness and therefore in promoting compliance. Again, both professionals can be enrolled in monitoring adherence and some endpoints of the risk-benefit profile during the therapy, even without the direct involvement of the physician, if appropriate local services are arranged.

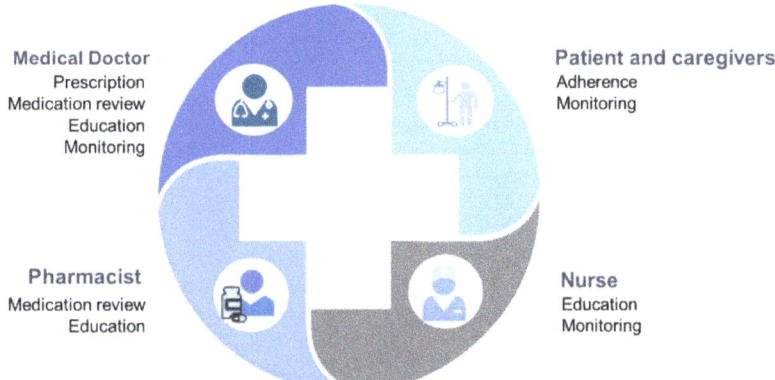

Figure 1. The shared effort toward appropriateness of drug use.

Nevertheless, a crucial point is interprofessional collaboration. General practitioners (GPs) represent most older individuals' principal contact with healthcare professionals, as they regularly monitor symptoms and oversee refilling prescriptions. However, specialists manage patients with chronic diseases and are often in charge of adding or stopping medicines for these conditions without consulting GPs. Many experiences of pharmacist-led service have been described in the literature, and its optimization represents a current challenge. Successful pharmacist interventions are regular consultation (for instance, at the time of prescription refill) for detecting possible drug-drug interactions and adverse drug reactions, strengthening education and the importance of adherence, as well as supporting the use of apps of reminders and, when feasible, providing the patient with personalized pillboxes (see below). Focusing on specific cohorts of patients (e.g., with diabetes or oncological diagnoses) seems to increase the impact on outcomes, especially for process endpoints, as the number of concomitant medications and adherence [65]. Nurse-led initiatives have been especially focused on specific cohorts of patients, for which specialized healthcare professionals are needed: medication self-management training programs for chronic psychiatric treatment and patient-navigator service for oral oncological therapies are currently promising topics [66,67]. The collaboration between GPs, specialists, pharmacists, and nurses enables the effective implementation of medication review in clinical practice. Nonetheless, the opportunity to work as a team for different healthcare professionals involved in the medication review process necessitates adjusting the current clinical practice for shared decision-making. Moreover, the economic sustainability and impact on clinical outcomes of each strategy are not yet strongly demonstrated [68].

4.1.3. Electronic Tools Supporting Appropriate Prescription

Current prescribing practice is frequently supported by electronic tools, which allow doctors to simultaneously include each prescription into the patient's electronic health record and provide them with their receipt. This habit urges specific computerized prescription support systems to help medication review and therapeutic choice, especially for patients with comorbidity and polypharmacy. These systems belong to the larger area of digital health interventions (DHIs), which are technologies facilitating the accomplishment of the health needs of individuals and populations, and include e-Health (e.g., informative websites, educational videogames, telehealth webinars) [69,70], and m-Health (e.g., mobile microsensors, apps to study voice markers) [71].

The potential role of DHIs is broad and not yet fully explored. Many online resources are available for physicians, from authoritative websites, such as deprescribing.org, which provide recommendations, videos and list useful apps for specific therapeutic areas and users, to software with the relevant app for computer or smartphone. They may be used for single cases during the visit or integrated with the electronic chart databases and used to automatically receive a warning on potential inappropriate prescriptions or to process all single patient prescription lists periodically. Some examples of these specific websites are medstopper.com, drugs.com [folder: interaction checker], and intercheckweb.marionegri.it (in Italian). As for integrating DHIs in the electronic chart, a typical example is represented by platforms that document and track patients' therapy and clinical conditions (e-medication history). Some of them put a red flag close to potential interactions and remember to prescribe the investigations for early detection of adverse reactions over the follow-up (e.g., lipidaemia in antipsychotics).

4.1.4. Web Resources on Adverse Reaction Prevention

Concerning side effects of medicines, digital tool development is strongly focused on their prevention and early detection. Drug-induced Torsades de Pointes (TdP) and Drug-Induced Liver Injury (DILI) are among the most frequent causes of drug attrition during drug development and drug withdrawal in the post-marketing setting [72,73]. These adverse drug reactions share several similarities; though erroneously considered idiosyncratic, they actually occur in a dose-dependent manner in subjects with several host- and patient-related risk factors [74,75]. For instance, atrial fibrillation and previous myocardial infarction, which are highly prevalent in older adults, represent typical risk-factor for developing TdP in case of multiple drug treatments with antiarrhythmics, antipsychotics and some specific antimicrobials. Dedicated websites (www.crediblemeds.org, accessed on 27 July 2022; for TdP) and bookshelves (https://www.ncbi.nlm.nih.gov/books/NBK547852/ accessed on 27 July 2022; for DILI) have been implemented to support researchers and prescribers in therapy optimization, namely risk assessment in the individual patient [76].

Notwithstanding these efforts, our understanding, prediction and prevention in clinical practice are still unsatisfactory, especially for DILI, where the mechanistic basis and the *primum movens* are still uncertain. In this scenario, the question arises as to whether digital tools can actually support appropriateness, especially in older adults, or, conversely, are disregarded by clinicians due to alert fatigue.

With regard to TdP, cardio-oncology is an emerging rapidly-evolving area where a proactive medication review should be targeted as a preventive strategy to counteract the so-called reduced repolarization reserve caused by multiple drugs possibly interacting through pharmacokinetic and pharmacodynamic mechanisms [77]. A recent systematic review analyzed the use of risk assessment tools (RATs), including risk scores, computerized physician order entry systems and clinical decision support systems, as a strategy to identify patients at risk of TdP for repetitive or continuous electrocardiogram monitoring, discontinuation of pro-arrhythmic drugs, or serum electrolyte concentration monitoring [78]. The various RATs have peculiarities, including the heterogeneous setting of use and validation (e.g., intensive care units, hospital wards with different specialties). They are still suboptimal in terms of predictive performance, thus making combined use of RATs a candidate approach to reduce unnecessary alerts. Future studies are warranted to verify the potential adaptation in the outpatient setting and assess the actual impact on these DHIs, especially on hard endpoints such as hospitalization.

Regarding DILI, there are no recognized predictive DHIs. The opportunity for a medication review and stringent monitoring of transaminases remains pivotal strategies to reduce the burden of (inappropriate) co-medications and perform a timely diagnosis on a case-by-case basis. In this context, considering DILI diagnosis requires careful exclusion of alternative (non-pharmacological) causes, Hayashi et al. recently updated, simplified and computerized the Roussel Uclaf Causality Assessment Method (RUCAM), a current standard diagnostic algorithm, and developed an electronic evidence-based version, called RECAM, which is a promising user-friendly practice-changing tool also for clinicians without consolidated experience in DILI diagnosis [79]. Although further validation and refinement of criteria are needed, RECAM is an additional step in the era of digital medicine. It can also be implemented by adding pharmacokinetic substantiation to support the underlying pharmacological basis.

4.2. Patient'S Tools
4.2.1. Digital Tools for The Patient

Medicine digitalization also represents an opportunity for the patients. Some DHIs may primarily target the patients or their caregivers, indeed. For example, they may remind the patient that a pill should be taken at a specific time or make more accessible information included in the package insert or the electronic healthcare record. Many new mobile applications focus on monitoring body parameters using microsensors (e.g., physical activity, blood pressure, vocal markers). They may facilitate communications between patients and physicians, for example, reporting suspect adverse reactions, adherence information, and vital signs parameters directly to the electronic healthcare record.

Nonetheless, the heterogeneity and diversity of the available DHIs make their choice difficult for unsupervised patients. In 2021, an extended search of the Apple and Google Play Stores for apps conceived to increase medication adherence found more than 2000 heterogeneous, mostly uncertified, mobile applications [80]. To drive the systematization of digital health, the WHO implemented the classification of digital health interventions (DHIs, version 1.0), distinguishing between different users and functions. However, this classification was targeted at app developers and not the patients, so the difficulties met when choosing a DHI remain.

A second problem concerns the accessibility to older adults: most the DHIs, especially those not specifically designed for older adults, are poorly accessible to them [81]. But digital interventions specifically thought for primary prevention in older adults have been developed, including tools to gather health data for goal planning, video consults and online webinars [70].

In the attempt to drive the development of more accessible and effective interventions, Matthew-Maich et al. performed a scoping review to collect lessons specific for designing, implementing, and evaluating mHealth support for older adults at home and their caregivers [82]. Currently, many DHIs are characterized by low scientific quality and patient appreciation, and Backes et al. concluded that none of the more than 2000 apps investigated should be recommended by health providers [80]. Following accruing lessons –focusing on motivation (goal-setting and rewards), remote help, support by other patients, feedback by healthcare providers, and accessibility (native language and printable material) [70], will plausibly result in higher adherence. In particular, when addressing older adults population, it is of the upmost importance to account for digital inequalities related to sociodemographic gaps, in informatics skills and resources, together with cognitive decline and visual impairment [83].

Another promising option concerns the possibility of developing apps that allow information sharing among different stakeholders, providing role-specific interfaces. The same app, for example, may automatically remind the patients to take their drug, alert the caregiver in case of omission, and show the adherence interpolated with biomarker data in the electronic healthcare record for the physician (e.g., showing the relationship of the blood pressure of the patients and their adherence to antihypertensive drugs). Further, future apps may be personalized based on the patient's health conditions and the setting. For example, for non-compliant patients, it may be advisable to document to the caregiver the drug assumption by recording it on a video.

Finally, it is easier to develop effective interventions if specific populations are targeted, for example, patients with frailty (e.g., cognitive impairment, disability, chronic conditions) [71].

4.2.2. Dose-Dispensing Tools

As mentioned above, poor medication adherence is a common issue for older individuals. Even when the patient has accepted their treatment and the communication between healthcare professionals and the patient is good (see below), unintentional non-adherence may still occur. It occurs indeed when the patients forget to take their medications or they do not well understand the provider's indications [84]. Sometimes, especially in older adults, unintentional non-adherence occurs because of physical, mental, or psychological barriers leading to the inability to manage their treatment [85]. A peculiar problem is the complexity of the therapeutic regimen, a common issue in patients with multimorbidity and polypharmacy.

Dose-dispensing services are especially useful for older patients experiencing unintentional non-adherence [86]. The purpose of dosing aids is thus to assist patients in taking their medications and improve their adherence to medication [87]. These dose-dispensing tools (also known as dosettes or pillboxes) are storage devices for oral medications that also serve as a medication aide-mémoire to remind patients to take their medications at the right time [88,89]. The simplest ones have seven compartments for each day of the week, but they come in different sizes and shapes with subcompartments for different times of the day [87]. They can be filled by physicians, pharmacists, nurses or even by patients themselves or their caregivers [90]. In addition to making medication self-administration easier, these tools can improve unintentional adherence caused by forgetfulness and confusion [91–93]. These services are commonly implemented in hospitals and community pharmacies in many countries In an effort to better support patients, families, and caregivers, with new technologies, new dose-dispensing tools (smart pill dispensers) have been developed to help manage complex pharmacotherapies, such as pillboxes with visual and sound alarms that will alert the user to take the medication at the time it must be taken, or other sending email or notifications if a dose is skipped or taken at the wrong time [94]. Nevertheless, despite new technologies and tools being implemented in recent years, all dose-dispensing services should be subject to a medication review at the beginning and repeated regularly. Moreover, patient communication and coaching should accompany these tools or services with close cooperation among all actors involved in patient care (physicians, nurses, pharmacists, and caregivers) [95]. Table 1 summarizes the main tools available to support the appropriateness of drug utilization in older individuals.

Table 1. Main tools supporting the appropriate drug use.

Tools	Description	Examples
Prescriber's tools		
Lists and indexes	Lists of medications to be or not to be used based on efficacy, safety, and appropriateness; General appropriateness indexes	Beers criteria; START/STOPP * criteria; FORTA * list; REMEDI[e]S *; PRISCUS list; NORGEP-NH criteria; Eu(7)-PIM list; MAI *
Electronic tools	DHIs * providing recommendations, videos, and apps for specific therapeutic areas	www.deprescribing.org, accessed on 27 July 2022
	Websites and bookshelves supporting patients and prescribers in therapy optimization	www.medstopper.com, accessed on 27 July 2022; www.drugs.com, accessed on 27 July 2022 [folder: interaction checker]; www.intercheckweb.marionegri.it, accessed on 27 July 2022
Web resources on adverse drug reactions	Websites and bookshelves supporting patients and prescribers in therapy optimization	www.crediblemeds.org, accessed on 27 July 2022; www.ncbi.nlm.nih.gov/books/NBK547852/, accessed on 27 July 2022
	RATs * and diagnostic algorithms to identify patients at risk for adverse reactions	Risk scores; computerized physician order entry systems; clinical decision support systems; RECAM *
Patient's tools		
Digital tools for the patients	Mobile applications facilitating communications between patients and physicians	Apps reporting suspect adverse reactions, adherence information, and vital signs parameters directly to the electronic healthcare record
	DHIs * helping patients and caregivers adhering to treatment	Apps reminding the patient that a pill should be taken at a specific time; apps making more accessible information included in the package insert
	DHIs * for information sharing among different stakeholders	Apps that remind the patient to take pills, alert the caregiver in case of omission, and show the adherence interpolated with biomarker data in the electronic healthcare record for the physician
Dose-dispensing tools	Dose-dispensing services for patients experiencing unintentional non-adherence	Pillboxes with seven compartments for each day of the week; pillboxes with visual and sound alarms

* DHIs: digital health interventions; FORTA:Fit fOR The Aged; MAI: Medication appropriateness index; RATs: risk assessment tools; RECAM: Revised Electronic Causality Assessment Method; REMEDI[e]S: REview of potentially inappropriate MEDIcation pr[e]scribing in Seniors; START/STOPP: Screening Tool to Alert to Right Treatment/Screening Tool of Older Persons'Prescriptions.

5. Communication between Physician and Patient

As anticipated above, communicating with the patient is the first step to ensuring high adherence to medical recommendations. The term communication comes from Latin, and its original meaning is "to share". In the physician-patient interaction, there is a bidirectional sharing, not only of medical information from the physician to the patient but also of doubts and experiences from the patient to the physician. However, not always adequate attention is paid to this issue in daily clinical practice.

In an interesting study evaluating the interface between physicians and patients, only around 20% of patients had the opportunity to fully explain their concerns. In comparison, in almost 70% of cases, physicians prematurely interrupted the open statement of the patient to direct specific questions [96].

In line with this result, other primary or secondary care studies found that physicians tend to interrupt patients after a median time ranging from 11 to 23 s [97,98]. Conversely, giving them the possibility to fully express their concerns without interruptions would have only taken up to two minutes and given physicians most of the needed information [97]. Although physicians may be reluctant to ask open-ended questions due to limited time to dedicate to the visits, leaving patients free to express their concerns and open statements seems to be the most appropriate strategy and may limit the loss of useful information to drive physicians' diagnosis and treatment choices. Adding leaflets and online educational programs can further improve patient awareness and empowerment.

As far as physician-related factors influencing communication with the patient are concerned, some sociodemographic characteristics have shown to play substantial roles. For instance, in primary and secondary care, female physicians tended to spend approximately two minutes more than men in medical visits and establish a more patient-centered communication [99], with a higher emotional involvement [100]. Ethnicity may be an additional factor influencing some communication aspects. A previous work conducted in the United States found that patients undergoing a medical visit with a physician of the same ethnicity were more satisfied and perceived higher physician participation than those undergoing an ethnicity-discordant visit [101]. The length of work experience might also interfere with the ability to spend enough time with the patient. In a study focused on the communication of bad news to older patients, in fact, physicians with a longer work experience appeared to be more likely to dedicate an adequate amount of time to talk with the patient than those with fewer working years [100].

Considering patient-related factors influencing communication, poor health literacy could affect the comprehension of the medical recommendations. This aspect is particularly important for older people affected by multiple chronic conditions, who often take several drugs. In a study evaluating medication errors reported by patients, almost 80% of the involved patients reported at least one mistake, and in most cases, errors were due to difficulties in identifying the medication or understanding medical instructions. The presence of multiple chronic diseases, multidrug regimens, and changes in medical prescriptions emerged as factors associated with the probability of reporting medication errors [102]. In addition, older patients frequently suffer from conditions that can impair their ability to understand and correctly follow medical recommendations, such as vision or hearing impairments, cognitive deficits, or mobility restrictions [103]. The physician should recognize these problems and adapt the communication style to overcome these possible obstacles to a correct understanding of medical recommendations.

Identifying and acting on the factors that may affect the communication with the patient is of great relevance in consideration of the impact of such aspects on several health-related outcomes. First of all, enhancing communication between patients and healthcare professionals is the key to ensuring that patient preferences are taken into consideration, thereby patient adherence and their experience are improved [104]. This means exposing the patient to a lower risk of having new hospitalizations for unbalances of chronic diseases, poor quality of life and mortality, and reducing the costs for the healthcare systems [44,46,47,105]. A crucial moment to ensure good physician-patient communication is the transition between different care settings, such as hospital discharge. In this context, discrepancies between the usual and new prescribed therapies, in the absence of adequate communication and explanation of the medical recommendations, could predispose to medication errors and poor adherence. Although trials on the effectiveness of educational/behavioural and reminder/simplification interventions have given promising results, further investigations should be devoted to undercover the patients' point of view of communication on medical recommendations, in specific care settings or during transitions between them [106].

6. Conclusions

Physicians, especially geriatricians, strongly agree on the importance of periodic medication reviews and their advantage for the patient in terms of adherence as well as overall health outcomes. It's also established that other healthcare professionals, namely pharmacists and nurses, should be included in the medication review process, maintaining their roles and supporting both patients and prescribers. Digital health interventions represent useful solutions to help professionals identify inappropriate prescriptions and maintain patient adherence to prescribed therapies. The efficacy of every single strategy is far from being well demonstrated, especially in terms of main clinical outcomes and health and economic sustainability. However, the need for integrated strategies is largely shared among physicians, patients and policymakers.

Identifying the most appropriate approach requires defining the specific setting of care (hospital, ambulatory or primary care) and if a particular cohort of patients should be prioritized.

As a general framework, three main steps should be considered in implementing measures to improve appropriateness: prescription, acceptance by the patient, and continuous monitoring of adherence and the risk-benefit profile. Each step needs efforts from specific actors (doctors, patients, caregivers, healthcare personnel) and dedicated supporting tools. Moreover, how to support the appropriateness also strictly depends on the particular setting of care (hospital, ambulatory or primary care) and available economic resources. Therefore, it is urgent assigning to each approach proposed in the literature the following characteristics: level of effectiveness, the strength of evidence, setting of implementation, needed resources, and issues for its sustainability.

Author Contributions: Conceptualization, C.L., C.T. and E.P.; writing—original draft preparation, C.L., C.T., E.R., M.F., M.D. and V.G.; writing—review and editing, E.S., F.D.P., M.D. and S.V. All authors have read and agreed to the published version of the manuscript.

Funding: This research received no external funding.

Institutional Review Board Statement: Not applicable.

Informed Consent Statement: Not applicable.

Data Availability Statement: Not applicable.

Acknowledgments: Research activities of C.L. and V.G. have been supported by funds from The Italian Ministry of University and Research, "PON Ricerca e Innovazione-Istruzione e ricerca per il recupero-REACT-EU". Figure 1 was prepared using a template provided by Infograpia.com.

Conflicts of Interest: The authors declare no conflict of interest.

References

1. Lenzi, J.; Avaldi, V.M.; Rucci, P.; Pieri, G.; Fantini, M.P. Burden of multimorbidity in relation to age, gender and immigrant status: A cross-sectional study based on administrative data. *BMJ Open* **2016**, *6*, e012812. [CrossRef]
2. Sirois, C.; Domingues, N.S.; Laroche, M.L.; Zongo, A.; Lunghi, C.; Guénette, L.; Kröger, E.; Émond, V. Polypharmacy Definitions for Multimorbid Older Adults Need Stronger Foundations to Guide Research, Clinical Practice and Public Health. *Pharmacy* **2019**, *7*, E126. [CrossRef]
3. Midão, L.; Giardini, A.; Menditto, E.; Kardas, P.; Costa, E. Polypharmacy prevalence among older adults based on the survey of health, ageing and retirement in Europe. *Arch. Gerontol. Geriatr.* **2018**, *78*, 213–220. [CrossRef]
4. Molino, C.d.G.R.C.; Chocano-Bedoya, P.O.; Sadlon, A.; Theiler, R.; Orav, J.E.; Vellas, B.; Rizzoli, R.; Kressig, R.W.; Kanis, J.A.; Guyonnet, S.; et al. Prevalence of polypharmacy in community-dwelling older adults from seven centres in five European countries: A cross-sectional study of DO-HEALTH. *BMJ Open* **2022**, *12*, e051881. [CrossRef]
5. Onder, G.; Bonassi, S.; Abbatecola, A.M.; Folino-Gallo, P.; Lapi, F.; Marchionni, N.; Pani, L.; Pecorelli, S.; Sancarlo, D.; Scuteri, A.; et al. High Prevalence of Poor Quality Drug Prescribing in Older Individuals: A Nationwide Report From the Italian Medicines Agency (AIFA). *J. Gerontol. Ser. Biomed. Sci. Med. Sci.* **2014**, *69*, 430–437. [CrossRef]
6. Guerriero, F.; Orlando, V.; Tari, D.U.; Di Giorgio, A.; Cittadini, A.; Trifirò, G.; Menditto, E. How healthy is community-dwelling elderly population? Results from Southern Italy. *Transl. Med. UniSa* **2015**, *13*, 59–64.
7. Valent, F. Polypharmacy in the general population of a Northern Italian area: analysis of administrative data. *Ann. Dell'istituto Super. Sanitá* **2019**, *55*, 233–239. [CrossRef]
8. Fickweiler, F.; Fickweiler, W.; Urbach, E. Interactions between physicians and the pharmaceutical industry generally and sales representatives specifically and their association with physicians' attitudes and prescribing habits: A systematic review. *BMJ Open* **2017**, *7*, e016408. [CrossRef] [PubMed]
9. Bell, S.E.; Figert, A.E. Medicalization and pharmaceuticalization at the intersections: Looking backward, sideways and forward. *Soc. Sci. Med.* **2012**, *75*, 775–783. [CrossRef] [PubMed]

10. Abraham, J. Pharmaceuticalization of Society in Context: Theoretical, Empirical and Health Dimensions. *Sociology* **2010**, *44*, 603–622. [CrossRef]
11. Ailabouni, N.J.; Hilmer, S.N.; Kalisch, L.; Braund, R.; Reeve, E. COVID-19 Pandemic: Considerations for Safe Medication Use in Older Adults with Multimorbidity and Polypharmacy. *J. Gerontol. Ser. A* **2021**, *76*, 1068–1073. [CrossRef] [PubMed]
12. Elbeddini, A.; Prabaharan, T.; Almasalkhi, S.; Tran, C.; Zhou, Y. Barriers to conducting deprescribing in the elderly population amid the COVID-19 pandemic. *Res. Soc. Adm. Pharm.* **2021**, *17*, 1942–1945. [CrossRef] [PubMed]
13. Campitelli, M.A.; Bronskill, S.E.; Maclagan, L.C.; Harris, D.A.; Cotton, C.A.; Tadrous, M.; Gruneir, A.; Hogan, D.B.; Maxwell, C.J. Comparison of Medication Prescribing Before and After the COVID-19 Pandemic Among Nursing Home Residents in Ontario, Canada. *JAMA Netw. Open* **2021**, *4*, e2118441. [CrossRef] [PubMed]
14. Enners, S.; Gradl, G.; Kieble, M.; Böhm, M.; Laufs, U.; Schulz, M. Utilization of drugs with reports on potential efficacy or harm on COVID-19 before, during, and after the first pandemic wave. *Pharmacoepidemiol. Drug Saf.* **2021**, *30*, 1493–1503. [CrossRef] [PubMed]
15. Fried, T.R.; O'Leary, J.; Towle, V.; Goldstein, M.K.; Trentalange, M.; Martin, D.K. Health Outcomes Associated with Polypharmacy in Community-Dwelling Older Adults: A Systematic Review. *J. Am. Geriatr. Soc.* **2014**, *62*, 2261–2272. [CrossRef]
16. Steinman, M.A.; Seth Landefeld, C.; Rosenthal, G.E.; Berthenthal, D.; Sen, S.; Kaboli, P.J. Polypharmacy and Prescribing Quality in Older People: Polypharmacy and prescribing quality. *J. Am. Geriatr. Soc.* **2006**, *54*, 1516–1523. [CrossRef]
17. Onder, G.; Vetrano, D.L.; Palmer, K.; Trevisan, C.; Amato, L.; Berti, F.; Campomori, A.; Catalano, L.; Corsonello, A.; Kruger, P.; et al. Italian guidelines on management of persons with multimorbidity and polypharmacy. *Aging Clin. Exp. Res.* **2022**, *34*, 989–996. [CrossRef]
18. Chisaki, Y.; Aoji, S.; Yano, Y. Analysis of Adverse Drug Reaction Risk in Elderly Patients Using the Japanese Adverse Drug Event Report (JADER) Database. *Biol. Pharm. Bull.* **2017**, *40*, 824–829. [CrossRef]
19. Oscanoa, T.J.; Lizaraso, F.; Carvajal, A. Hospital admissions due to adverse drug reactions in the elderly: A meta-analysis. *Eur. J. Clin. Pharmacol.* **2017**, *73*, 759–770. [CrossRef]
20. Bloomfield, H.E.; Greer, N.; Linsky, A.M.; Bolduc, J.; Naidl, T.; Vardeny, O.; MacDonald, R.; McKenzie, L.; Wilt, T.J. Deprescribing for Community-Dwelling Older Adults: A Systematic Review and Meta-analysis. *J. Gen. Intern. Med.* **2020**, *35*, 3323–3332. [CrossRef]
21. Kua, C.H.; Yeo, C.Y.Y.; Tan, P.C.; Char, C.W.T.; Tan, C.W.Y.; Mak, V.; Leong, I.Y.O.; Lee, S.W.H. Association of Deprescribing With Reduction in Mortality and Hospitalization: A Pragmatic Stepped-Wedge Cluster-Randomized Controlled Trial. *J. Am. Med. Dir. Assoc.* **2021**, *22*, 82–89.e3. [CrossRef] [PubMed]
22. Muth, C.; Blom, J.W.; Smith, S.M.; Johnell, K.; Gonzalez-Gonzalez, A.I.; Nguyen, T.S.; Brueckle, M.S.; Cesari, M.; Tinetti, M.E.; Valderas, J.M. Evidence supporting the best clinical management of patients with multimorbidity and polypharmacy: A systematic guideline review and expert consensus. *J. Intern. Med.* **2019**, *285*, 272–288. [CrossRef] [PubMed]
23. Mucalo, I.; Hadžiabdić, M.O.; Brajković, A.; Lukić, S.; Marić, P.; Marinović, I.; Bačić-Vrca, V. Potentially inappropriate medicines in elderly hospitalised patients according to the EU(7)-PIM list, STOPP version 2 criteria and comprehensive protocol. *Eur. J. Clin. Pharmacol.* **2017**, *73*, 991–999. [CrossRef] [PubMed]
24. Debacq, C.; Bourgueil, J.; Aidoud, A.; Bleuet, J.; Mennecart, M.; Dardaine-Giraud, V.; Fougère, B. Persistence of Effect of Medication Review on Potentially Inappropriate Prescriptions in Older Patients Following Hospital Discharge. *Drugs Aging* **2021**, *38*, 243–252. [CrossRef] [PubMed]
25. Kiesel, E.K.; Drey, M.; Pudritz, Y.M. Influence of a ward-based pharmacist on the medication quality of geriatric inpatients: A before–after study. *Int. J. Clin. Pharm.* **2022**, *44*, 480–488. [CrossRef]
26. Shiber, S.; Zuker-Herman, R.; Drescher, M.J.; Glezerman, M. Gender differences in the comprehension of care plans in an emergency department setting. *Isr. J. Health Policy Res.* **2018**, *7*, 50. [CrossRef]
27. Kerse, N.; Buetow, S.; Mainous, A.G.; Young, G.; Coster, G.; Arroll, B. Physician-patient relationship and medication compliance: A primary care investigation. *Ann. Fam. Med.* **2004**, *2*, 455–461. [CrossRef]
28. Neri, L.; Peris, K.; Longo, C.; Calvieri, S.; Frascione, P.; Parodi, A.; Eibenschuz, L.; Bottoni, U.; Pellacani, G. Physician-patient communication and patient-reported outcomes in the actinic keratosis treatment adherence initiative (AK-TRAIN): A multicenter, prospective, real-life study of treatment satisfaction, quality of life and adherence to topical field-directed therapy for the treatment of actinic keratosis in Italy. *J. Eur. Acad. Dermatol. Venereol.* **2019**, *33*, 93–107. [CrossRef]
29. Hong, S.H. Potential for physician communication to build favorable medication beliefs among older adults with hypertension: A cross-sectional survey. *PLoS ONE* **2019**, *14*, e0210169. [CrossRef]
30. Calkins, D.R.; Davis, R.B.; Reiley, P.; Phillips, R.S.; Pineo, K.L.; Delbanco, T.L.; Iezzoni, L.I. Patient-physician communication at hospital discharge and patients' understanding of the postdischarge treatment plan. *Arch. Intern. Med.* **1997**, *157*, 1026–1030. [CrossRef]
31. Makaryus, A.N.; Friedman, E.A. Patients' understanding of their treatment plans and diagnosis at discharge. *Mayo Clin. Proc.* **2005**, *80*, 991–994. [CrossRef]
32. Samuels-Kalow, M.E.; Stack, A.M.; Porter, S.C. Effective Discharge Communication in the Emergency Department. *Ann. Emerg. Med.* **2012**, *60*, 152–159. [CrossRef] [PubMed]
33. Williams, D.M.; Counselman, F.L.; Caggiano, C.D. Emergency department discharge instructions and patient literacy: A problem of disparity. *Am. J. Emerg. Med.* **1996**, *14*, 19–22. [CrossRef]

34. McInnes, G.T. Integrated approaches to management of hypertension: Promoting treatment acceptance. *Am. Heart J.* **1999**, *138*, S252–S255. [CrossRef]
35. Shariff, Z.B.; Dahmash, D.T.; Kirby, D.J.; Missaghi, S.; Rajabi-Siahboomi, A.; Maidment, I.D. Does the Formulation of Oral Solid Dosage Forms Affect Acceptance and Adherence in Older Patients? A Mixed Methods Systematic Review. *J. Am. Med. Dir. Assoc.* **2020**, *21*, 1015–1023.e8. [CrossRef]
36. World Health Organization. *Adherence to Long-Term Therapies: Evidence for Action*; Sabaté, E., Ed.; World Health Organization: Geneva, Switzerland, 2003.
37. Lindquist, L.A.; Go, L.; Fleisher, J.; Jain, N.; Friesema, E.; Baker, D.W. Relationship of Health Literacy to Intentional and Unintentional Non-Adherence of Hospital Discharge Medications. *J. Gen. Intern. Med.* **2012**, *27*, 173–178. [CrossRef]
38. Baker, R.; Mainous Iii, A.G.; Gray, D.P.; Love, M.M. Exploration of the relationship between continuity, trust in regular doctors and patient satisfaction with consultations with family doctors. *Scand. J. Prim. Health Care* **2003**, *21*, 27–32. [CrossRef]
39. Ridd, M.; Shaw, A.; Lewis, G.; Salisbury, C. The patient–doctor relationship: A synthesis of the qualitative literature on patients' perspectives. *Br. J. Gen. Pract.* **2009**, *59*, e116–e133. [CrossRef]
40. Thom, D.H.; Kravitz, R.L.; Bell, R.A.; Krupat, E.; Azari, R. Patient trust in the physician: Relationship to patient requests. *Fam. Pract.* **2002**, *19*, 476–483. [CrossRef]
41. Clyne, B.; Cooper, J.A.; Boland, F.; Hughes, C.M.; Fahey, T.; Smith, S.M. Beliefs about prescribed medication among older patients with polypharmacy: A mixed methods study in primary care. *Br. J. Gen. Pract.* **2017**, *67*, e507–e518. [CrossRef]
42. Leonard, M.B.; Pursley, D.M.; Robinson, L.A.; Abman, S.H.; Davis, J.M. The importance of trustworthiness: Lessons from the COVID-19 pandemic. *Pediatr. Res.* **2022**, *91*, 482–485. [CrossRef] [PubMed]
43. Mielke, N.; Huscher, D.; Douros, A.; Ebert, N.; Gaedeke, J.; van der Giet, M.; Kuhlmann, M.K.; Martus, P.; Schaeffner, E. Self-reported medication in community-dwelling older adults in Germany: Results from the Berlin Initiative Study. *BMC Geriatr.* **2020**, *20*, 22. [CrossRef] [PubMed]
44. DiMatteo, M.R.; Giordani, P.J.; Lepper, H.S.; Croghan, T.W. Patient adherence and medical treatment outcomes: A meta-analysis. *Med. Care* **2002**, *40*, 794–811. [CrossRef]
45. Marcum, Z.A.; Hanlon, J.T.; Murray, M.D. Improving Medication Adherence and Health Outcomes in Older Adults: An Evidence-Based Review of Randomized Controlled Trials. *Drugs Aging* **2017**, *34*, 191–201. [CrossRef] [PubMed]
46. Marcum, Z.A.; Gellad, W.F. Medication Adherence to Multidrug Regimens. *Clin. Geriatr. Med.* **2012**, *28*, 287–300. [CrossRef]
47. Osterberg, L.; Blaschke, T. Adherence to medication. *N. Engl. J. Med.* **2005**, *353*, 487–497. [CrossRef]
48. Cooper, V.; Metcalf, L.; Versnel, J.; Upton, J.; Walker, S.; Horne, R. Patient-reported side effects, concerns and adherence to corticosteroid treatment for asthma, and comparison with physician estimates of side-effect prevalence: A UK-wide, cross-sectional study. *Npj Prim. Care Respir. Med.* **2015**, *25*, 1–6. [CrossRef]
49. Kimura, Y.; Koya, T.; Hasegawa, T.; Ueno, H.; Yoshizawa, K.; Kimura, Y.; Hayashi, M.; Watanabe, S.; Kikuchi, T. Characterization of low adherence population in asthma patients from Japan using Adherence Starts with Knowledge-12. *Allergol. Int.* **2020**, *69*, 61–65. [CrossRef]
50. Pazan, F.; Kather, J.; Wehling, M. A systematic review and novel classification of listing tools to improve medication in older people. *Eur. J. Clin. Pharmacol.* **2019**, *75*, 619–625. [CrossRef]
51. American Geriatrics Society. American Geriatrics Society 2019 Updated AGS Beers Criteria® for Potentially Inappropriate Medication Use in Older Adults. *J. Am. Geriatr. Soc.* **2019**, *67*, 674–694. [CrossRef]
52. O'Mahony, D.; O'Sullivan, D.; Byrne, S.; O'Connor, M.N.; Ryan, C.; Gallagher, P. STOPP/START criteria for potentially inappropriate prescribing in older people: Version 2. *Age Ageing* **2014**, *44*, 213–218. [CrossRef] [PubMed]
53. Chang, C.M.; Chen, M.J.; Tsai, C.Y.; Ho, L.H.; Hsieh, H.L.; Chau, Y.L.; Liu, C.Y. Medical conditions and medications as risk factors of falls in the inpatient older people: A case–control study. *Int. J. Geriatr. Psychiatry* **2011**, *26*, 602–607. [CrossRef] [PubMed]
54. Holt, S.; Schmiedl, S.; Thürmann, P.A. Potentially Inappropriate Medications in the Elderly: The PRISCUS List. *Dtsch. Arztebl. Int.* **2010**, *107*, 543–551. [CrossRef] [PubMed]
55. Laroche, M.L.; Charmes, J.P.; Merle, L. Potentially inappropriate medications in the elderly: A French consensus panel list. *Eur. J. Clin. Pharmacol.* **2007**, *63*, 725–731. [CrossRef] [PubMed]
56. Lavan, A.H.; Gallagher, P.; Parsons, C.; O'Mahony, D. STOPPFrail (Screening Tool of Older Persons Prescriptions in Frail adults with limited life expectancy): Consensus validation. *Age Ageing* **2017**, *46*, 600–607. [CrossRef]
57. Rancourt, C.; Moisan, J.; Baillargeon, L.; Verreault, R.; Laurin, D.; Grégoire, J.P. Potentially inappropriate prescriptions for older patients in long-term care. *BMC Geriatr.* **2004**, *4*, 9. [CrossRef]
58. Renom-Guiteras, A.; Meyer, G.; Thürmann, P.A. The EU(7)-PIM list: A list of potentially inappropriate medications for older people consented by experts from seven European countries. *Eur. J. Clin. Pharmacol.* **2015**, *71*, 861–875. [CrossRef]
59. Maher, R.L.; Hanlon, J.; Hajjar, E.R. Clinical consequences of polypharmacy in elderly. *Expert Opin. Drug Saf.* **2014**, *13*, 57–65. [CrossRef]
60. Kuhn-Thiel, A.M.; Weiß, C.; Wehling, M.; FORTA Authors/Expert Panel Members. Consensus validation of the FORTA (Fit fOR The Aged) List: A clinical tool for increasing the appropriateness of pharmacotherapy in the elderly. *Drugs Aging* **2014**, *31*, 131–140. [CrossRef]

61. Perpétuo, C.; Plácido, A.I.; Rodrigues, D.; Aperta, J.; Piñeiro-Lamas, M.; Figueiras, A.; Herdeiro, M.T.; Roque, F. Prescription of Potentially Inappropriate Medication in Older Inpatients of an Internal Medicine Ward: Concordance and Overlap Among the EU(7)-PIM List and Beers and STOPP Criteria. *Front. Pharmacol.* **2021**, *12*, 676020. [CrossRef]
62. Roux, B.; Berthou-Contreras, J.; Beuscart, J.B.; Charenton-Blavignac, M.; Doucet, J.; Fournier, J.P.; de la Gastine, B.; Gautier, S.; Gonthier, R.; Gras, V.; et al. REview of potentially inappropriate MEDIcation pr[e]scribing in Seniors (REMEDI[e]S): French implicit and explicit criteria. *Eur. J. Clin. Pharmacol.* **2021**, *77*, 1713–1724. [CrossRef] [PubMed]
63. Nyborg, G.; Straand, J.; Klovning, A.; Brekke, M. The Norwegian General Practice–Nursing Home criteria (NORGEP-NH) for potentially inappropriate medication use: A web-based Delphi study. *Scand. J. Prim. Health Care* **2015**, *33*, 134–141. [CrossRef] [PubMed]
64. Fialová, D.; Brkić, J.; Laffon, B.; Reissigová, J.; Grešáková, S.; Dogan, S.; Doro, P.; Tasić, L.; Marinković, V.; Valdiglesias, V.; et al. Applicability of EU(7)-PIM criteria in cross-national studies in European countries. *Ther. Adv. Drug Saf.* **2019**, *10*, 2042098619854014. [CrossRef] [PubMed]
65. Alshehri, A.A.; Jalal, Z.; Cheema, E.; Haque, M.S.; Jenkins, D.; Yahyouche, A. Impact of the pharmacist-led intervention on the control of medical cardiovascular risk factors for the primary prevention of cardiovascular disease in general practice: A systematic review and meta-analysis of randomised controlled trials. *Br. J. Clin. Pharmacol.* **2020**, *86*, 29–38. [CrossRef] [PubMed]
66. Loots, E.; Goossens, E.; Vanwesemael, T.; Morrens, M.; Van Rompaey, B.; Dilles, T. Interventions to Improve Medication Adherence in Patients with Schizophrenia or Bipolar Disorders: A Systematic Review and Meta-Analysis. *Int. J. Environ. Res. Public Health* **2021**, *18*, 10213. [CrossRef]
67. Tho, P.C.; Ang, E. The effectiveness of patient navigation programs for adult cancer patients undergoing treatment: A systematic review. *JBI Evid. Synth.* **2016**, *14*, 295–321. [CrossRef]
68. Laberge, M.; Sirois, C.; Lunghi, C.; Gaudreault, M.; Nakamura, Y.; Bolduc, C.; Laroche, M.L. Economic Evaluations of Interventions to Optimize Medication Use in Older Adults with Polypharmacy and Multimorbidity: A Systematic Review. *Clin. Interv. Aging* **2021**, *16*, 767–779. [CrossRef]
69. Eysenbach, G. What is e-health? *J. Med. Internet Res.* **2001**, *3*, e20. [CrossRef]
70. Kampmeijer, R.; Pavlova, M.; Tambor, M.; Golinowska, S.; Groot, W. The use of e-health and m-health tools in health promotion and primary prevention among older adults: A systematic literature review. *BMC Health Serv. Res.* **2016**, *16*, 290. [CrossRef]
71. Linn, N.; Goetzinger, C.; Regnaux, J.P.; Schmitz, S.; Dessenne, C.; Fagherazzi, G.; Aguayo, G.A. Digital Health Interventions among People Living with Frailty: A Scoping Review. *J. Am. Med. Dir. Assoc.* **2021**, *22*, 1802–1812.e21. [CrossRef]
72. Laverty, H.; Benson, C.; Cartwright, E.; Cross, M.; Garland, C.; Hammond, T.; Holloway, C.; McMahon, N.; Milligan, J.; Park, B.; et al. How can we improve our understanding of cardiovascular safety liabilities to develop safer medicines?: Cardiovascular toxicity of medicines. *Br. J. Pharmacol.* **2011**, *163*, 675–693. [CrossRef] [PubMed]
73. Onakpoya, I.J.; Heneghan, C.J.; Aronson, J.K. Post-marketing withdrawal of 462 medicinal products because of adverse drug reactions: A systematic review of the world literature. *BMC Med.* **2016**, *14*, 10. [CrossRef] [PubMed]
74. Andrade, R.J.; Aithal, G.P.; Björnsson, E.S.; Kaplowitz, N.; Kullak-Ublick, G.A.; Larrey, D.; Karlsen, T.H. EASL Clinical Practice Guidelines: Drug-induced liver injury. *J. Hepatol.* **2019**, *70*, 1222–1261. [CrossRef] [PubMed]
75. Schwartz, P.J.; Woosley, R.L. Predicting the Unpredictable. *J. Am. Coll. Cardiol.* **2006**, *67*, 1639–1650. [CrossRef]
76. Poluzzi, E.; Raschi, E.; Diemberger, I.; De Ponti, F. Drug-Induced Arrhythmia: Bridging the Gap Between Pathophysiological Knowledge and Clinical Practice. *Drug Saf.* **2017**, *40*, 461–464. [CrossRef]
77. Gatti, M.; Raschi, E.; Poluzzi, E.; Martignani, C.; Salvagni, S.; Ardizzoni, A.; Diemberger, I. The Complex Management of Atrial Fibrillation and Cancer in the COVID-19 Era: Drug Interactions, Thromboembolic Risk, and Proarrhythmia. *Curr. Heart Fail. Rep.* **2020**, *17*, 365–383. [CrossRef]
78. Skullbacka, S.; Airaksinen, M.; Puustinen, J.; Toivo, T. Risk assessment tools for QT prolonging pharmacotherapy in older adults: A systematic review. *Eur. J. Clin. Pharmacol.* **2022**, *78*, 765–779. [CrossRef]
79. Hayashi, P.H.; Lucena, M.I.; Fontana, R.J.; Bjornsson, E.S.; Aithal, G.P.; Barnhart, H.; Gonzalez-Jimenez, A.; Yang, Q.; Gu, J.; Andrade, R.J.; et al. A revised electronic version of RUCAM for the diagnosis of DILI. *Hepatology* **2022**, *76*, 18–31. [CrossRef]
80. Backes, C.; Moyano, C.; Rimaud, C.; Bienvenu, C.; Schneider, M.P. Digital Medication Adherence Support: Could Healthcare Providers Recommend Mobile Health Apps? *Front. Med. Technol.* **2021**, *2*, 616242. [CrossRef]
81. Sourbati, M.; Loos, E.F. Interfacing age: Diversity and (in)visibility in digital public service. *J. Digit. Media Policy* **2019**, *10*, 275–293. [CrossRef]
82. Matthew-Maich, N.; Harris, L.; Ploeg, J.; Markle-Reid, M.; Valaitis, R.; Ibrahim, S.; Gafni, A.; Isaacs, S. Designing, Implementing, and Evaluating Mobile Health Technologies for Managing Chronic Conditions in Older Adults: A Scoping Review. *JMIR mHealth uHealth* **2016**, *4*, e29. [CrossRef] [PubMed]
83. Gulliford, M.; Alageel, S. Digital health intervention at older ages. *Lancet Digit. Health* **2019**, *1*, e382–e383. [CrossRef]
84. Mukhtar, O.; Weinman, J.; Jackson, S.H.D. Intentional Non-Adherence to Medications by Older Adults. *Drugs Aging* **2014**, *31*, 149–157. [CrossRef]
85. Amorim, W.W.; Passos, L.C.; Gama, R.S.; Souza, R.M.; Oliveira, M.G. Factors associated with older patients' misunderstandings of medication dosage regimen instructions after consultation in primary care in Brazil. *J. Eval. Clin. Pract.* **2021**, *27*, 817–825. [CrossRef]

86. Mertens, B.J.; Kwint, H.F.; van Marum, R.J.; Bouvy, M.L. Are multidose drug dispensing systems initiated for the appropriate patients? *Eur. J. Clin. Pharmacol.* **2018**, *74*, 1159–1164. [CrossRef]
87. Hersberger, K.E.; Boeni, F.; Arnet, I. Dose-dispensing service as an intervention to improve adherence to polymedication. *Expert Rev. Clin. Pharmacol.* **2013**, *6*, 413–421. [CrossRef]
88. Levings, B.; Szep, S.; Helps, S. Towards the safer use of dosettes. *J. Qual. Clin. Pract.* **1999**, *19*, 69–72. [CrossRef]
89. Smith, D.L. Compliance Packaging: A Patient Education Tool. *Am. Pharm.* **1989**, *29*, 42–53. [CrossRef]
90. Schwartz, J.K. Pillbox use, satisfaction, and effectiveness among persons with chronic health conditions. *Assist. Technol.* **2017**, *29*, 181–187. [CrossRef]
91. Barton, E.; Twining, L.; Walters, L. Understanding the decision to commence a dose administration aid. *Aust. Fam. Physician* **2017**, *46*, 943–947.
92. Straka, I.; Minar, M.; Grofik, M.; Skorvanek, M.; Bolekova, V.; Gazova, A.; Kyselovic, J.; Valkovic, P. Effect of Pillbox Organizers with Alarms on Adherence to Pharmacotherapy in Parkinson Disease Patients Taking Three and More Daily Doses of Dopaminergic Medications. *J. Pers. Med.* **2022**, *12*, 179. [CrossRef] [PubMed]
93. Boeni, F.; Spinatsch, E.; Suter, K.; Hersberger, K.E.; Arnet, I. Effect of drug reminder packaging on medication adherence: A systematic review revealing research gaps. *Syst. Rev.* **2014**, *3*, 29. [CrossRef] [PubMed]
94. Stip, E.; Vincent, P.D.; Sablier, J.; Guevremont, C.; Zhornitsky, S.; Tranulis, C. A randomized controlled trial with a Canadian electronic pill dispenser used to measure and improve medication adherence in patients with schizophrenia. *Front. Pharmacol.* **2013**, *4*, 100. [CrossRef]
95. Zedler, B.K.; Kakad, P.; Colilla, S.; Murrelle, L.; Shah, N.R. Does Packaging with a Calendar Feature Improve Adherence to Self-Administered Medication for Long-Term Use? A Systematic Review. *Clin. Ther.* **2011**, *33*, 62–73. [CrossRef] [PubMed]
96. Beckman, H.B. The Effect of Physician Behavior on the Collection of Data. *Ann. Intern. Med.* **1984**, *101*, 692. [CrossRef] [PubMed]
97. Di Palma, J.A.; Herrera, J.L. The Role of Effective Clinician-Patient Communication in the Management of Irritable Bowel Syndrome and Chronic Constipation. *J. Clin. Gastroenterol.* **2012**, *46*, 748–751. [CrossRef]
98. Singh Ospina, N.; Phillips, K.A.; Rodriguez-Gutierrez, R.; Castaneda-Guarderas, A.; Gionfriddo, M.R.; Branda, M.E.; Montori, V.M. Eliciting the Patient's Agenda- Secondary Analysis of Recorded Clinical Encounters. *J. Gen. Intern. Med.* **2019**, *34*, 36–40. [CrossRef]
99. Roter, D.L.; Hall, J.A.; Aoki, Y. Physician Gender Effects in Medical Communication: A Meta-analytic Review. *JAMA* **2002**, *288*, 756. [CrossRef]
100. Vogliotti, E.; Pintore, G.; Zoccarato, F.; Biasin, M.; Sergi, G.; Inelmen, E.M.; Trevisan, C. Communicating Bad News to Older Patients from the Physician's Point of View: Focus on the Influence of Gender and Length of Work Experience. *Gerontology* **2021**, 1–7. [CrossRef]
101. Cooper, L.A.; Roter, D.L.; Johnson, R.L.; Ford, D.E.; Steinwachs, D.M.; Powe, N.R. Patient-Centered Communication, Ratings of Care, and Concordance of Patient and Physician Race. *Ann. Intern. Med.* **2003**, *139*, 907. [CrossRef]
102. Mira, J.J.; Orozco-Beltran, D.; Perez-Jover, V.; Martinez-Jimeno, L.; Gil-Guillen, V.F.; Carratala-Munuera, C.; Sanchez-Molla, M.; Pertusa-Martinez, S.; Asencio-Aznar, A. Physician patient communication failure facilitates medication errors in older polymedicated patients with multiple comorbidities. *Fam. Pract.* **2013**, *30*, 56–63. [CrossRef] [PubMed]
103. Advinha, A.M.; Lopes, M.J.; de Oliveira-Martins, S. Assessment of the elderly's functional ability to manage their medication: A systematic literature review. *Int. J. Clin. Pharm.* **2017**, *39*, 1–15. [CrossRef] [PubMed]
104. Lee, W.; Noh, Y.; Kang, H.; Hong, S.H. The mediatory role of medication adherence in improving patients' medication experience through patient-physician communication among older hypertensive patients. *Patient Prefer. Adherence* **2017**, *11*, 1119–1126. [CrossRef]
105. Marcum, Z.A.; Pugh, M.J.V.; Amuan, M.E.; Aspinall, S.L.; Handler, S.M.; Ruby, C.M.; Hanlon, J.T. Prevalence of Potentially Preventable Unplanned Hospitalizations Caused by Therapeutic Failures and Adverse Drug Withdrawal Events among Older Veterans. *J. Gerontol. A Biol. Sci. Med. Sci.* **2012**, *67*, 867–874. [CrossRef]
106. Ozavci, G.; Bucknall, T.; Woodward-Kron, R.; Hughes, C.; Jorm, C.; Joseph, K.; Manias, E. A systematic review of older patients' experiences and perceptions of communication about managing medication across transitions of care. *Res. Soc. Adm. Pharm.* **2021**, *17*, 273–291. [CrossRef]

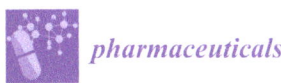

Article

Use of an Electronic Medication Management Support System in Patients with Polypharmacy in General Practice: A Quantitative Process Evaluation of the AdAM Trial

Robin Brünn [1,*], Dorothea Lemke [1], Jale Basten [2], Petra Kellermann-Mühlhoff [3], Juliane Köberlein-Neu [4], Christiane Muth [1,5], Marjan van den Akker [1,6,7] and on behalf of the AdAM Study Group [†]

1 Institute of General Practice, Goethe University, 60590 Frankfurt am Main, Germany; lemke@allgemeinmedizin.uni-frankfurt.de (D.L.); christiane.muth@uni-bielefeld.de (C.M.); m.vandenakker@allgemeinmedizin.uni-frankfurt.de (M.v.d.A.)
2 Department of Medical Informatics, Biometry and Epidemiology, Ruhr University, 44789 Bochum, Germany; basten@amib.ruhr-uni-bochum.de
3 BARMER, Statutory Health Insurance, 42285 Wuppertal, Germany; petra.kellermann-muehlhoff@barmer.de
4 Center for Health Economics and Health Services Research, Schumpeter School of Business and Economics, University of Wuppertal, 42119 Wuppertal, Germany; koeberlein@wiwi.uni-wuppertal.de
5 Department of General Practice and Family Medicine, Medical Faculty East-Westphalia, University of Bielefeld, 33515 Bielefeld, Germany
6 Department of Family Medicine, Care and Public Health Research Institute, Maastricht University, 6200 Maastricht, The Netherlands
7 Department of Public Health and Primary Care, Academic Centre of General Practice, KU Leuven, 3000 Leuven, Belgium
* Correspondence: bruenn@allgemeinmedizin.uni-frankfurt.de
† Membership of the AdAM study group is provided in the Acknowledgments.

Citation: Brünn, R.; Lemke, D.; Basten, J.; Kellermann-Mühlhoff, P.; Köberlein-Neu, J.; Muth, C.; van den Akker, M.; on behalf of the AdAM Study Group. Use of an Electronic Medication Management Support System in Patients with Polypharmacy in General Practice: A Quantitative Process Evaluation of the AdAM Trial. *Pharmaceuticals* **2022**, *15*, 759. https://doi.org/10.3390/ph15060759

Academic Editors: Charlotte Vermehren and Niels Westergaard

Received: 10 May 2022
Accepted: 16 June 2022
Published: 17 June 2022

Publisher's Note: MDPI stays neutral with regard to jurisdictional claims in published maps and institutional affiliations.

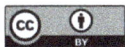

Copyright: © 2022 by the authors. Licensee MDPI, Basel, Switzerland. This article is an open access article distributed under the terms and conditions of the Creative Commons Attribution (CC BY) license (https://creativecommons.org/licenses/by/4.0/).

Abstract: Polypharmacy is associated with a risk of negative health outcomes. Potentially inappropriate medications, interactions resulting from contradicting medical guidelines, and inappropriate monitoring, all increase the risk. This process evaluation (PE) of the AdAM study investigates implementation and use of a computerized decision-support system (CDSS). The CDSS analyzes medication appropriateness by including claims data, and hence provides general practitioners (GPs) with full access to patients' medical treatments. We based our PE on pseudonymized logbook entries into the CDSS and used the four dimensions of the Medical Research Council PE framework. Reach, which examines the extent to which the intended study population was included, and Dose, Fidelity, and Tailoring, which examine how the software was actually used by GPs. The PE was explorative and descriptive. Study participants were representative of the target population, except for patients receiving a high level of nursing care, as they were treated less frequently. GPs identified and corrected inappropriate prescriptions flagged by the CDSS. The frequency and intensity of interventions documented in the form of logbook entries lagged behind expectations, raising questions about implementation barriers to the intervention and the limitations of the PE. Impossibility to connect the CDSS to GPs' electronic medical records (EMR) of GPs due to technical conditions in the German healthcare system may have hindered the implementation of the intervention. Data logged in the CDSS may underestimate medication changes in patients, as documentation was voluntary and already included in EMR.

Keywords: polypharmacy; medication review; digital decision-support; health services research; general practice; process evaluation

1. Introduction

Life expectancy around the world has risen as a result of improvements in the diagnosis and treatment of chronic and acute diseases, and better living conditions and hygiene [1]. Longer lives increase the likelihood of developing chronic diseases—if more than one disease occurs in one person at the same time—a condition known as multimorbidity [2]. As increasingly specialized clinical experts use increasingly complex pharmacotherapies to treat individual diseases, while insufficiently taking into account a patient's multimorbidity, polypharmacy—usually defined as the concurrent intake of at least five different chronic medications [3]—is becoming ever more common [4,5]. There is growing awareness that polypharmacy should itself be treated as a risk factor, since the parallel treatment of different diseases with pharmacotherapy can have contradicting or reinforcing effects that are potentially life-threatening [6]. Polypharmacy is, for example, associated with higher rates of hospitalization [7–9] and death [9], as well as decreased quality of life and higher symptom burden [10].

The use of computerized decision-support systems (CDSS) to prevent or manage problematic polypharmacy has been evaluated in previous studies, and been shown to improve prescribing quality and reduce the prescription of potentially inappropriate medication [11,12]. However, the results have not always been significant [13], and their impact has frequently only been considered independently of patient-relevant outcomes. When they have been linked to patient-relevant outcomes, results have been inconsistent and have lacked robustness [14,15]. Since such interventions are generally complex, knowledge is lacking on what parameters lead to what outcomes, and on whether interventions have actually been implemented as intended. To gain a better understanding of the processes underlying complex interventions, it is recommended that they are accompanied by a preplanned process evaluation [16–18]. A comprehensive process evaluation is also very helpful when complex interventions do not show the anticipated effects. In these cases, the aim of process evaluations is to find the reason(s) for the observed lack of effectiveness. However, few trials follow this advice [19,20].

To circumvent these problems in the AdAM study, a process evaluation based on data logged by a CDSS named "eMMa" (a detailed explanation of the functioning can be found in the Methods section) was carried out with the aim of gaining an insight into how and why the AdAM intervention works the way it does. The study protocol has been published elsewhere a priori [21]. This paper presents the results of the process evaluation of the AdAM intervention, whereby the recommendations of the Medical Research Council (MRC) framework for process evaluations of complex interventions [18] helped us decide on which results to present and on how to structure our report. They also enabled us to provide a multidimensional view of the actual interventions. We ultimately settled on the following research questions: (1) How many and what were the typical characteristics of the GPs and patients that took part in the intervention (i.e., the Intervention "Reach")? (2) What proportion of medication alerts were handled by GPs, and which were considered high priority (Intervention "Dose", not to be confused with the dosage of a specific drug)? (3) What proportion of participants received the intervention as intended, thus increasing the likelihood of success (Intervention "Fidelity")? (4) How did GPs integrate the intervention into their daily routines (Intervention "Tailoring")?

2. Results

2.1. Intervention Reach

The "Reach" intervention dimension refers to the participants that were actually reached by the intervention. Overall, 42,719 patients were considered potentially eligible in the main intention-to-treat analysis, of whom 9268 patients enrolled and 9261 (22%) showed up in the software (here called the "active population": AP). The remaining 33,451 patients (78%) did not enroll in the study and made up the non-enrolled potentials (NEP), along with their respective GPs ($n = 351$, 34%) and practices ($n = 248$, 37%), if they agreed to participate in the trial (see Figure 1). Table 1 shows a comparison between the AP and NEP groups for patients. As only 7 of the enrolled patients did not appear in the software ("inactive population": IP), statistical analysis was not feasible for them. Of 925 eligible GPs from 676 practices, 574 GPs (62%) from 428 practices (63%) agreed to participate in the AdAM study. Of these, 465 GPs (50%) from 347 practices (51%) were identified as having actively used the software program and thus comprised the AP. The remaining 109 GPs (12%) and 81 practices (12%) belonged to the IP. Since this analysis focuses on the data gathered from the CDSS, no comparison with potentially eligible GPs and practices in the study region could be conducted. Tables 2 and 3 compare the AP to the IP and NEP for GPs and practices.

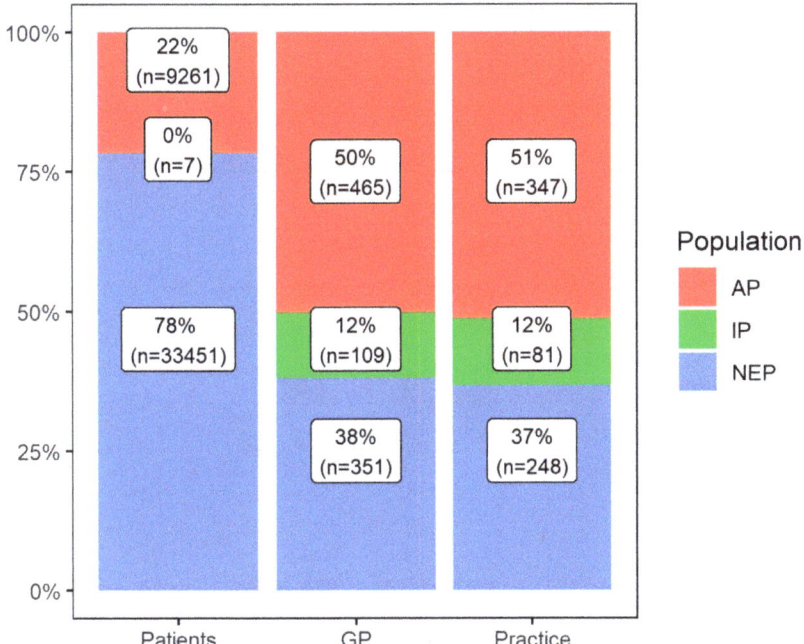

Figure 1. Distribution of patients, GPs, and practices in the defined populations (AP: active population, IP: inactive population, NEP: non-enrolled potentials).

Table 1. Group comparison of AP and NEP patients.

Predictors	OR	95% CI	p-Value
(Intercept)	0.17	0.14–0.19	<0.001
Age	1.01	1.01–1.01	<0.001
Sex (ref: male)			
Female	0.93	0.89–0.98	0.004
medCDS *	1.04	0.98–1.09	0.177
Nursing care level (ref: 0)			
Nursing care level 1	0.76	0.65–0.88	<0.001
Nursing care level 2	0.74	0.68–0.80	<0.001
Nursing care level 3	0.52	0.46–0.57	<0.001
Nursing care level 4	0.34	0.29–0.40	<0.001
Nursing care level 5	0.27	0.21–0.35	<0.001
R^2 Tjur		0.011	

* medCDS is a chronic disease score [22].

Table 2. Factors related to the chance of belonging to AP versus IP and AP versus NEP GPs.

	AP vs. IP			AP vs. NEP		
Predictors	OR	95% CI	p-Value	OR	95% CI	p-Value
(Intercept)	24.93	5.11–129.84	**<0.001**	5.31	1.97–14.51	**0.001**
Specialization (ref: Specialized in general practice)						
Without specialist qualification	0.48	0.18–1.35	0.145	1.05	0.45–2.42	0.909
Internist active in general practice	0.86	0.55–1.36	0.519	1.27	0.93–1.73	0.137
Other	0.34	0.03–7.45	0.384	1.1	0.10–23.83	0.94
Age GP	0.97	0.94–0.99	**0.018**	0.97	0.95–0.98	**<0.001**
Sex GP (ref: male)						
Female	1.03	0.65–1.63	0.906	1.02	0.75–1.38	0.9
GP network (ref: no)						
Yes	0.95	0.61–1.51	0.825	1.21	0.89–1.66	0.232
Randomization group (ref: control)						
Intervention	1.36	0.89–2.08	0.157	1.93	1.45–2.57	**<0.001**
R^2 Tjur	0.023			0.051		

Table 3. Factors related to the chance of belonging to AP versus IP and AP versus NEP practices.

	AP vs. IP			AP vs. NEP		
Predictors	OR	95% CI	p-Value	OR	95% CI	p-Value
(Intercept)	2.41	1.05–5.52	**0.037**	1.02	0.61–1.72	0.933
Number of GPs	1.22	0.88–1.78	0.277	0.99	0.81–1.22	0.915
Duration of practice	1	0.98–1.03	0.735	0.99	0.97–1.01	0.278
Type of practice (ref: single practice)						
Group practice	0.95	0.48–1.87	0.878	1.75	1.10–2.79	**0.018**
Medical care center	-	-	0.987	1.12	0.15–9.86	0.913
Randomization group (ref: control)						
Intervention	1.34	0.82–2.18	0.24	2.02	1.45–2.82	**<0.001**
R^2 Tjur	0.009			0.046		

Compared to the NEP patient population, the AP patient group contains more men and is slightly older. The nursing care level is defined in German social security laws and specifies the need for nursing services and the welfare payment a patient is entitled to. A higher nursing care level indicates a greater need for nursing services and a higher welfare payment. With an increasing nursing care level, it was less likely that patients would receive the intervention.

On average, GPs that actively used the software were younger than those that had only inactive or non-enrolled patients. Group practices and practices that were randomized to the intervention group from the beginning were also more frequent users than practices that switched to the intervention group in later waves. No other characteristics had a significant impact on CDSS usage.

2.2. Intervention Dose

The "Dose" intervention dimension provides an insight into the extent to which the intervention was adopted and implemented, i.e., refers to the "dose" of the intervention the participants actually received. Figures 2 and 3 show the distribution of the number of alerts per patient and GP, as tracked by eMMa before and after the intervention. Overall, the numbers remained constant, indicating no improvement in prescribed medications. An analysis of cases in which a complete anamnesis had been performed and confirmed by GPs, showed a modest reduction in the median number of alerts per patient.

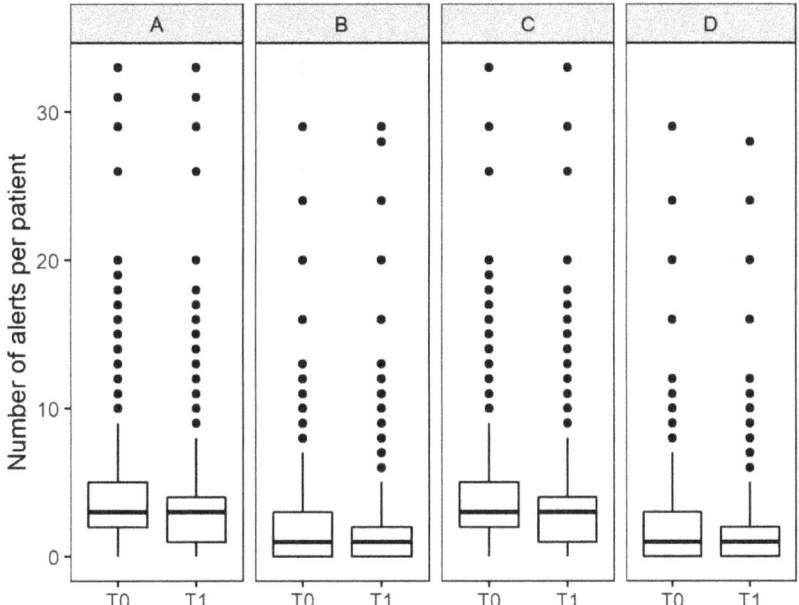

Figure 2. Box plot showing the number of alerts per patient at T_0 and T_1 (**A**), stratified according to the subgroups "severe alerts" (**B**), "completed anamnesis" (**C**), and a combination of both subgroups (**D**).

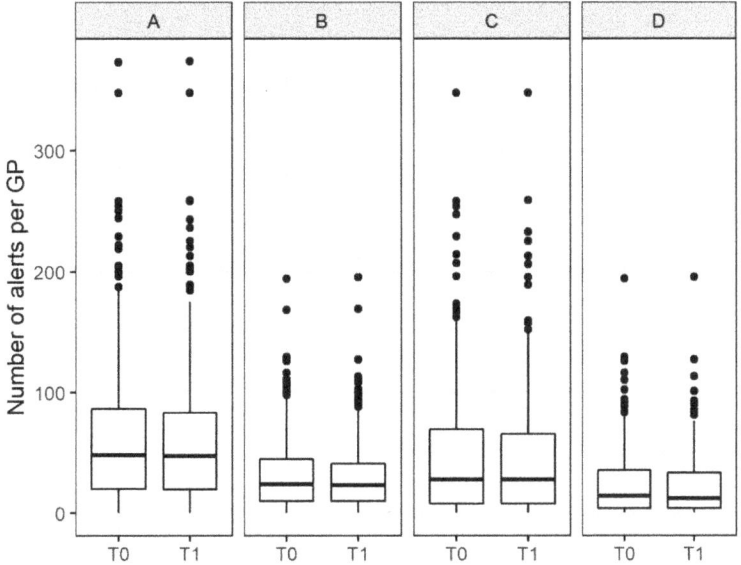

Figure 3. Box plot showing the number of alerts per GP at T_0 and T_1 (**A**), stratified according to the subgroups "severe alerts" (**B**), "completed anamnesis" (**C**) and a combination of both subgroups (**D**).

After adjusting the number of alerts per GP to take account of the number of treated patients (Figure 4), the alert count remained virtually constant (mostly a max. of +/− 1 alert per patient), but there is an inverse correlation between the overall number of patients treated by a GP and the change in the number of alerts.

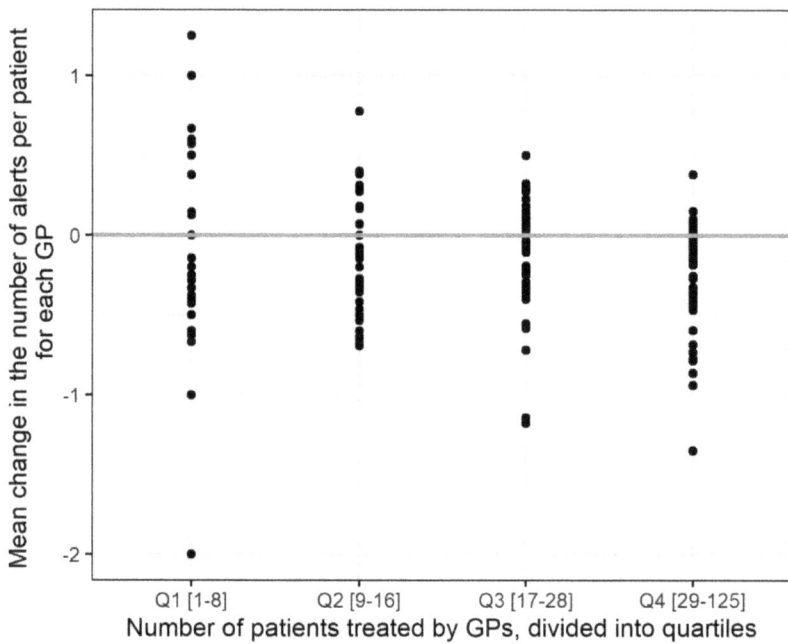

Figure 4. Average change in the number of alerts per GP, stratified according to the number of patients from the active study population treated by the GP (expressed in quartiles).

Stratifying by alert category gives an insight into the kinds of potential inappropriateness that were assessed with a higher priority (Table 4). Since the software did not generate alerts for Dear Doctor Letters, no analysis was conducted in this category. The number of alerts warning of an inappropriate dosage or the unsuitability of a medication in view of a patient's kidney function declined most frequently. GPs did not appear to pay much attention to alerts relating to potential allergies or duplicate prescriptions, and these actually increased.

Table 4. Overall number of alerts per category at T_0 and change over the course of the study.

Analysis	Alert Category	Number of Alerts at T_0 (Proportion of Total Alerts)	Change at T_1 (%)	Number of Alerts of Severity 1 at T_0 (Proportion of Total Alerts)	Change at T_1 (%) (Severity 1 Alerts Only)
Main	Dosage	15,790 (56%)	−5.0	9530 (66%)	−6.2
	Kidney	2625 (9%)	−6.2	2625 (18%)	−6.2
	Interaction	5836 (21%)	−0.5	449 (3%)	−6.1
	Duplicate prescription	2323 (8%)	3.2	1615 (11%)	3.8
	Age	1653 (6%)	−0.1	N/A	N/A
	Allergy	143 (1%)	3.4	143 (1%)	3.4

Table 4. Cont.

Analysis	Alert Category	Number of Alerts at T_0 (Proportion of Total Alerts)	Change at T_1 (%)	Number of Alerts of Severity 1 at T_0 (Proportion of Total Alerts)	Change at T_1 (%) (Severity 1 Alerts Only)
Sensitivity "completed anamnesis"	Dosage	8879 (55%)	−9.6	5337 (66%)	−11.9
	Kidney	1489 (9%)	−11.5	1489 (18%)	−11.5
	Interaction	3400 (21%)	−1.6	250 (3%)	−11.6
	Duplicate prescription	1417 (9%)	3.2	990 (12%)	4.2
	Age	944 (6%)	−1.2	N/A	N/A
	Allergy	83 (1%)	3.4	83 (1%)	3.4

The reduction was greatest when severe alerts and patients that had received a complete anamnesis were the only groups taken into consideration. Potential drug–drug interactions are reacted to much more frequently when the CDSS rates them as "severity level 1".

Poisson regression analysis resulted in the incidence rate ratios shown in Table 5. Sensitivity analysis for justified alerts is depicted in Table 6. Significant differences in incidence rate ratios are shown in bold.

Table 5. Incidence rate ratio of alerts before and after the intervention, stratified by age, sex, alert category, and severity level.

		Incidence Rate Ratio (T_1 vs. T_0)					
Severity	Category	Female			Male		
		<65 Years	≥65 <85	≥85	<65 Years	≥65 <85	≥85
1 & 2	Dosage	0.95 (0.88–1.01)	**0.94 (0.92–0.99)** **	0.95 (0.90–1.00)	0.96 (0.89–1.03)	0.96 (0.91–1.00)	0.96 (0.88–1.06)
	Kidney	0.93 (0.77–1.13)	0.95 (0.87–1.04)	0.92 (0.81–1.03)	0.94 (0.76–1.14)	0.95 (0.85–1.07)	0.96 (0.78–1.18)
	Interaction	1.01 (0.90–1.13)	1.00 (0.94–1.06)	0.98 (0.89–1.09)	0.99 (0.88–1.12)	0.99 (0.92–1.07)	1.01 (0.87–1.18)
	Duplicate prescription	1.03 (0.90–1.19)	1.04 (0.94–1.15)	1.01 (0.84–1.21)	1.04 (0.88–1.22)	1.04 (0.92–1.17)	1.01 (0.78–1.41)
	Age	1.13 (0.67–1.72)	1.04 (0.99–1.06)	0.99 (0.84–1.15)	1.14 (0.56–1.87)	1.01 (0.88–1.17)	1.00 (0.74–1.43)
	Allergy	1.00 (0.55–1.83)	1.05 (0.74–1.50)	1.05 (0.59–1.85)	1.00 (0.42–2.40)	1.0 (0.57–1.76)	1.17 (0.39–3.47)
1	Dosage	0.93 (0.85–1.02)	**0.94 (0.90–0.99)** *	**0.92 (0.86–0.99)** *	0.95 (0.90–1.02)	0.95 (0.90–1.01)	0.94 (0.84–1.07)
	Kidney	0.93 (0.77–1.13)	0.95 (0.87–1.04)	0.92 (0.81–1.03)	0.94 (0.76–1.14)	0.95 (0.85–1.07)	0.96 (0.78–1.18)
	Interaction	0.94 (0.62–1.46)	0.93 (0.76–1.17)	0.93 (0.64–1.30)	0.96 (0.64–1.45)	0.93 (0.71–1.21)	1.04 (0.51–1.89)
	Duplicate prescription	1.04 (0.88–1.23)	1.05 (0.94–1.19)	1.01 (0.81–1.25)	1.05 (0.87–1.28)	1.03 (0.90–1.19)	1.01 (0.74–1.49)
	Allergy	1.00 (0.55–1.83)	1.05 (0.74–1.50)	1.05 (0.59–1.85)	1.00 (0.42–2.40)	1.00 (0.57–1.76)	1.23 (0.43–3.46)

** $p < 0.01$. * $p < 0.05$.

Table 6. Incidence rate ratio of unjustified alerts before and after the intervention, stratified by age, sex, alert category, and severity level.

		Incidence Rate Ratio (T1 vs. T0)					
Severity	Category	Female			Male		
		<65 Years	≥65 <85	≥85	<65 Years	≥65 <85	≥85
1 & 2	Dosage	**0.85 (0.79–0.91)** ***	**0.87 (0.84–0.90)** ***	**0.86 (0.82–0.91)** ***	**0.86 (0.80–0.93)** ***	**0.89 (0.85–0.93)** ***	**0.89 (0.81–0.98)** *
	Kidney	**0.78 (0.65–0.95)** **	**0.83 (0.76–0.95)** ***	**0.83 (0.73–0.94)** **	0.83 (0.67–1.03)	**0.86 (0.76–0.97)** *	0.89 (0.72–1.10)
	Interaction	0.96 (0.86–1.08)	**0.92 (0.87–0.98)** **	0.90 (0.81–1.00)	0.93 (0.83–1.06)	0.93 (0.86–1.00)	0.93 (0.80–1.09)
	Duplicate prescription	1.00 (0.87–1.14)	1.01 (0.91–1.11)	0.94 (0.79–1.14)	1.02 (0.86–1.20)	1.01 (0.89–1.15)	0.97 (0.74–1.27)
	Age	1.01 (0.78–1.46)	0.95 (0.85–1.02)	0.92 (0.79–1.07)	1.13 (0.59–1.90)	0.94 (0.82–1.11)	0.91 (0.67–1.23)
	Allergy	1.00 (0.55–1.83)	1.02 (0.71–1.46)	0.96 (0.53–1.82)	1.00 (0.42–2.40)	0.92 (0.51–1.63)	1.17 (0.39–3.47)
1	Dosage	**0.81 (0.77–0.82)** ***	**0.85 (0.81–0.89)** ***	**0.83 (0.77–0.89)** ***	**0.84 (0.81–0.86)** ***	**0.87 (0.82–0.93)** ***	**0.87 (0.82–0.93)** ***
	Kidney	**0.783 (0.64–0.95)** **	**0.83 (0.76–0.91)** ***	**0.83 (0.73–0.94)** **	0.83 (0.67–1.03)	**0.86 (0.76–0.97)** *	0.89 (0.72–1.10)
	Interaction	0.86 (0.55–1.34)	0.85 (0.67–1.07)	0.84 (0.60–1.19)	0.80 (0.52–1.24)	0.79 (0.60–1.04)	0.92 (0.53–1.61)
	Duplicate prescription	1.00 (0.85–1.19)	1.02 (0.91–1.15)	0.94 (0.76–1.18)	1.03 (0.85–1.25)	1.02 (0.88–1.17)	0.99 (0.73–1.36)
	Allergy	0.96 (0.53–1.72)	1.02 (0.71–1.46)	0.96 (0.53–1.72)	1.00 (0.42–2.40)	0.92 (0.51–1.63)	1.17 (0.39–3.47)

*** $p < 0,001$, ** $p < 0,01$, * $p < 0,05$.

Overall, there were only a few significant reductions in alerts, and these were solely in the dosage category (Table 5). However, when alerts flagged as "justified" were left out of the analysis, the picture changed, and a significant reduction in dosage alerts could be detected in all subgroups (Table 6). The same is true for almost all kidney alert subgroups. Point estimates for severity level 1 alerts are equal or lower than those of alerts overall, but the significance of the reduction was limited by low case numbers.

2.3. Intervention Fidelity

The "Fidelity" intervention dimension evaluates how frequently the intervention was implemented in such a way that it was actually possible to achieve the aim of the intervention. Table 7 shows how many patients had severe alerts at T_0 and how many of these cases were satisfactorily dealt with according to the criteria defined in the methods section (confirmed completed anamnesis and zero unjustified alerts of severity level 1 at T_1). The alerts were stratified by category. On a GP level, no participant fulfilled the Fidelity criteria in any given category for all their patients.

Table 7. Proportion of patients fulfilling the Fidelity criteria.

Alert Category	Number of Patients for Whom the Number of Severe Alerts is >0 at T_0	Number of Patients Fulfilling Fidelity Criteria	Proportion of Patients Fulfilling Fidelity Criteria
Dosage	3210	780	24.3%
Kidney	1322	383	29.0%
Interaction	246	71	28.9%
Duplicate prescription	787	57	7.2%
Allergy	64	4	6.2%

As in the case of the Dose dimension findings, duplicate prescriptions and allergies received little attention in comparison to the other categories.

As far as the more highly prioritized categories are concerned, the GPs acknowledged and dealt with all the severe alerts in fewer than 30% of patients, indicating that the intervention goal was only moderately fulfilled.

Summarizing over all categories, severe alerts were only fully resolved or justified in 889 patients. Figure 5 compares this number to the number of potentially eligible patients, enrolled patients, patients receiving the intervention from their GPs, as well as the number of patients that were treated with an intensity that would have made complete fidelity possible. Figure 5 indicates the steps that had to be accomplished to fulfil Fidelity criteria and shows that many patients were lost on the way.

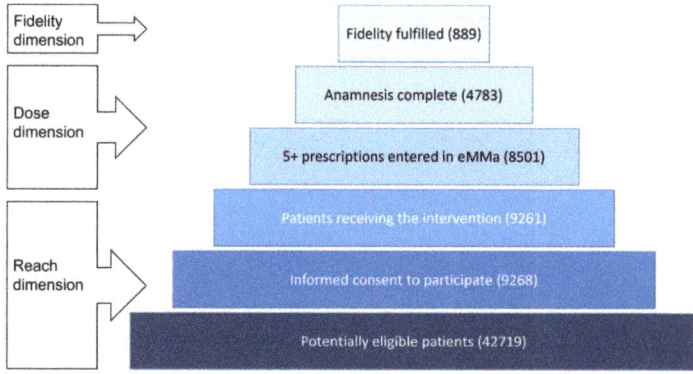

Figure 5. Steps to be climbed in order to achieve Intervention Fidelity. The left-hand legend shows the dimensions impacted by the steps.

2.4. Intervention Tailoring

The "Tailoring" intervention dimension describes how participating GPs handled the intervention, and gives an indication how the intervention could be adapted to fit better into daily routines. Figure 6 shows on which days of the week T_0 was triggered for patients, i.e., when the first GP assessment appeared in the software. In Figure 7, the same distribution is shown for the months of the year and in Figure 8, for the whole intervention period.

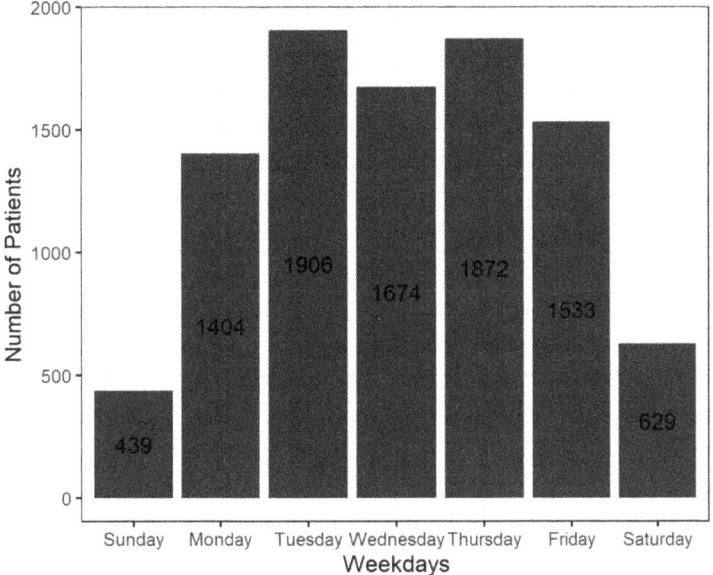

Figure 6. Number of patients, stratified by the day in the week when T_0 was triggered.

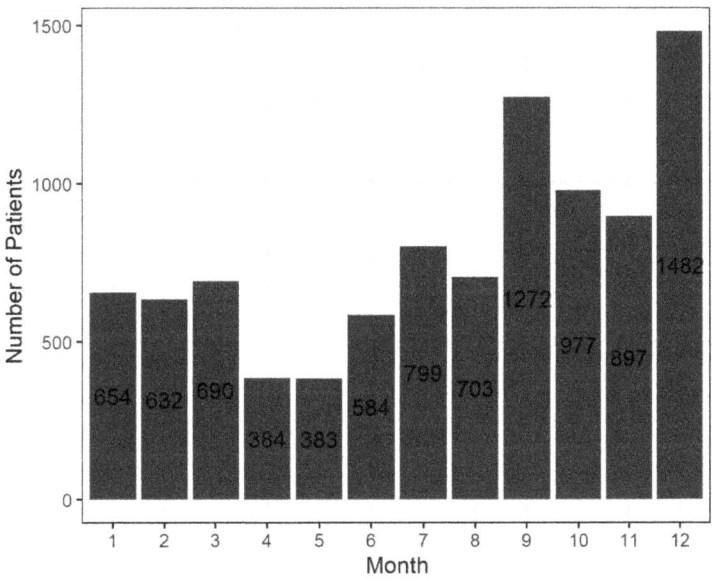

Figure 7. Number of patients stratified by month of the year when T_0 was triggered.

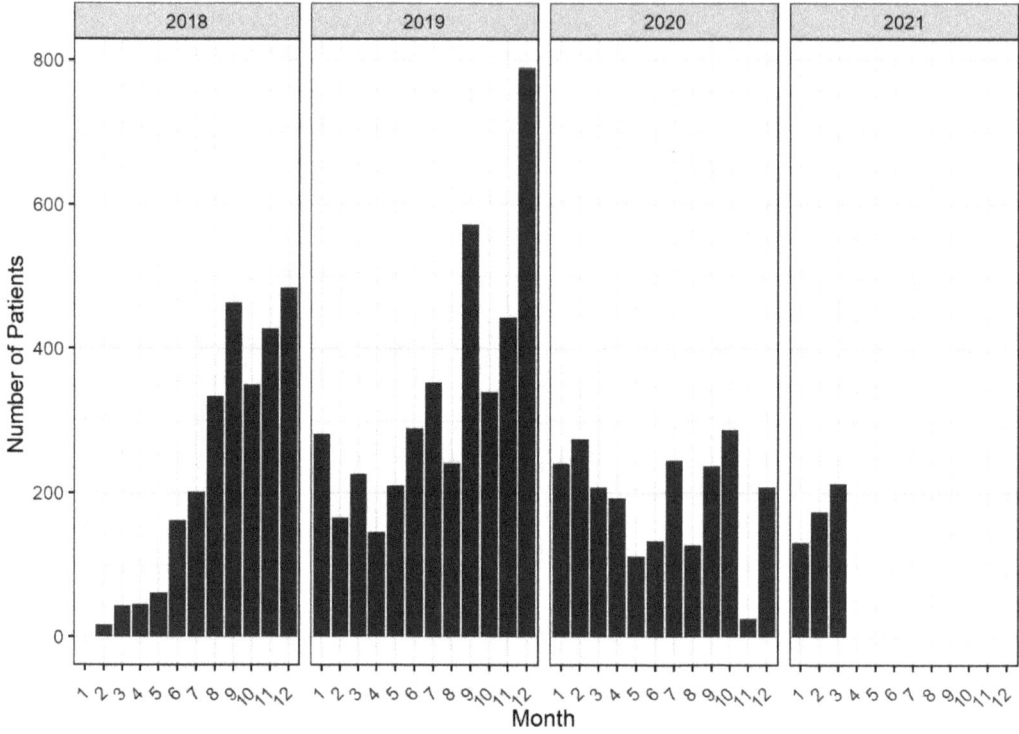

Figure 8. Number of patients, stratified by the month and year when T_0 was triggered over the course of the study.

These analyses show when GPs preferred or had the chance to conduct medication reviews. The vast majority of cases (89%) were initiated between Monday and Friday, with peaks on Tuesdays and Thursdays. Only a small portion (11%) were initiated on Saturdays, Sundays, and public holidays, when practices are usually closed. In terms of months, the CDSS was used more often in the second half of the year, and especially in September and December. This pattern remains similar when the whole intervention period is examined, except for 2020, when the rise in patient cases was dampened by the COVID-19 pandemic.

Since the intervention software was in a test phase and on several occasions had to be updated, we initially planned to conduct sensitivity analyses to account for major software releases and lengthy software inaccessibility due to technical problems. However, as no error logbook was available, these analyses could not be conducted.

3. Discussion

3.1. Main Findings

Our process evaluation showed no relevant selection bias on either a patient, GP, or practice level in the participants included in the AdAM trial, compared to the eligible population in the study region (Intervention Reach). The reduction in the number of alerts was minimal (Intervention Dose) and all severe alerts were dealt with in only a modest number of participating patients, which was the final measure of a successful intervention (Intervention Fidelity). An analysis showed that the CDSS was most frequently used on days with long practice hours (Intervention Tailoring).

3.2. Our Findings in the Context of Existing Research

The inclusion criteria for our study were broad and the patient group correspondingly heterogeneous. Unlike other similar studies, the group was not preselected according to medication, disease, or age group [23,24]. As a result, the focus of GP training was on dealing with polypharmacy in general, and did not attempt to provide in-depth instruction on how to optimize specific cases, as is the case in polypharmacy trials with narrower inclusion criteria [25,26]. Moreover, some of the included patients did not profit from the intervention because there were very few or sometimes even no alerts that could be reacted to. This problem has also occurred in previous interventions [27].

Existing research into time-consuming documentation has shown that time efficiency is crucial for GPs, which was an implementation barrier in our study [28]. It is therefore plausible that a significant number of participating GPs failed to document all changes in the software. Previous studies have also indicated that integrating CDSS into the electronic health records of patients would improve the usefulness of medication reviews [23].

Furthermore, a recent systematic review found that physicians considered most alerts generated by CDSS to be unhelpful or inappropriate and therefore ignored them [29], which is confirmed by the low rate of documentation in eMMa. Moreover, a significant number of alerts required monitoring certain parameters such as blood potassium levels and cardiac rhythm, or changing drug intake schedules, at the same time as using the CDSS [30,31]. The software only registered the use of such strategies when the alert under consideration was marked as justified. The sensitivity analysis indicated that some GPs made use of this possibility, albeit only few, which was probably because the additional documentation time was not reflected in any improvement in the patient's medication.

Difficulties in making medication changes arise when specialists are involved, as GPs are unwilling to interfere with their colleagues' decisions [32], not least because patients like their specialists to be consulted before such decisions are made [33]. One solution may be to improve interdisciplinary cooperation so that complicated medication regimens, that require both time and practice, can be jointly assessed and improved. The involvement of pharmacists was not part of this intervention, but their support in conducting medication reviews would appear to be plausible, especially in view of the discussed implementation barriers, and existing literature, which indicates benefits in terms of both medication appropriateness [34] and patient-relevant outcomes such as quality of life [35]. Qualitative studies conducted in the AdAM trial suggest that the expertise of pharmacists is also appreciated by GPs [36] and patients [37]. In addition, as the AdAM intervention comprised only one voluntary two-hour education session, with accompanying online videos and FAQs, it is quite possible that better results could have been generated if training in polypharmacy and use of the software had been better, as can be seen in comparable trials [32,38,39].

3.3. Strengths and Limitations

The fact that the design of the AdAM study included an underlying process evaluation that had been planned and published beforehand, improves the methodological quality of the trial. Furthermore, this process evaluation addresses each step of the CDSS application process and responds to the urgent need for a deeper understanding of CDSS uptake reported in a recently published systematic review [40]. We could show that GPs attached more importance to severe alerts, and that alerts relating to medication dosage and kidney function were more frequently dealt with than those concerning e.g., drug–drug interactions or possible unsuitability due to a patient's age (Intervention Dose). However, it should be taken into account that the software also generated alerts when a drug was entered into the system without additional information on the daily dosage or a patient's renal function. The management of these alerts would not necessarily have resulted in any improvement in medication but simply have indicated that missing information had been entered into eMMa.

Our analyses also help understand the characteristics of participating GPs, and the kind of patients whose medication reviews they prioritized. Participating patients had a slightly lower average level of nursing care, indicating a barrier to the use of the intervention tools in nursing home patients and for home visits.

Overall, the documented changes were rather small, and all severe alerts were removed or justified in only few patients (Intervention Fidelity). However, it was not possible to distinguish between a patient's medication having been left unchanged, or a change not having been documented in the software. As both the intended intensity of the intervention (Intervention Dose) and the desired intervention goal (Intervention Fidelity) were rarely fulfilled, conclusions about the potential risk reduction attributable to the intervention can only be drawn to a limited extent. Since the CDSS could not be linked with the practice management systems, GPs had to document all changes twice, which time constraints may have prevented, resulting in an underestimation of the use of eMMa.

Results in the Intervention Tailoring dimension showed that in the beginning of the intervention period, when updates and technical difficulties frequently occurred, the enrollment of patients in eMMa was low. GPs that were involved in the early stages of the intervention may have given up on the software after encountering technical problems early on. Furthermore, only few patients enrolled in the early months of each year, which coincided with the flu season. To the best of our knowledge, little research has been conducted into the impact of seasonal fluctuations on implementing a real-world study, so further analysis of the data gathered in the AdAM study may help in the planning of future interventions in clinical settings. Additionally, the COVID-19 pandemic struck during the intervention period. This unforeseeable event was a major, but certainly not the only disruption to the daily care of patients with polypharmacy that was observed during the course of this intervention, which makes the interpretation of results even more difficult.

3.4. Recommendations for Research and Clinical Practice

It is necessary to conduct more in-depth training before beginning such an intervention. An integration of the intervention tool in the practice management system and further measures to increase time efficiency would also facilitate adaptation and implementation for GPs and generate more robust data for scientific analysis. It is necessary to investigate whether the integration of further healthcare professionals, such as specialized physicians and pharmacists, would result in more effective medication reviews, especially in complex cases.

4. Materials and Methods

4.1. Background Information on the AdAM Study

The approach of the AdAM intervention ("*Anwendung für ein digital gestütztes Arzneimitteltherapie- und Versorgungsmanagement*", or "application of digitally supported drug-therapy and care management") is described in detail elsewhere [41]. In short, the intervention foresees that GPs perform at least one medication review in adult patients receiving five or more chronic medications with the help of a CDSS (software was developed under the name "eMMa", which is an abbreviation for electronic medication management) that has been fed with all relevant medical information in the form of claims data from the statutory health insurance company BARMER. The primary aim is to decrease hospitalization and death rates among polypharmacy patients compared to a patient group receiving usual care.

4.2. eMMA

The AdAM intervention involved the application of a CDSS that examined the medication of patients with polypharmacy after claims data provided by the patients' statutory health insurance company had been entered into the system, and after GPs had confirmed the claims data and fed additional relevant information into the system themselves. The underlying software then generated alerts that were categorized by severity (of which only the two highest of four levels overall are analyzed here, since the two lower levels do not pose clinical significance) and type of potential inappropriateness. The alerts that could be seen by GPs and that were analyzed in this study are displayed in Figure 9. GPs then had the possibility to make medication changes and to discuss them with their patients. A detailed breakdown of the steps conducted by GPs is depicted in Figure 10, whereby both figures were previously published in our study protocol [21].

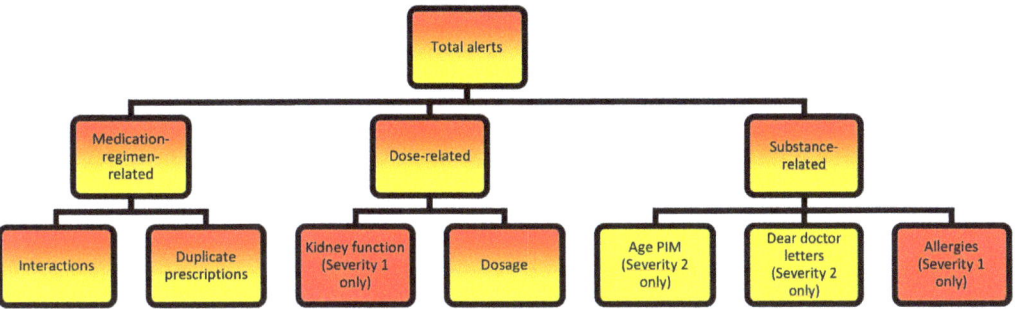

Figure 9. Alert categories documented by the software. Red font indicates alerts of the highest severity, and yellow font indicates medium severity.

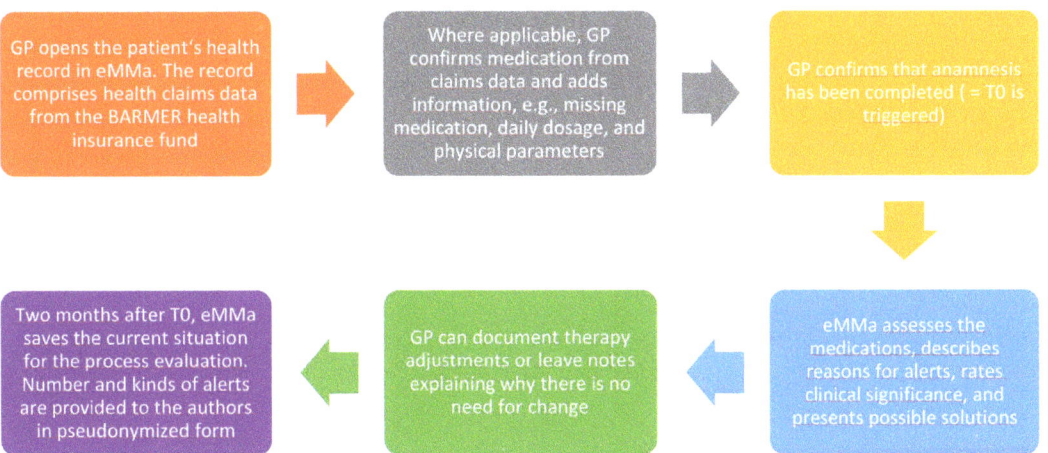

Figure 10. Schematic working process for GPs that use eMMa. The final step (purple field) defines T_1.

4.3. Theoretical Background of the Process Evaluation

The process evaluation is based on consensus recommendations in accordance with MRC guidance and the MRC process evaluation framework [18] and assesses four dimensions (Intervention Reach, Dose, Fidelity, Tailoring) of the implementation and application process. The defined dimensions and their adaptation to suit the implementation of the AdAM software are briefly explained below. A more detailed description can be found elsewhere [21].

4.4. Inclusion and Exclusion Criteria for Log Data Analysis

All patients to whom one of the following criteria applied, were included in the analysis of data extracted from the AdAM software:

1. The GP confirmed in the software that an anamnesis had been completed (referred to as "completed anamnesis").
2. The software was used to print a medication plan.
3. At least five medications were entered into the software.

The inclusion criteria were prioritized in descending order: The first day on which criterion 1 was met was defined as T_0. If this was never the case, criterion 2 and, if necessary, criterion 3 were treated analogously. Duplicates, i.e., patients whose pseudonym was included twice, were excluded after verification. In addition, patients were excluded if their GP only participated in the piloting test phase or had ceased to participate in the study before randomization (e.g., had retired). Patients that enrolled in eMMa after completion of the project were also excluded.

The Intervention Reach compares participants that fulfil the criteria to those that do not. All potentially eligible participants are therefore included in the analyses for that dimension.

4.5. Population and Outcomes

(a) Intervention Reach

This dimension deals with the "reach" of the intervention, i.e., whether the selection and inclusion of study participants was carried out as foreseen in the study protocol, and how the study population differed from the defined population in terms of the variables given in Appendix A, Table A1. These comparisons were conducted at the level of patients, physicians, and practices, and were used to determine structural similarity between the groups, and whether, for example, any particular group of patients was prioritized in the intervention.

For this purpose, all patients receiving the eMMa intervention (=active population, AP) were compared to:

- Study participants that had enrolled but did not receive the intervention (=inactive population, IP);
- Persons that fulfilled the entry criteria for the intention-to-treat population and were on the list of patients provided to participating GPs but did not take part in the intervention (=non-enrolled potentials, NEP).

Analogously, all GPs and practices enrolled in the AdAM study that cared for at least one AP patient, irrespective of whether they also treated patients in the IP or NEP groups were compared to:

- Enrolled GPs and practices that cared for at least one IP patient, but no AP patient;
- Enrolled GPs and practices that cared for at least one NEP patient, but no AP or IP patient.

An overview can be found in Figure 11.

Pseudonymized data for patient comparisons originated from BARMER's data warehouse (a database in which all claims data are stored pseudonymously). Comparisons at GP and practice level were carried out using pseudonymized data from the association of statutory healthcare physicians in the study region (KVWL). Group comparisons were carried out using logistic regression and two-sided tests carried out with a significance level of alpha = 5%. Group membership was defined as the dependent variable.

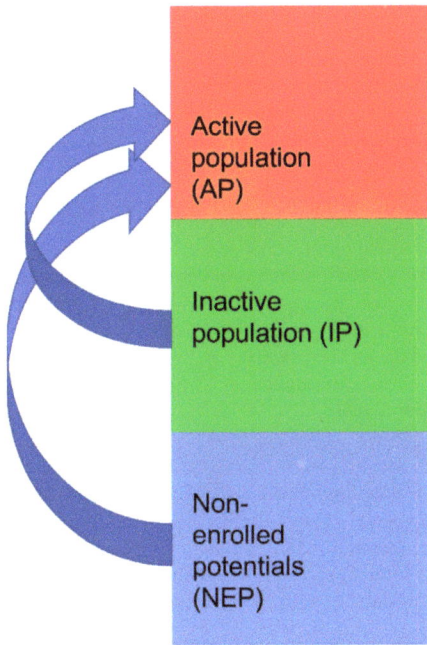

Figure 11. Populations that were compared for the Reach dimension.

(b) Intervention Dose

This dimension applies to the AP group only and assesses the extent of reductions in alerts in patients that received the AdAM intervention two months after patient data were originally entered into the software. In addition, prioritization associated with the severity and categories of alerts were also analyzed (Figure 9). The alerts were divided into justified (marked as processed or commented on by the GP) and unjustified alerts (not marked as processed or commented on by the GP). The number of alerts was measured at two points in time: the first timestamp (date) occurred when T_0 is triggered, and automatically two months later (referred to as T_1).

In this dimension, the main analysis is of the reduction in alerts between T_0 and T_1, stratified by severity and the category of alerts. In addition, sensitivity analyses were performed that only included unjustified alerts at T_1.

Further sensitivity analyses only included the population for which GPs had confirmed that the anamnesis of the patient had been completed and that all medication been entered into the software. This was the original plan, whereby T_0 was to be triggered in the software by pressing a button, and only then was it possible to deal with alerts. Before release, the software developers decided against making this process compulsory.

In order to adjust for clustering at a GP level, a multilevel Poisson model was calculated using the pseudonymized GP ID as a random effect. The total number of alerts was the dependent variable in the model, and T_0 and T_1 were the predictors. All models were stratified by age and sex.

(c) Intervention Fidelity

This dimension applies only to the AP group and examines the trustworthiness of the intervention, i.e., whether the software was used in such a way that a successful intervention (reduction in hospitalization and death) was possible. Alerts rated at the highest severity level were used to operationalize this dimension, as they were considered strongly indicative of a need for action. Furthermore, the GP had to have completed the anamnesis to show the software was being used as intended.

As long as all alerts at this level had been resolved or justified at T_1, they were considered to have been successfully dealt with in terms of Fidelity.

For this dimension, we reported the proportion of patients whose serious warnings were completely resolved at T_1. In addition, the analyses were stratified according to alert category.

(d) Intervention Tailoring

In contrast to the other dimensions, the focus here was on the individual adjustments GPs made in order to better integrate the intervention into daily practice routines. For this purpose, the temporal dimension of software use was investigated. Consequently, data are only analyzed for the AP group. Specifically, we looked at the number of patients whose data were called up for the first time on particular days of the week or in particular months, and looked for a concentration of such events during certain periods (e.g., at the weekend), or seasonal dependencies.

5. Conclusions

There are indications that the CDSS helped participating physicians prescribe fewer high-risk medications by encouraging them to adjust dosages, and to modify prescriptions to take account of renal function impairment. However, the intervention does not appear to have been used intensively, whereby it should be taken into consideration that utilization may have been under-reported in the log data. Overall, the results of the process evaluation indicate that the extent of the implementation of the AdAM intervention was weaker than anticipated.

Author Contributions: Conceptualization, C.M. and M.v.d.A.; methodology, R.B., D.L., J.K.-N., C.M. and M.v.d.A.; formal analysis, D.L.; investigation, R.B., D.L. and M.v.d.A.; data curation, D.L. and J.B.; writing—original draft preparation, R.B. and D.L.; writing—review and editing, R.B., D.L., J.B., P.K.-M., J.K.-N., C.M. and M.v.d.A.; visualization, R.B. and D.L.; supervision, M.v.d.A.; project administration, P.K.-M., J.K.-N., C.M. and M.v.d.A.; funding acquisition, P.K.-M., J.K.-N. and C.M. All authors have read and agreed to the published version of the manuscript.

Funding: This research was funded by INNOVATIONSONDS NEUE VERSORGUNGSFORMEN (Innovation Fund of the German Federal Joint Committee), grant number 01NVF16006. The APC was funded by the open access publication fund of Goethe University, Frankfurt am Main, Germany.

Institutional Review Board Statement: The study was conducted in accordance with the Declaration of Helsinki, and approved by the Ethics Committee of ÄRZTEKAMMER NORDRHEIN (Association of Physicians in the German region North Rhine) (protocol code 2017184, 26 July 2017).

Informed Consent Statement: Informed consent was obtained from all subjects involved in the study.

Data Availability Statement: The data presented in this study are available on request from the corresponding author. The data are not publicly available due to data protection regulations.

Acknowledgments: We would like to thank Phillip Elliott for the professional language review, and the whole AdAM study group for their cooperative and productive work in the past years. Members of the Adam study group include: Lara Düvel (BARMER, Wuppertal, Germany), Till Beckmann (BARMER, Wuppertal, Germany), Reinhard Hammerschmidt (KVWL, Dortmund, Germany), Julia Jachmich (KVWL, Dortmund, Germany), Eva Leicher (KVWL, Dortmund, Germany), Benjamin Brandt (KVWL, Dortmund, Germany), Johanna Richard (KVWL, Dortmund, Germany), Frank Meyer (KVWL, Dortmund, Germany), Mathias Flume (KVWL, Dortmund, Germany), Thomas Müller (KVWL, Dortmund, Germany), Ferdinand M. Gerlach (Institute of General Practice, Goethe-University, Frankfurt am Main, Germany), Beate S. Müller (Institute of General Practice, Goethe-University, Frankfurt am Main, Germany), Benno Flaig (Institute of General Practice, Goethe University, Frankfurt am Main, Germany), Ana Isabel González-González (Institute of General Practice, Goethe-University, Frankfurt am Main, Germany), Truc Sophia Dinh (Institute of General Practice, Goethe-University, Frankfurt am Main, Germany), Kiran Chapidi (formerly Institute of General Practice, Goethe-University, Frankfurt am Main, Germany), Peter Ihle (PMV research group, University of Cologne, Cologne, Germany), Ingo Meyer (PMV research group, University of Cologne, Cologne, Germany), Hans Joachim Trampisch (Department of Medical Informatics, Biometry and Epidemiology, Ruhr University, Bochum, Germany), Renate Klaaßen-Mielke (Department of Medical Informatics, Biometry and Epidemiology, Ruhr University, Bochum, Germany), Nina Timmesfeld (Department of Medical Informatics, Biometry and Epidemiology, Ruhr University, Bochum, Germany), Wolfgang Greiner (Department of Health Economics and Health Care Management, Faculty of Health Science, Bielefeld University, Bielefeld, Germany), Bastian Surmann (Department of Health Economics and Health Care Management, Faculty of Health Science, Bielefeld University, Bielefeld, Germany), Holger Pfaff (Institute for Medical Sociology, Health Services Research and Rehabilitation Science, Department of Health Services Research, University of Cologne, Cologne, Germany), Ute Karbach (Technical University Dortmund, Department of Rehabilitation Sociology, Faculty of Rehabilitation Sciences, Dortmund, Germany), Alexandra Piotrowski (Center for Health Economics and Health Services Research, University of Wuppertal, Germany), Karolina Beifuß (Center for Health Economics and Health Services Research, University of Wuppertal, Germany), Sarah Meyer (Center for Health Economics and Health Services Research, University of Wuppertal, Germany), Sara Söling (Center for Health Economics and Health Services Research, University of Wuppertal, Germany), Daniel Grandt (Department of Internal Medicine. Clinic Saarbrücken, Germany), Simone Grandt (RpDoc Solutions GmbH, Saarbrücken, Germany).

Conflicts of Interest: The authors declare no conflict of interest. The funders had no role in the design of the study; in the collection, analyses, or interpretation of data; in the writing of the manuscript, or in the decision to publish the results.

Appendix A

Table A1. Variables for the Reach dimension (ref = reference category in logistic regression).

Comparison 1	Comparison 2	Patients	GPs	Factor Levels	Practices	Factor Levels
		Age (years)	Age (years)		Type of practice	Single practice (ref)
						Group practice
						Medical care center
		Sex	Sex		Number of employed GPs	
				Male (ref)	Time since practice inception (years)	
				Female	Randomization group	
		medCDS	Specialization type			Intervention
AP versus IP	AP versus NEP	Nursing care level care (0 (ref), 1–5)		Specialized in general practice (ref)		Control (ref)
				GP without specialization		
				Internist active in general practice		
				Other		
			Participation in a GP network			
				Yes		
				No (ref)		
			Randomization group			
				Intervention		
				Control (ref)		

References

1. United Nations; Department of Economic and Social Affairs; Population Division. World Population Ageing 2019: Highlights. 2019. Available online: https://www.un.org/en/development/desa/population/publications/pdf/ageing/WorldPopulationAgeing2019-Highlights.pdf (accessed on 10 May 2022).
2. Van den Akker, M.; Buntinx, F.; Knottnerus, J.A. Comorbidity or multimorbidity. *Eur. J. Gen. Pract.* **1996**, *2*, 65–70. [CrossRef]
3. Masnoon, N.; Shakib, S.; Kalisch-Ellett, L.; Caughey, G.E. What is polypharmacy? A systematic review of definitions. *BMC Geriatr.* **2017**, *17*, 230. [CrossRef] [PubMed]
4. Guthrie, B.; Makubate, B.; Hernandez-Santiago, V.; Dreischulte, T. The rising tide of polypharmacy and drug-drug interactions: Population database analysis 1995–2010. *BMC Med.* **2015**, *13*, 74. [CrossRef]

5. Franchi, C.; Tettamanti, M.; Pasina, L.; Djignefa, C.D.; Fortino, I.; Bortolotti, A.; Merlino, L.; Nobili, A. Changes in drug prescribing to Italian community-dwelling elderly people: The EPIFARM-Elderly Project 2000–2010. *Eur. J. Clin. Pharmacol.* **2014**, *70*, 437–443. [CrossRef]
6. Duerden, M.; Avery, T.; Payne, R. *Polypharmacy and Medicines Optimisation: Making it Safe and Sound*; The King's Fund: London, UK, 2013.
7. Lu, W.-H.; Wen, Y.-W.; Chen, L.-K.; Hsiao, F.-Y. Effect of polypharmacy, potentially inappropriate medications and anticholinergic burden on clinical outcomes: A retrospective cohort study. *CMAJ* **2015**, *187*, E130–E137. [CrossRef]
8. Sganga, F.; Landi, F.; Ruggiero, C.; Corsonello, A.; Vetrano, D.L.; Lattanzio, F.; Cherubini, A.; Bernabei, R.; Onder, G. Polypharmacy and health outcomes among older adults discharged from hospital: Results from the CRIME study. *Geriatr. Gerontol. Int.* **2015**, *15*, 141–146. [CrossRef] [PubMed]
9. Franchi, C.; Marcucci, M.; Mannucci, P.M.; Tettamanti, M.; Pasina, L.; Fortino, I.; Bortolotti, A.; Merlino, L.; Nobili, A. Changes in clinical outcomes for community-dwelling older people exposed to incident chronic polypharmacy: A comparison between 2001 and 2009. *Pharmacoepidemiol. Drug Saf.* **2016**, *25*, 204–211. [CrossRef]
10. Schenker, Y.; Park, S.Y.; Jeong, K.; Pruskowski, J.; Kavalieratos, D.; Resick, J.; Abernethy, A.; Kutner, J.S. Associations Between Polypharmacy, Symptom Burden, and Quality of Life in Patients with Advanced, Life-Limiting Illness. *J. Gen. Intern. Med.* **2019**, *34*, 559–566. [CrossRef]
11. Yourman, L.; Concato, J.; Agostini, J.V. Use of computer decision support interventions to improve medication prescribing in older adults: A systematic review. *Am. J. Geriatr. Pharmacother.* **2008**, *6*, 119–129. [CrossRef]
12. Scott, I.A.; Pillans, P.I.; Barras, M.; Morris, C. Using EMR-enabled computerized decision support systems to reduce prescribing of potentially inappropriate medications: A narrative review. *Ther. Adv. Drug Saf.* **2018**, *9*, 559–573. [CrossRef]
13. Pearson, S.-A.; Moxey, A.; Robertson, J.; Hains, I.; Williamson, M.; Reeve, J.; Newby, D. Do computerised clinical decision support systems for prescribing change practice? A systematic review of the literature (1990–2007). *BMC Health Serv. Res.* **2009**, *9*, 154. [CrossRef] [PubMed]
14. Garg, A.X.; Adhikari, N.K.J.; McDonald, H.; Rosas-Arellano, M.P.; Devereaux, P.J.; Beyene, J.; Sam, J.; Haynes, R.B. Effects of computerized clinical decision support systems on practitioner performance and patient out-comes: A systematic review. *JAMA* **2005**, *293*, 1223–1238. [CrossRef] [PubMed]
15. Clyne, B.; Bradley, M.C.; Hughes, C.; Fahey, T.; Lapane, K.L. Electronic prescribing and other forms of technology to reduce inappropriate medication use and polypharmacy in older people: A review of current evidence. *Clin. Geriatr. Med.* **2012**, *28*, 301–322. [CrossRef] [PubMed]
16. Steckler, A.; Linnan, L.; Israel, B.A. (Eds.) *Process Evaluation for Public Health Interventions and Research*; Jossey-Bass a Wiley Imprint: San Francisco, CA, USA, 2002; ISBN 978-1-119-02248-0.
17. Möhler, R.; Köpke, S.; Meyer, G. Criteria for Reporting the Development and Evaluation of Complex Interventions in healthcare: Revised guideline (CReDECI 2). *Trials* **2015**, *16*, 204. [CrossRef] [PubMed]
18. Moore, G.F.; Audrey, S.; Barker, M.; Bond, L.; Bonell, C.; Hardeman, W.; Moore, L.; O'Cathain, A.; Tinati, T.; Wight, D.; et al. Process evaluation of complex interventions: Medical Research Council guidance. *BMJ* **2015**, *350*, h1258. [CrossRef] [PubMed]
19. Scott, S.D.; Rotter, T.; Flynn, R.; Brooks, H.M.; Plesuk, T.; Bannar-Martin, K.H.; Chambers, T.; Hartling, L. Systematic review of the use of process evaluations in knowledge translation research. *Syst. Rev.* **2019**, *8*, 266. [CrossRef]
20. Grant, A.; Treweek, S.; Dreischulte, T.; Foy, R.; Guthrie, B. Process evaluations for cluster-randomised trials of complex interventions: A proposed framework for design and reporting. *Trials* **2013**, *14*, 15. [CrossRef]
21. Brünn, R.; Lemke, D.; Chapidi, K.; Köberlein-Neu, J.; Piotrowski, A.; Söling, S.; Greiner, W.; Kellermann-Mühlhoff, P.; Timmesfeld, N.; van den Akker, M.; et al. Use of an electronic medication management support system in patients with polypharmacy in general practice: Study protocol of a quantitative process evaluation of the AdAM trial. *Ther. Adv. Drug Saf.* **2022**, *13*, 1–14. [CrossRef]
22. Quinzler, R.; Freitag, M.H.; Wiese, B.; Beyer, M.; Brenner, H.; Dahlhaus, A.; Döring, A.; Freund, T.; Heier, M.; Knopf, H.; et al. A novel superior medication-based chronic disease score predicted all-cause mortality in in-dependent geriatric cohorts. *J. Clin. Epidemiol.* **2019**, *105*, 112–124. [CrossRef]
23. Taheri Moghadam, S.; Sadoughi, F.; Velayati, F.; Ehsanzadeh, S.J.; Poursharif, S. The effects of clinical decision support system for prescribing medication on patient outcomes and physician practice performance: A systematic review and meta-analysis. *BMC Med. Inform. Decis. Mak.* **2021**, *21*, 98. [CrossRef]
24. El Asmar, M.L.; Dharmayat, K.I.; Vallejo-Vaz, A.J.; Irwin, R.; Mastellos, N. Effect of computerised, knowledge-based, clinical decision support systems on patient-reported and clinical outcomes of patients with chronic disease managed in primary care settings: A systematic review. *BMJ Open* **2021**, *11*, e054659. [CrossRef] [PubMed]
25. Dreischulte, T.; Donnan, P.; Grant, A.; Hapca, A.; McCowan, C.; Guthrie, B. Safer Prescribing—A Trial of Education, Informatics, and Financial Incentives. *N. Engl. J. Med.* **2016**, *374*, 1053–1064. [CrossRef]
26. Thiem, U.; Wilm, S.; Greiner, W.; Rudolf, H.; Trampisch, H.-J.; Müller, C.; Theile, G.; Thürmann, P.A. Reduction of potentially inappropriate medication in the elderly: Design of a cluster-randomised controlled trial in German primary care practices (RIME). *Ther. Adv. Drug Saf.* **2020**, *12*, 2042098620918459. [CrossRef]

27. Muth, C.; Uhlmann, L.; Haefeli, W.E.; Rochon, J.; van den Akker, M.; Perera, R.; Güthlin, C.; Beyer, M.; Oswald, F.; Valderas, J.M.; et al. Effectiveness of a complex intervention on Prioritising Multimedication in Multimor-bidity (PRIMUM) in primary care: Results of a pragmatic cluster randomised controlled trial. *BMJ Open* **2018**, *8*, e017740. [CrossRef] [PubMed]
28. Rieckert, A.; Sommerauer, C.; Krumeich, A.; Sönnichsen, A. Reduction of inappropriate medication in older populations by electronic decision support (the PRIMA-eDS study): A qualitative study of practical implementation in primary care. *BMC Fam. Pract.* **2018**, *19*, 110. [CrossRef] [PubMed]
29. Poly, T.N.; Islam, M.M.; Yang, H.-C.; Li, Y.-C.J. Appropriateness of Overridden Alerts in Computerized Physician Order Entry: Systematic Review. *JMIR Med. Inform.* **2020**, *8*, e15503. [CrossRef] [PubMed]
30. Bergk, V.; Gasse, C.; Rothenbacher, D.; Loew, M.; Brenner, H.; Haefeli, W.E. Drug interactions in primary care: Impact of a new algorithm on risk determination. *Clin. Pharmacol. Ther.* **2004**, *76*, 85–96. [CrossRef]
31. Seidling, H.M.; Klein, U.; Schaier, M.; Czock, D.; Theile, D.; Pruszydlo, M.G.; Kaltschmidt, J.; Mikus, G.; Haefeli, W.E. What, if all alerts were specific—Estimating the potential impact on drug interaction alert burden. *Int. J. Med. Inform.* **2014**, *83*, 285–291. [CrossRef] [PubMed]
32. Leiva-Fernández, F.; Prados-Torres, J.D.; Prados-Torres, A.; Del-Cura-González, I.; Castillo-Jimena, M.; López-Rodríguez, J.A.; Rogero-Blanco, M.E.; Lozano-Hernández, C.M.; López-Verde, F.; Bujalance-Zafra, M.J.; et al. Training primary care professionals in multimorbidity management: Educational assessment of the eMULTI-PAP course. *Mech. Ageing Dev.* **2020**, *192*, 111354. [CrossRef]
33. Reeve, E.; Low, L.-F.; Hilmer, S.N. Beliefs and attitudes of older adults and carers about deprescribing of medications: A qualitative focus group study. *Br. J. Gen. Pract.* **2016**, *66*, e552–e560. [CrossRef]
34. Martin, P.; Tamblyn, R.; Benedetti, A.; Ahmed, S.; Tannenbaum, C. Effect of a Pharmacist-Led Educational Intervention on Inappropriate Medication Prescriptions in Older Adults: The D-PRESCRIBE Randomized Clinical Trial. *JAMA* **2018**, *320*, 1889–1898. [CrossRef] [PubMed]
35. Schulz, M.; Griese-Mammen, N.; Anker, S.D.; Koehler, F.; Ihle, P.; Ruckes, C.; Schumacher, P.M.; Trenk, D.; Böhm, M.; Laufs, U. Pharmacy-based interdisciplinary intervention for patients with chronic heart failure: Results of the PHARM-CHF randomized controlled trial. *Eur. J. Heart Fail.* **2019**, *21*, 1012–1021. [CrossRef] [PubMed]
36. Söling, S.; Köberlein-Neu, J.; Müller, B.S.; Dinh, T.S.; Muth, C.; Pfaff, H.; Karbach, U. From sensitization to adoption? A qualitative study of the implementation of a digitally supported intervention for clinical decision making in polypharmacy. *Implement. Sci.* **2020**, *15*, 82. [CrossRef] [PubMed]
37. Brünn, R.; Müller, B.; Flaig, B.; Kellermann-Mühlhoff, P.; Karbach, U.; Söling, S.; Muth, C.; van den Akker, M. I must, and I can live with that: A thematic analysis of patients perspectives on polypharmacy and a digital decision support system for GPs. *BMC Fam. Pract.* **2021**, *22*, 168. [CrossRef] [PubMed]
38. Die Leitliniengruppe Hessen. S3-Leitlinie Multimedikation, Langfassung: AWMF-Registernummer: 053-043. Available online: https://www.awmf.org/uploads/tx_szleitlinien/053-043l_S3_Multimedikation_2021-08.pdf (accessed on 1 October 2021).
39. Mann, C.; Shaw, A.R.G.; Guthrie, B.; Wye, L.; Man, M.-S.; Chaplin, K.; Salisbury, C. Can implementation failure or intervention failure explain the result of the 3D multimorbidity trial in general practice: Mixed-methods process evaluation. *BMJ Open* **2019**, *9*, e031438. [CrossRef]
40. Kouri, A.; Yamada, J.; Lam Shin Cheung, J.; van de Velde, S.; Gupta, S. Do providers use computerized clinical decision support systems? A systematic review and meta-regression of clinical decision support uptake. *Implement. Sci.* **2022**, *17*, 21. [CrossRef]
41. Müller, B.S.; Klaaßen-Mielke, R.; Gonzalez-Gonzalez, A.I.; Grandt, D.; Hammerschmidt, R.; Köberlein-Neu, J.; Kellermann-Mühlhoff, P.; Trampisch, H.J.; Beckmann, T.; Düvel, L.; et al. Effectiveness of the application of an electronic medication management support system in patients with polypharmacy in general practice: A study protocol of cluster-randomised controlled trial (AdAM). *BMJ Open* **2021**, *11*, e048191. [CrossRef]

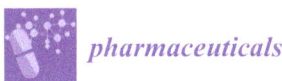 *pharmaceuticals*

Opinion

Clinical Utility of Medication-Based Risk Scores to Reduce Polypharmacy and Potentially Avoidable Healthcare Utilization

Armando Silva-Almodóvar [1,2] and Milap C. Nahata [1,3,*]

[1] Institute of Therapeutic Innovations and Outcomes (ITIO), College of Pharmacy, Ohio State University, Columbus, OH 43210, USA; silvaalmodovar.1@osu.edu
[2] Tabula Rasa HealthCare, Tucson, AZ 85701, USA
[3] College of Medicine, Ohio State University, Columbus, OH 43210, USA
* Correspondence: nahata.1@osu.edu; Tel.: +1-614-292-2472

Abstract: The management of multiple chronic health conditions often requires patients to be exposed to polypharmacy to improve their health and enhance their quality of life. However, exposure to polypharmacy has been associated with an increased risk for adverse effects, drug-drug interactions, inappropriate prescribing, medication nonadherence, increased healthcare utilization such as emergency department visits and hospitalizations, and costs. Medication-based risk scores have been utilized to identify patients who may benefit from deprescribing interventions and reduce rates of inappropriate prescribing. These risk scores may also be utilized to prompt targeted discussions between patients and providers regarding medications or medication classes contributing to an individual's risk for harm, eventually leading to the deprescribing of the offending medication(s). This opinion will describe existing medication-based risk scores in the literature, their utility in identifying patients at risk for specific adverse events, and how they may be incorporated in healthcare settings to reduce rates of potentially inappropriate polypharmacy and avoidable healthcare utilization and costs.

Keywords: medication-based risk score; deprescribing; polypharmacy; health outcomes

1. Introduction

Patients with multiple chronic conditions may be exposed to several medications to improve health, enhance quality of life, and reduce healthcare utilization. The chronic exposure of multiple medications has been termed polypharmacy [1]. While the operational definition of polypharmacy may vary, from utilizing ≥2 to ≥11 medications [1], polypharmacy is associated with an increased risk of drug-drug interactions, drug-related problems, inappropriate prescribing, medication non-adherence, and increased healthcare utilization such as emergency department visits, hospitalizations, and medical costs [2].

Medication-based risk scores can be utilized by healthcare providers to identify patients who would benefit from deprescribing interventions to reduce rates of potentially inappropriate polypharmacy, adverse health outcomes, and avoidable healthcare utilization. The utilization of these tools is especially important due to the increasing proportions of adults with multiple chronic conditions, resulting in higher prevalence of polypharmacy [3]. The higher prevalence of polypharmacy has led to an increased risk for clinically relevant drug-drug and drug-disease interactions. This opinion will describe medication-based risk scores that can be used to identify patients at substantial risk for experiencing clinically significant adverse outcomes, propose their utility in identifying medication targets for deprescribing, and suggest how these tools can be incorporated into clinical practice or clinical decision support systems.

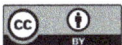

2. Medication-Based Risk Scores

2.1. Medication Regimen Complexity Index (MRCI)

The MRCI is a risk assessment tool that quantifies the complexity of an individual's medication regimen by taking into consideration the medication dosage form and route, dosing frequency, and unique directions provided to take certain medications [4]. This tool utilizes a continuous scale where higher scores suggest that an individual's medication regimen is more complex [4]. A systematic review found higher MRCI to be associated with medication nonadherence, hospital readmission, and lower quality of life [5]. While some studies found patients with scores greater than a certain number to be associated with worsening health outcomes in select populations [5], there are no validated parameters suggesting which values signal a clearly increased risk for adverse events. Future research is warranted to determine specific scores to be utilized as surrogate markers to identify patients likely to benefit most from deprescribing interventions. It is important to note that while the MRCI score is typically calculated manually due to the consideration of unique medication directions, a study by McDonald et al. [6] described how to automate the calculation of MRCI within an electronic health record.

2.2. Medication Complexity Score (MCS)

The development of the MRCI allowed clinicians and researchers to quantify the complexity of an individual's medication regimen. However, since part of the score requires the use of unique prescribing details [5], the score cannot be calculated using only prescription claims data. This is a potential weakness, as prescription claims data may be better suited to capture prescribing patterns across multiple health systems and prescribers [7]. The MCS was developed and modeled against the MRCI to demonstrate its comparability as a tool in identifying medication burden and risk for greater healthcare utilization with the use of just prescription claims [7]. The MCS utilizes a prescription claim's national drug code to infer the drug's dosage form and route; the days' supply and number of units are utilized to infer a dosing frequency. The final component of the MRCI, being unique medication instructions, was not adapted to the MCS. As with MRCI, future research identifying specific cut-off values of the MCS score signifying which patients would benefit most from deprescribing interventions would be beneficial.

2.3. Medication Fall Risk Score (MFRS)

Just under 1,000,000 patients fall within healthcare facilities each year in the United States (US) [8]. Reducing the prevalence of falls within facilities is necessary to ensure positive patient outcomes while reducing avoidable costs incurred by patients and healthcare facilities. Specific medications are important risk factors to consider when evaluating a patient's risk of falling due to their mechanisms of action being associated with greater risk of dizziness, sedation, impaired cognition, and changes in blood pressure [8]. The MFRS incorporates the prescribing of specific medication classes (e.g., antipsychotics, benzodiazepines, antiarrhythmics, antidepressants) to determine the associated risk of incurring a fall. Medications are weighted and summed to determine an individual's risk of falling. Patients with a score ≥ 6 are at "a higher risk for falling" and are further evaluated using medication fall risk evaluation tools [9]. In addition to the implementation of further medication reviews and local clinical interventions specific to healthcare settings, patients identified as being at an increased risk of falls may benefit from deprescribing interventions to reduce their risk of falls.

2.4. Medication-Based Index of Physical Function (MedIP)

Another tool used to measure fall risk is the MedIP. This tool was developed to overcome biases from tools that focus on specific medication classes [10]. The MedIP utilizes medications included in the Side Effect Resource (SIDER) dataset, a resource that obtains side effect related information of medications from public sources such as package inserts [11]. The MedIP calculates a sum utilizing elementary matrix operations that take into consideration the drugs being used by a patient, their risk of side effects and the contribution of side effects to fall risk based on data found within SIDER. While higher scores indicate a greater risk of falling, the validation study estimated a score of 2764 to have optimal sensitivity and specificity in predicting fall risk [10].

2.5. Drug Burden Index (DBI)

The use of medications with sedative and anticholinergic properties has been associated with adverse events among older adults including cognitive impairment and falls [12]. The DBI score takes into consideration the dose and exposure of medications with anticholinergic and/or sedative effects on patients [13]. This score utilizes an algorithm that sums the sedative and anticholinergic weighted burden of each medication to generate a score. Each medication weight is calculated by dividing the daily dose with the sum of the minimum recommended daily dose and the daily dose [12]. Higher scores suggest a higher anticholinergic and sedative burden; studies have generally evaluated healthcare utilization risk comparing patients with scores greater than 0 or 1 versus lower scores [12].

While the findings of studies assessing the relationship between DBI and healthcare utilizations and outcomes such as falls have varied, higher DBI has been consistently shown to be associated with frailty, poorer quality of life, and physical impairment [12]. However, it is important to note the DBI score has several limitations: medications with relevant anticholinergic and sedative effects are considered equivalent (there is no adjustment for medications having stronger or weaker sedative or anticholinergic effects), and there is presently not an updated consensus document listing medications to consider for the determination of DBI. It is also important to note that the DBI was developed utilizing the minimum daily dose as indicated by the United States Food and Drug Administration. Given that minimum daily doses may vary among countries and with indications for use, a DBI algorithm was developed utilizing a defined daily dose published by the World Health Organization (WHO) to facilitate use of this algorithm across different countries [14].

2.6. Anticholinergic Burden Medication Based Risk Scores

Medications contributing to anticholinergic burden is a field of significant interest due to widely used drug classes with anticholinergic properties being associated with significant healthcare utilization and poor health outcomes. This has led to the publication of numerous scales, lists, and risk scores that quantify an individual's anticholinergic burden to estimate their risk of adverse outcomes. Furthermore, given the substantial interest and breadth of research examining anticholinergic burden, several systematic reviews have been published examining the utility of these scales to predict poor health outcomes such as adverse events, falls, mortality, delirium, and poor quality of life [15–24].

Scores, scales, and lists available to measure anticholinergic burden or identify exposure to anticholinergic medications include the anticholinergic drug scale [25] (ADS), anticholinergic burden classification [26] (ABC), anticholinergic effect on cognition [27] (AEC), anticholinergic risk scale [28] (ARS), anticholinergic cognitive burden scale [29] (ACBS), anticholinergic activity scale [30] (AAS), anticholinergic loading scale [31] (ALS), Korean anticholinergic burden scale [32], German anticholinergic burden score [33], Brazilian anticholinergic activity scale [34], Cancelli's ACH burden scale [35], Aizenberg's Anticholinergic Burden Scale [36], Duran's Anticholinergic Burden Scale [17], Salahudeen's Anticholinergic Burden Scale [15], Summers drug risk number [37], Whalleys Anticholinergic Burden Scale [38], Chew's list of anticholinergic drugs [39], Clinician-Rated Anticholinergic Score [40], Minzenberg's Clinical Index and Pharmacological Index [41], anticholinergic impregnation scale [42], a modified ARS [43], modified ACB [44], deliriogenic risk scale [45], and the anticholinergic toxicity scale [46].

These tools provide prescribers with an understanding of a patient's risks for specific adverse outcomes based on their cumulative exposure to medications with anticholinergic activity. However, despite the large number of tools available to highlight anticholinergic burden, there are several details to consider. Significant variability exists between tools, with some taking into consideration the dose of medications, and several tools identifying <30 medications and others considering >500 medications with expected anticholinergic activity [22]. Furthermore, while agreement on the level of anticholinergic activity may vary between tools, it is unclear which specific tool is best. Providers may benefit from using systematic reviews that have compiled lists of medications across multiple scales to comprehensively define which medications had low, moderate, and high anticholinergic activity [15,17,22]. Published systematic reviews of these tools have provided greater detail of the strengths and weaknesses of these tools and their associations with poor health outcomes [15–24].

2.7. Sedative Load Model (SLM)

The SLM was designed to characterize an individual's exposure to medications with sedative properties and to quantify their risk of impaired mobility [47,48]. This risk is calculated by summing the weights of medications contributing to an individual's sedative burden. Medications considered a primary sedative included a score of 2, while medications with a major side effect or with ingredients considered potentially sedating were given a score of 1 [47]. A higher sedative load is associated with impaired mobility [47]. While additional research is needed in diverse older adult populations, higher sedative load has been associated with incident delirium and falls among patients with Alzheimer's disease [49].

2.8. Sloan Sedative Risk Score

Sloan et al., modified the SLM to construct a sedative load risk score that incorporated the dose of a medication as well [50]. This risk score applies weights differently, with psychotropic medications intended to cause sedation receiving a weight of 6, while medications with sedation as a common side effect were given a weight of 3, and medications at a low-risk of sedation side effect were given a weight of 1 [50]. The dose of each medication is divided by the mean effective dose, which is then multiplied by the assigned weight and summed for a final score [50]. While the utilization of this model can describe the sedative risk of a population, with higher scores implying greater risk, it is unclear if there is a specific score associated with the significantly increased risk of falling or other adverse outcomes related to sedation.

2.9. Central Nervous System (CNS) Medication Burden

Another measure that was developed to quantify an individual's medication related risk for falls included the CNS medication burden [51]. This risk score is calculated by summing the daily dose of each CNS medication with each divided by the minimum effective geriatric daily dose [51]. Individuals with scores ≥ 3 are considered at greater risk of experiencing serious falls [51,52]. Future research would be beneficial to assess if medication-based interventions that reduce an individual's medication exposure subsequently reduce their risk of falls.

2.10. Medication Appropriateness Index (MAI)

A challenge in deprescribing medications is the identification of prescriptions that are appropriate and inappropriate. While the previously noted risk scores identified medications or medication classes that were potentially inappropriate for an individual, the MAI is a scoring system that determines if a medication is inappropriate and should be targeted for modification or deprescribing. The original tool utilizes 10 questions where a clinician assesses if a drug is indicated, effective, appropriately dosed, given with appropriate instructions, practical to use, prescribed with appropriate length of therapy, relatively affordable compared to similar drugs, and does not have any clinically significant drug-drug or drug-disease interactions [53]. A clinician must determine if a drug is appropriate (score = 1), inappropriate (score = 3), or marginally appropriate (score = 2), with each drug having a maximum score of 18; higher scores would suggest that a drug may be inappropriate. The sum of the scores is used to determine an individual's exposure to inappropriate medications [53]. The tool has been validated in multiple settings comparing responses among clinicians to ensure consistency in its application across various practitioners [54]. Additionally, the MAI has been modified to a three-item survey and adapted and validated in various settings [55].

Despite the advantages of utilizing an individual clinician's knowledge to determine the inappropriateness of a medication or medication regimen, there are important limitations of MAI. Agreement between clinicians on the determination of the inappropriateness of a medication may improve after discussion, suggesting that interpretation of inappropriateness based on patient specific factors and identification of clinically relevant drug-drug or drug-disease interactions can differ based on a provider's experience and background [56]. Furthermore, assessing for the appropriateness of medications based on price or practicality may benefit from patient input. Finally, the tool may take up to 10 min to properly evaluate one drug, therefore it may not be practical to use for patients on multiple medications in most settings [53].

2.11. MedWise Risk Score

Previous medication-based risk scores may be limited in their utility given that they are used to track one or two specific risk factors in a patient's medication regimen, such as fall risk, anticholinergic burden, sedative load, complexity, or appropriateness. In contrast, the MedWise Risk Score measures an individual's risk for adverse events based on specific risk factors including sedative load, anticholinergic burden, competitive CYP450 drug interaction burden, risk of QT prolongation, and risk for adverse events utilizing the FDA Adverse Event Reporting System [57]. This score exists on a continuous scale with higher scores being associated with adverse events, healthcare related costs, emergency room visits, falls, and mortality [57–59]. Furthermore, use of the MedWise Risk Score as part of medication risk mitigation services may significantly reduce healthcare costs related to emergency room visits, hospital admissions, and skilled nursing visits for organizations providing services for older adults that require nursing facility level care [60].

2.12. Medication Intensity Scale (MIS)

An important goal of care among patients with asthma is to improve quality of life and reduce healthcare utilization such as emergency room visits and hospitalizations. In 2013, asthma was associated with approximately $50 billion in medical costs in the United States [61]. The MIS is one means of identifying patients with suboptimal control of their asthma to target resources and reduce the prevalence of potentially avoidable healthcare costs. The MIS is a four-point scale (0–3) that ascribes a point to a patient for having 5–13 beta-agonists canisters, >13 beta-agonist canisters, and having greater than two dispensations of oral corticosteroids within a year [62]. Validation of this tool demonstrated that higher scores were associated with greater emergency department utilization [62]. The validation study of this tool recommends that the cut-off chosen for intervention be determined by the cost of the intervention; when it was given using lower cut-offs it substantially increased the false positive rate of patients with asthma at risk for utilizing the emergency department [62]. The automated monitoring of prescription claims could identify patients with asthma at greatest need of intervention to improve asthma control and reduce potentially avoidable healthcare utilization.

3. Implementation within Healthcare Systems

Medication-based risk scores are a set of tools that can be utilized at the healthcare system level and the individual prescriber level to identify patients at significant risk for experiencing specific adverse events or potentially avoidable healthcare utilization. While risk scores have been traditionally utilized as tools for risk adjustment and prediction of healthcare utilization [63], medication-based risk scores can be utilized by providers to identify patients at greater risk for specific adverse events and reduce potentially inappropriate polypharmacy. The use of medication-based risk scores may prompt discussions between patients and providers regarding medications contributing to an individual's risk for harm, eventually leading to the deprescribing of the offending medication. Furthermore, given their dependence on only medication-related information, these risk scores can be operationalized in settings where prescribing occurs, or prescription claims data is accessible. However, prior to the incorporation of medication-based risk scores into healthcare services, there are important details to consider.

The use of medication-based risk scores should be used with resources that facilitate deprescribing interventions. While most medication-based risk scores are validated to detect an increased risk of specific adverse events or healthcare utilization, they have not been studied extensively in their efficiency in identifying medications that should be deprescribed nor have they been compared to each other in this respect. It is important to note that medication-based risk scores should not solely be used to determine the appropriateness or inappropriateness of a medication. They should be used to complement a comprehensive evaluation of an individual's medications. These tools are used to identify potential targets for deprescribing and enhance the quality of information contributing to the risk-benefit assessment of an individual's prescriptions. Within primary care and outpatient settings, these risk scores can be used to identify patients who may benefit from deprescribing before a potentially avoidable event occurs, while hospital or emergency room settings can utilize these risk scores to compliment the identification of adverse events related to medication use. Hospital settings may benefit more from using risk scores that incorporate physiological data to identify emergent events that require prompt intervention.

Providers need to evaluate which risk scores are most useful in identifying patients at greatest risk for specific harms or healthcare utilization within their specific healthcare settings. Presently, each risk score describes the risk for exposure to certain medications and medication classes in relation to specific adverse outcomes. It is also important to realize that risk scores alone do not overcome barriers to deprescribing such as managing interprofessional relationships, increasing provider workload, the reluctance to discontinue chronic medications, or differences in knowledge between providers [64]. Some of these barriers can be overcome with the use of deprescribing algorithms and guidelines that provide steps and rationale to safely and efficiently deprescribe certain medications [65].

Primary care and outpatient healthcare settings may want to utilize medication management programs or pharmacovigilance services to monitor the use and prescribing of medications without additional work and burden for prescribers. Alternatively, insurance plan providers can utilize prescription claims data to identify patients at greater risk of adverse events based on their prescribing data. Medication management programs can be utilized to communicate with the providers of these patients to prompt review of their medications to consider deprescribing interventions. The implementation of medication reviews at the insurance claims level can overcome challenges associated with patient fragmentation of data across various healthcare and dispensing settings. Additionally, having personnel specialized in the deprescribing of medications can ensure that medication-based risk scores and deprescribing tools are used optimally and efficiently among patient populations. Patients with higher risk for medication related adverse events may benefit from periodic medication reviews where medications with the lowest benefit to harm ratio are targeted for deprescribing [66].

4. Conclusions

Medication-based risk scores are useful in identifying patients potentially at risk for suboptimal health outcomes and avoidable healthcare utilization and adverse events. To ensure that healthcare settings are able to efficiently reduce harms associated with exposure to the medications, combining these tools with deprescribing algorithms and guidelines may facilitate the discontinuation of medications that provide the least benefit and most harm to patients. The utilization of pharmacovigilance and medication management programs may be implemented within healthcare settings to identify opportunities for deprescribing and reduce potentially avoidable healthcare utilization.

Author Contributions: Conceptualization, A.S.-A. and M.C.N.; writing—original draft preparation, A.S.-A. and M.C.N.; writing—review and editing, A.S.-A. and M.C.N. All authors have read and agreed to the published version of the manuscript.

Funding: Milap Nahata was supported in part by the Avatar Foundation. Armando Silva Almodóvar is supported in part by the National Institute on Aging (R24AG064025).

Institutional Review Board Statement: Not applicable.

Data Availability Statement: Data is contained within the article.

Conflicts of Interest: The authors declare that they have no conflicts of interest. The funders had no role in the design of the study; in the collection, analyses, or interpretation of data; in the writing of the manuscript, or in the decision to publish the results. The opinions expressed herein are solely those of the authors and do not reflect the opinions or views of TRHC, its companies, or its employees.

References

1. Masnoon, N.; Shakib, S.; Kalisch-Ellett, L.; Caughey, G.E. What is polypharmacy? A systematic review of definitions. *BMC Geriatr.* **2017**, *17*, 230. [CrossRef] [PubMed]
2. Davies, L.E.; Spiers, G.; Kingston, A.; Todd, A.; Adamson, J.; Hanratty, B. Adverse outcomes of polypharmacy in older people: Systematic review of reviews. *J. Am. Med. Dir. Assoc.* **2020**, *21*, 181–187. [CrossRef] [PubMed]
3. World Health Organization. *Multimorbidity: Technical Series on Safer Primary Care*; World Health Organization: Geneva, Switzerland, 2016.
4. George, J.; Phun, Y.T.; Bailey, M.J.; Kong, D.C.; Stewart, K. Development and validation of the medication regimen complexity index. *Ann. Pharm.* **2004**, *38*, 1369–1376. [CrossRef] [PubMed]
5. Alves-Conceição, V.; Rocha, K.S.S.; Silva, F.V.N.; Silva, R.O.S.; Silva, D.T.D.; Lyra, D.P., Jr. Medication Regimen Complexity Measured by MRCI: A Systematic Review to Identify Health Outcomes. *Ann. Pharmacother.* **2018**, *52*, 1117–1134. [CrossRef] [PubMed]
6. McDonald, M.V.; Peng, T.R.; Sridharan, S.; Foust, J.B.; Kogan, P.; Pezzin, L.E.; Feldman, P.H. Automating the medication regimen complexity index. *J. Am. Med. Inf. Assoc.* **2013**, *20*, 499–505. [CrossRef] [PubMed]
7. Kitchen, C.A.; Chang, H.Y.; Bishop, M.A.; Shermock, K.M.; Kharrazi, H.; Weiner, J.P. Comparing and validating medication complexity from insurance claims against electronic health records. *J. Manag. Care Spec. Pharm.* **2022**, *28*, 473–484. [CrossRef]
8. Preventing Falls in Hospitals. Content Last Reviewed March 2021. Agency for Healthcare Research and Quality, Rockville, MD. Available online: https://www.ahrq.gov/patient-safety/settings/hospital/fall-prevention/toolkit/index.html (accessed on 27 April 2022).
9. Beasley, B.; Patatanian, E. Development and Implementation of a Pharmacy Fall Prevention Program. *Hosp. Pharm.* **2009**, *44*, 1095–1102. [CrossRef]
10. Hall, C.D.; Karpen, S.C.; Odle, B.; Panus, P.C.; Walls, Z.F. Development and evaluation of the medication-based index of physical function (MedIP). *Age Ageing* **2017**, *46*, 761–766. [CrossRef]
11. Kuhn, M.; Campillos, M.; Letunic, I.; Jensen, L.J.; Bork, P. A side effect resource to capture phenotypic effects of drugs. *Mol. Syst. Biol.* **2010**, *6*, 343. [CrossRef]
12. Wouters, H.; van der Meer, H.; Taxis, K. Quantification of anticholinergic and sedative drug load with the Drug Burden Index: A review of outcomes and methodological quality of studies. *Eur. J. Clin. Pharmacol.* **2017**, *73*, 257–266. [CrossRef]
13. Hilmer, S.N.; Mager, D.E.; Simonsick, E.M.; Cao, Y.; Ling, S.M.; Windham, B.G.; Harris, T.B.; Hanlon, J.T.; Rubin, S.M.; Shorr, R.I.; et al. A drug burden index to define the functional burden of medications in older people. *Arch. Intern. Med.* **2007**, *167*, 781–787. [CrossRef] [PubMed]
14. Faure, R.; Dauphinot, V.; Krolak-Salmon, P.; Mouchoux, C. A standard international version of the Drug Burden Index for cross-national comparison of the functional burden of medications in older people. *J. Am. Geriatr. Soc.* **2013**, *61*, 1227–1228. [CrossRef] [PubMed]
15. Salahudeen, M.S.; Duffull, S.B.; Nishtala, P.S. Anticholinergic burden quantified by anticholinergic risk scales and adverse outcomes in older people: A systematic review. *BMC Geriatr.* **2015**, *15*, 31. [CrossRef] [PubMed]
16. Stewart, C.; Taylor-Rowan, M.; Soiza, R.L.; Quinn, T.J.; Loke, Y.K.; Myint, P.K. Anticholinergic burden measures and older people's falls risk: A systematic prognostic review. *Adv. Drug Saf.* **2021**, *12*, 20420986211016645. [CrossRef]
17. Durán, C.E.; Azermai, M.; Vander Stichele, R.H. Systematic review of anticholinergic risk scales in older adults. *Eur. J. Clin. Pharmacol.* **2013**, *69*, 1485–1496. [CrossRef]
18. Graves-Morris, K.; Stewart, C.; Soiza, R.L.; Taylor-Rowan, M.; Quinn, T.J.; Loke, Y.K.; Myint, P.K. The prognostic value of anticholinergic burden measures in relation to mortality in older individuals: A systematic review and meta-analysis. *Front. Pharmacol.* **2020**, *11*, 570. [CrossRef]

19. Georgiou, R.; Lamnisos, D.; Giannakou, K. Anticholinergic burden and cognitive performance in patients with schizophrenia: A systematic literature review. *Front. Psychiatry* **2021**, *12*, 779607. [CrossRef]
20. Egberts, A.; Moreno-Gonzalez, R.; Alan, H.; Ziere, G.; Mattace-Raso, F.U.S. Anticholinergic Drug Burden and Delirium: A Systematic Review. *J. Am. Med. Dir. Assoc.* **2021**, *22*, 65–73.e4. [CrossRef]
21. Lisibach, A.; Benelli, V.; Ceppi, M.G.; Waldner-Knogler, K.; Csajka, C.; Lutters, M. Quality of anticholinergic burden scales and their impact on clinical outcomes: A systematic review. *Eur. J. Clin. Pharmacol.* **2021**, *77*, 147–162. [CrossRef]
22. Al Rihani, S.B.; Deodhar, M.; Darakjian, L.I.; Dow, P.; Smith, M.K.; Bikmetov, R.; Turgeon, J.; Michaud, V. Quantifying Anticholinergic Burden and Sedative Load in Older Adults with Polypharmacy: A Systematic Review of Risk Scales and Models. *Drugs Aging* **2021**, *38*, 977–994. [CrossRef]
23. Stewart, C.; Yrjana, K.; Kishor, M.; Soiza, R.L.; Taylor-Rowan, M.; Quinn, T.J.; Loke, Y.K.; Myint, P.K. Anticholinergic Burden Measures Predict Older People's Physical Function and Quality of Life: A Systematic Review. *J. Am. Med. Dir. Assoc.* **2021**, *22*, 56–64. [CrossRef] [PubMed]
24. Welsh, T.J.; van der Wardt, V.; Ojo, G.; Gordon, A.L.; Gladman, J.R.F. Anticholinergic Drug Burden Tools/Scales and Adverse Outcomes in Different Clinical Settings: A Systematic Review of Reviews. *Drugs Aging* **2018**, *35*, 523–538. [CrossRef] [PubMed]
25. Carnahan, R.M.; Lund, B.C.; Perry, P.J.; Pollock, B.G.; Culp, K.R. The Anticholinergic Drug Scale as a measure of drug-related anticholinergic burden: Associations with serum anticholinergic activity. *J. Clin. Pharmacol.* **2006**, *46*, 1481–1486. [CrossRef] [PubMed]
26. Ancelin, M.L.; Artero, S.; Portet, F.; Dupuy, A.M.; Touchon, J.; Ritchie, K. Non-degenerative mild cognitive impairment in elderly people and use of anticholinergic drugs: Longitudinal cohort study. *BMJ* **2006**, *332*, 455–459. [CrossRef] [PubMed]
27. Bishara, D.; Harwood, D.; Sauer, J.; Taylor, D.M. Anticholinergic effect on cognition (AEC) of drugs commonly used in older people. *Int. J. Geriatr. Psychiatry* **2017**, *32*, 650–656. [CrossRef]
28. Rudolph, J.L.; Salow, M.J.; Angelini, M.C.; McGlinchey, R.E. The anticholinergic risk scale and anticholinergic adverse effects in older persons. *Arch. Intern. Med.* **2008**, *168*, 508–513. [CrossRef]
29. Boustani, M.; Campbell, N.; Munger, S.; Maidment, I.; Fox, C. Impact of anticholinergics on the aging brain: A review and practical application. *Aging Health* **2008**, *4*, 311–320. [CrossRef]
30. Ehrt, U.; Broich, K.; Larsen, J.P.; Ballard, C.; Aarsland, D. Use of drugs with anticholinergic effect and impact on cognition in Parkinson's disease: A cohort study. *J. Neurol. Neurosurg. Psychiatry* **2010**, *81*, 160–165. [CrossRef]
31. Sittironnarit, G.; Ames, D.; Bush, A.; Faux, N.; Flicker, L.; Foster, J.; Hilmer, S.; Lautenschlager, N.T.; Maruff, P.; Masters, C.L.; et al. Effects of anticholinergic drugs on cognitive function in older Australians: Results from the AIBL study. *Dement. Geriatr. Cogn. Disord.* **2011**, *31*, 173–178. [CrossRef]
32. Jun, K.; Hwang, S.; Ah, Y.M.; Suh, Y.; Lee, J.Y. Development of an Anticholinergic Burden Scale specific for Korean older adults. *Geriatr. Gerontol. Int.* **2019**, *19*, 628–634. [CrossRef]
33. Kiesel, E.K.; Hopf, Y.M.; Drey, M. An anticholinergic burden score for German prescribers: Score development. *BMC Geriatr.* **2018**, *18*, 239. [CrossRef] [PubMed]
34. Nery, R.T.; Reis, A.M.M. Development of a Brazilian anticholinergic activity drug scale. *Einstein* **2019**, *17*, eAO4435. [CrossRef] [PubMed]
35. Cancelli, I.; Gigli, G.L.; Piani, A.; Zanchettin, B.; Janes, F.; Rinaldi, A.; Valente, M. Drugs with anticholinergic properties as a risk factor for cognitive impairment in elderly people: A population-based study. *J. Clin. Psychopharmacol.* **2008**, *28*, 654–659. [CrossRef]
36. Aizenberg, D.; Sigler, M.; Weizman, A.; Barak, Y. Anticholinergic burden and the risk of falls among elderly psychiatric inpatients: A 4-year case-control study. *Int. Psychogeriatr.* **2002**, *14*, 307–310. [CrossRef] [PubMed]
37. Summers, W.K. A clinical method of estimating risk of drug induced delirium. *Life Sci.* **1978**, *22*, 1511–1516. [CrossRef]
38. Whalley, L.J.; Sharma, S.; Fox, H.C.; Murray, A.D.; Staff, R.T.; Duthie, A.C.; Deary, I.J.; Starr, J.M. Anticholinergic drugs in late life: Adverse effects on cognition but not on progress to dementia. *J. Alzheimer's Dis.* **2012**, *30*, 253–261. [CrossRef]
39. Chew, M.L.; Mulsant, B.H.; Pollock, B.G.; Lehman, M.E.; Greenspan, A.; Mahmoud, R.A.; Kirshner, M.A.; Sorisio, D.A.; Bies, R.R.; Gharabawi, G. Anticholinergic activity of 107 medications commonly used by older adults. *J. Am. Geriatr. Soc.* **2008**, *56*, 1333–1341. [CrossRef]
40. Han, L.; Agostini, J.V.; Allore, H.G. Cumulative anticholinergic exposure is associated with poor memory and executive function in older men. *J. Am. Geriatr. Soc.* **2008**, *56*, 2203–2210. [CrossRef]
41. Minzenberg, M.J.; Poole, J.H.; Benton, C.; Vinogradov, S. Association of anticholinergic load with impairment of complex attention and memory in schizophrenia. *Am. J. Psychiatry* **2004**, *161*, 116–124. [CrossRef]
42. Briet, J.; Javelot, H.; Heitzmann, E.; Weiner, L.; Lameira, C.; D'Athis, P.; Corneloup, M.; Vailleau, J.-L. The anticholinergic impregnation scale: Towards the elaboration of a scale adapted to prescriptions in French psychiatric settings. *Therapie* **2017**, *72*, 427–437. [CrossRef]
43. Hwang, S.; Jun, K.; Ah, Y.M.; Han, E.; Chung, J.E.; Lee, J.Y. Impact of anticholinergic burden on emergency department visits among older adults in Korea: A national population cohort study. *Arch. Gerontol. Geriatr.* **2019**, *85*, 103912. [CrossRef] [PubMed]
44. Ah, Y.M.; Suh, Y.; Jun, K.; Hwang, S.; Lee, J.Y. Effect of anticholinergic burden on treatment modification, delirium and mortality in newly diagnosed dementia patients starting a cholinesterase inhibitor: A population-based study. *Basic Clin. Pharm. Toxicol.* **2019**, *124*, 741–748. [CrossRef] [PubMed]

45. Hefner, G.; Shams, M.; Wenzel-Seifert, K. Rating the delirogenic potential of drugs for prediction of side effects in elderly psychiatric inpatients. *J. Pharm. Pharm.* **2015**, *1*. Available online: https://www.academia.edu/37901010/Rating_The_Delirogenic_Potential_of_Drugs_for_Prediction_of_Side_Effects_in_Elderly_Psychiatric_Inpatients (accessed on 27 April 2022).
46. Xu, D.; Anderson, H.D.; Tao, A.; Hannah, K.L.; Linnebur, S.A.; Valuck, R.J.; Culbertson, V.L. Assessing and predicting drug-induced anticholinergic risks: An integrated computational approach. *Adv. Drug Saf.* **2017**, *8*, 361–370. [CrossRef]
47. Taipale, H.T.; Bell, J.S.; Gnjidic, D.; Sulkava, R.; Hartikainen, S. Sedative load among community-dwelling people aged 75 years or older: Association with balance and mobility. *J. Clin. Psychopharmacol.* **2012**, *32*, 218–224. [CrossRef]
48. Linjakumpu, T.; Hartikainen, S.; Klaukka, T.; Koponen, H.; Kivelä, S.L.; Isoaho, R. A model to classify the sedative load of drugs. *Int. J. Geriatr. Psychiatry* **2003**, *18*, 542–544. [CrossRef]
49. Dyer, A.H.; Murphy, C.; Lawlor, B.; Kennelly, S.P.; NILVAD StudyGroup. Sedative Load in Community-Dwelling Older Adults with Mild-Moderate Alzheimer's Disease: Longitudinal Relationships with Adverse Events, Delirium and Falls. *Drugs Aging* **2020**, *37*, 829–837. [CrossRef]
50. Sloane, P.; Ivey, J.; Roth, M.; Roederer, M.; Williams, C.S. Accounting for the sedative and analgesic effects of medication changes during patient participation in clinical research studies: Measurement development and application to a sample of institutionalized geriatric patients. *Contemp. Clin. Trials.* **2008**, *29*, 140–148. [CrossRef]
51. Hanlon, J.T.; Zhao, X.; Naples, J.G.; Aspinall, S.L.; Perera, S.; Nace, D.A.; Castle, N.G.; Greenspan, S.L.; Thorpe, C.T. Central Nervous System Medication Burden and Serious Falls in Older Nursing Home Residents. *J. Am. Geriatr. Soc.* **2017**, *65*, 1183–1189. [CrossRef]
52. Hanlon, J.T.; Boudreau, R.M.; Roumani, Y.F.; Newman, A.B.; Ruby, C.M.; Wright, R.M.; Hilmer, S.N.; Shorr, R.I.; Bauer, D.C.; Simonsick, E.M.; et al. Number and dosage of central nervous system medications on recurrent falls in community elders: The Health, Aging and Body Composition study. *J. Gerontol. A Biol. Sci. Med. Sci.* **2009**, *64*, 492–498. [CrossRef]
53. Hanlon, J.T.; Schmader, K.E.; Samsa, G.P.; Weinberger, M.; Uttech, K.M.; Lewis, I.K.; Cohen, H.J.; Feussner, J.R. A method for assessing drug therapy appropriateness. *J. Clin. Epidemiol.* **1992**, *45*, 1045–1051. [CrossRef]
54. Hanlon, J.T.; Schmader, K.E. The medication appropriateness index at 20: Where it started, where it has been, and where it may be going. *Drugs Aging* **2013**, *30*, 893–900. [CrossRef] [PubMed]
55. Hanlon, J.T.; Schmader, K.E. The medication appropriateness index: A clinimetric measure. *Psychother. Psychosom.* **2022**, *91*, 78–83. [CrossRef] [PubMed]
56. Spinewine, A.; Dumont, C.; Mallet, L.; Swine, C. Medication appropriateness index: Reliability and recommendations for future use. *J. Am. Geriatr. Soc.* **2006**, *54*, 720–722. [CrossRef] [PubMed]
57. Bankes, D.; Jin, H.; Finnel, S.; Michaud, V.; Knowlton, C.; Turgeon, J.; Stein, A. Association of a Novel Medication Risk Score with Adverse Drug Events and Other Pertinent Outcomes Among Participants of the Programs of All-Inclusive Care for the Elderly. *Pharmacy* **2020**, *8*, 87. [CrossRef]
58. Michaud, V.; Smith, M.K.; Bikmetov, R.; Dow, P.; Johnson, J.; Stein, A. Association of the MedWise Risk Score with health care outcomes. *Am. J. Manag. Care* **2021**, *27* (Suppl. 16), S280–S291. [CrossRef]
59. Ratigan, A.R.; Michaud, V.; Turgeon, J.; Bikmetov, R.; Villarreal, G.G.; Anderson, H.D.; Pulver, G.; Pace, W.D. Longitudinal association of a medication risk score with mortality among ambulatory patients acquired through electronic health record data. *J. Patient Saf.* **2021**, *17*, 249. [CrossRef]
60. Jin, H.; Yang, S.; Bankes, D.; Finnel, S.; Turgeon, J.; Stein, A.; Finnel, S.; Jin, H.; Turgeon, J. Evaluating the Impact of Medication Risk Mitigation Services in Medically Complex Older Adults. *Healthcare* **2022**, *10*, 551. [CrossRef]
61. Nurmagambetov, T.; Kuwahara, R.; Garbe, P. The Economic Burden of Asthma in the United States, 2008–2013. *Ann. Am. Thorac. Soc.* **2018**, *15*, 348–356. [CrossRef]
62. Schatz, M.; Zeiger, R.S.; Vollmer, W.M.; Mosen, D.; Apter, A.J.; Stibolt, T.B.; Leong, A.; Johnson, M.S.; Mendoza, G.; Cook, E.F. Development and validation of a medication intensity scale derived from computerized psharmacy data that predicts emergency hospital utilization for persistent asthma. *Am. J. Manag. Care* **2006**, *12*, 478–484.
63. Mehta, H.B.; Wang, L.; Malagaris, I.; Duan, Y.; Rosman, L.; Alexander, G.C. More than two-dozen prescription drug-based risk scores are available for risk adjustment: A systematic review. *J. Clin. Epidemiol.* **2021**, *137*, 113–125. [CrossRef] [PubMed]
64. Cullinan, S.; Raae Hansen, C.; Byrne, S.; O'Mahony, D.; Kearney, P.; Sahm, L. Challenges of deprescribing in the multimorbid patient. *Eur. J. Hosp. Pharm.* **2017**, *24*, 43–46. [CrossRef] [PubMed]
65. Canadian Deprescribing Network. Deprescribing Guidelines and Algorithms. Deprescribing.org Web Site. Available online: https://deprescribing.org/resources/deprescribing-guidelines-algorithms/ (accessed on 26 April 2022).
66. Scott, I.A.; Hilmer, S.N.; Reeve, E.; Potter, K.; Le Couteur, D.; Rigby, D.; Gnjidic, D.; Del Mar, C.B.; Roughead, E.E.; Page, A.; et al. Reducing inappropriate polypharmacy: The process of deprescribing. *JAMA Intern. Med.* **2015**, *175*, 827–834. [CrossRef] [PubMed]

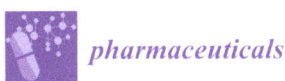

Article

Exploration of Symptom Scale as an Outcome for Deprescribing: A Medication Review Study in Nursing Homes

Dagmar Abelone Dalin [1], Sara Frandsen [1], Gitte Krogh Madsen [2] and Charlotte Vermehren [1,3,*]

1. Department of Clinical Pharmacology, Copenhagen University Hospital Bispebjerg, DK-2400 Copenhagen, Denmark; dagmar.abelone.dalin@regionh.dk (D.A.D.); sara.frandsen@regionh.dk (S.F.)
2. General practice "Roskilde Lægehus", Roskilde, DK-4000 Roskilde, Denmark; gitte.madsen@dadlnet.dk
3. Department of Drug Design and Pharmacology, PHARMA, Faculty of Health and Medical Sciences, University of Copenhagen, DK-2100 Copenhagen, Denmark
* Correspondence: charlotte.vermehren@regionh.dk; Tel.: +45-38-63-52-09

Citation: Dalin, D.A.; Frandsen, S.; Madsen, G.K.; Vermehren, C. Exploration of Symptom Scale as an Outcome for Deprescribing: A Medication Review Study in Nursing Homes. *Pharmaceuticals* 2022, 15, 505. https://doi.org/10.3390/ph15050505

Academic Editor: Márcia Carvalho

Received: 15 March 2022
Accepted: 18 April 2022
Published: 21 April 2022

Publisher's Note: MDPI stays neutral with regard to jurisdictional claims in published maps and institutional affiliations.

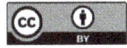

Copyright: © 2022 by the authors. Licensee MDPI, Basel, Switzerland. This article is an open access article distributed under the terms and conditions of the Creative Commons Attribution (CC BY) license (https://creativecommons.org/licenses/by/4.0/).

Abstract: The use of inappropriate medication is an increasing problem among the elderly, leading to hospitalizations, mortality, adverse effects, and lower quality of life (QoL). Deprescribing interventions (e.g., medication reviews (MRs)) have been examined as a possible remedy for this problem. In order to be able to evaluate the potential benefits and harms of a deprescribing intervention, quality of life (QoL) has increasingly been used as an outcome. The sensitivity of QoL measurements may, however, not be sufficient to detect a change in specific disease symptoms, e.g., a flair-up in symptoms or relief of side effects after deprescribing. Using symptom assessments as an outcome, we might be able to identify and evaluate the adverse effects of overmedication and deprescribing alike. The objective of this study was to explore whether symptom assessment is a feasible and valuable method of evaluating outcomes of MRs among the elderly in nursing homes. To the best of our knowledge, this has not been investigated before. We performed a feasibility study based on an experimental design and conducted MRs for elderly patients in nursing homes. Their symptoms were registered at baseline and at a follow-up 3 months after performing the MR. In total, 86 patients, corresponding to 68% of the included patients, received the MR and completed the symptom questionnaires as well as the QoL measurements at baseline and follow-up, respectively. Forty-eight of these patients had at least one deprescribing recommendation implemented. Overall, a tendency towards the improvement of most symptoms was seen after deprescribing, which correlated with the tendencies observed for the QoL measurements. Remarkably, deprescribing did not cause a deterioration of symptoms or QoL, which might otherwise be expected for patients of this age group, of whom the health is often rapidly declining. In conclusion, it was found that symptom assessments were feasible among nursing home residents and resulted in additional relevant information about the potential benefits and harms of deprescribing. It is thus recommended to further explore the use of symptom assessment as an outcome of deprescribing interventions, e.g., in a controlled trial.

Keywords: medication review; deprescriptions; quality of life; aged; aged, 80 and over; nursing homes; deprescribing

1. Introduction

The prevalence of chronic diseases increases with age, and the elderly therefore have a higher risk of polypharmacy [1,2]. Polypharmacy is often defined as taking at least five different medications regularly [2,3] and has been shown to increase the risk of inappropriate medication and hospitalizations among elderly patients [4–6]. In addition, the risk of adverse effects and drug interactions [2,5,7], mortality [8], and reduced quality of life (QoL) [9] have been correlated with polypharmacy.

Medications that were appropriate at the time of prescription may become inappropriate over time and with age, either because the patient's health condition improves or the harms outweighs the benefits [10,11]. As an example of the latter, the use of preventive medication, e.g., statins, in the last years of life can cause considerable muscle pain without any preventive effect being expected [12].

Medication review (MR) interventions are considered to be a valuable tool to combat inappropriate polypharmacy through deprescribing recommendations [13]. Deprescribing is defined as the planned and supervised process of dose reduction or stopping of medications that might be causing harm, or which may no longer have a benefit [14]. During an MR, the patient's complete medication list is critically and structurally reviewed in relation to indications, effects, side effects, and compliance. In MR studies, outcomes are frequently either medication-related, e.g., a decrease in the number of medications, or resource-related, e.g., cost, number of general practitioner (GP) visits, or hospitalization, rather than patient-related [15–17]. The use of patient-related outcomes such as QoL is steadily increasing in medication review studies [15] to investigate whether the intervention brings a relevant benefit to the patient. Currently, there is no convincing evidence that a medication review leads to an improved QoL [18]. The QoL scales might not have sufficient sensitivity to be able to detect improvements in QoL, especially not among nursing home residents, for whom a natural rapid deterioration in their condition is expected. However, it is crucial to be able to assess whether a medication review leads to improved patient outcomes upon deprescribing medications. A recent review analyzed the various outcomes of MR studies and found a lack of reporting of potential harm (e.g., adverse events) caused by the interventions [15], making it difficult to evaluate the benefit–risk ratio of MRs. It is our hypothesis that the assessment of symptoms as an outcome of MR could be a feasible and valuable additional approach in order to identify and report the potential benefits and harms of MR. Some specific symptoms, e.g., dizziness, have been used as outcomes in MR, but to our knowledge a systematic symptom assessment has not previously been used as an outcome in MR. The objective of this study was to explore whether symptom assessment is a feasible and a potential valid outcome measure of deprescribing when performing MRs of elderly patients in nursing homes. Additionally, symptom measurements are compared with QoL values in order to investigate whether symptom measurements can contribute further knowledge about the patient-relevant effects of MRs.

2. Results

2.1. Patients

In Hvidovre Municipality, Denmark, 322 residents living in the three participating nursing homes were screened for participation in the project. Of these residents, 234 were found to be eligible according to the inclusion criteria. Of these, 135 patients were included in the study (see for further information on inclusion and exclusion). Nine patients (6.7%) died before the intervention; hence, 126 patients in total received the MR intervention. Ten patients (7.9%) died before follow-up and 30 patients (23.8%) did not complete the symptom and QoL questionnaires, resulting in 86 patients who completed the questionnaires both at baseline and follow-up, and 48 patients who had a deprescribing intervention implemented and who completed the symptom and QoL questionnaires (Figure 1).

The participating patients were divided into three investigational groups according to the degree of their study participation: the Medication Review Group (patients who received an MR), the Follow-Up Group (patients who, in addition, completed the symptom and QoL questionnaires), and the Deprescribing Subgroup (patients who had a deprescribing recommendation implemented and who completed the symptom and QoL questionnaires), respectively.

The 126 patients included in the Medication Review Group had an average age of 82 years (SD 7.8) and 32% were male. They had a total of 1575 medications and were affiliated with 18 different general practices. On average, each patient had a mean of 13 medications at baseline, of which 10 were regular medications, and 3 were as-needed medications. Table 1 summarizes the patient characteristics regarding age, medication, and scoring of symptoms and QoL, respectively, divided into the three investigational groups.

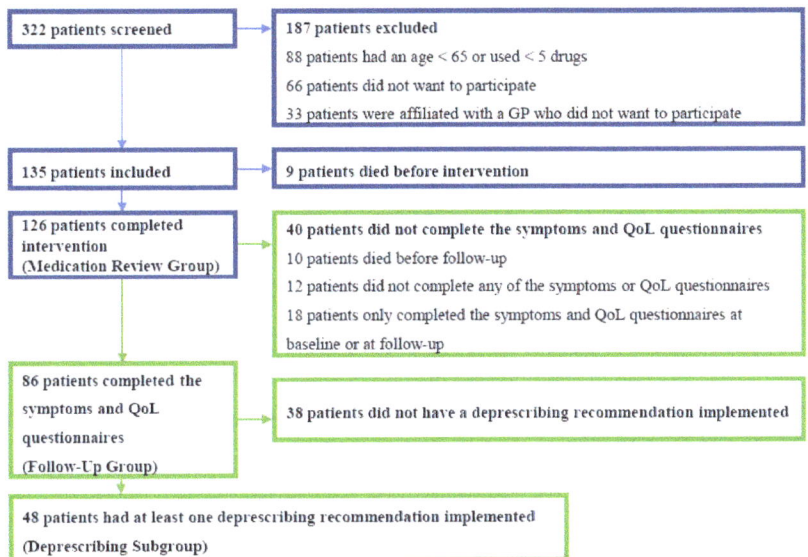

Figure 1. The flow of patients from screening to the inclusion of eligible patients in the Medication Review, Follow-Up, and Deprescribing Subgroup, respectively. The upper five boxes (blue) describe the inclusion process, as well as reasons for exclusion and dropout, whereas the lower four boxes (green) describe the subsets of patients relevant to the aim of this article, i.e., patients who completed the symptoms and quality of life (QoL) questionnaires both at baseline and follow-up were included in the Follow-Up Group. Subsequently, patients in the Follow-Up Group who had a deprescribing recommendation implemented were included in the Deprescribing Subgroup.

2.2. Medication Review

We recommended changes to 491 medications (31% of all medications) out of the total of 1.575 medications. The GPs agreed upon 460 of the recommendations (94% of recommendations), and 196 recommendations were implemented at follow-up (45%), of which 159 were deprescribing recommendations. For the 86 patients with completed QoL and symptoms' questionnaires (the Follow-Up Group), 55 patients had at least one implemented recommendation (both deprescribing and other recommendations) at follow-up, and 48 patients had at least one deprescribing recommendation implemented (the Deprescribing Subgroup). Deprescribing was the most frequent recommendation (78% of all recommendations), and we recommended deprescribing 24% of all 1575 medications. The GPs agreed to deprescribe 23% of all 1575 medications.

2.3. Symptoms

For the Follow-Up Group (n = 86), there was no significant difference in the mean of symptom scores before and after the intervention: pain (-0.34), tiredness (0.10), drowsiness (0.03), nausea (0.14), loss of appetite (0.42), shortness of breath (-0.03), depression (0.30), and anxiety (-0.02).

For the Deprescribing Subgroup (n = 48), no significant difference in the mean of symptom scores was found either. However, in this group a tendency towards an improvement of the average score within all symptoms, except loss of appetite and shortness of breath, was observed. The average symptom scores for the Deprescribing Subgroup before and after MR, i.e., deprescribing, are shown in Figure 2.

Table 1. Characteristics of the patients constituting the investigational groups—the Medication Review Group, Follow-Up Group and Deprescribing Subgroup—regarding age, gender, medication, and outcomes. The symptoms and quality of life (QoL) questionnaires were not completed by all patients belonging to the Medication Review Group, which is why this column is not completed (-).

Investigational groups	Medication Review Group, i.e., Patients Who Received MRs (n= 126)		
		Follow-up Group, i.e., patients who completed the symptoms and QoL questionnaires (n = 86)	Deprescribing Subgroup, i.e., patients from the Follow-Up Group who had a deprescribing recommendation implemented (n = 48)
Mean age/year (SD)	82.3 (7.8)	81.8 (7.0)	82.2 (7.1)
Male/%	32%	30%	25%
Medications at baseline			
No. of medications	1.575	1.084	670
Mean no. of medications per patient	13	12	14
No. of recommendations	491	315	221
Mean no. of recommendations per patient	3.9	3.7	4.6
Symptoms at baseline			
Pain (SD)	-	2.9 (2.7)	3.3 (3.0)
Tiredness (SD)	-	4.2 (2.8)	4.5 (2.8)
Drowsinesss (SD)	-	3.3 (2.8)	3.5 (2.8)
Nausea (SD)	-	0.5 (1.5)	0.5 (1.2)
Loss of appetite (SD)	-	1.6 (2.4)	1.5 (2.3)
Shortness of breath (SD)	-	1.4 (2.3)	1.2 (2.2)
Depression (SD)	-	2.1 (2.7)	2.2 (2.7)
Anxiety (SD)	-	1.7 (2.6)	1.9 (2.8)
Wellbeing (SD)	-	3.3 (2.2)	3.3 (2.2)
Quality of life at baseline			
EQ-5D index (SD)	-	0.5 (0.3)	0.5 (0.3)
VAS score (SD)	-	56.2 (21.4)	56.2 (19.9)

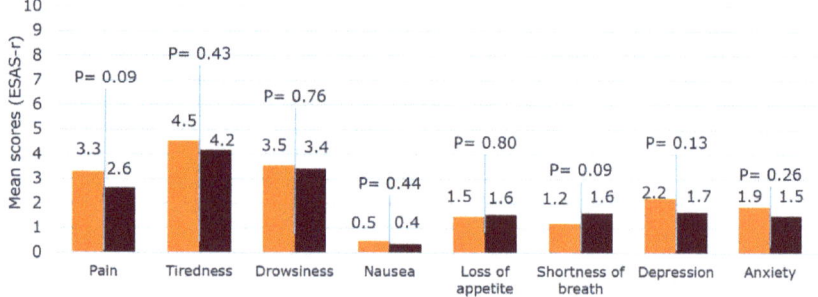

Figure 2. Mean scores of the Deprescribing Subgroup (n = 48) for each symptom, measured using the Edmonton Symptom Assessment System (revised version) (ESAS-r) scale, before deprescribing (orange) and after deprescribing (brown). The ESAS-r scale uses a numeric scale from 0–10, where 0 indicates no symptoms and 10 indicates the worst intensity of a symptom. There was no significant difference for any symptoms.

The results suggested that, among the patients in the Deprescribing Subgroup, there was a greater tendency towards the improvement of symptoms compared to a deterioration (Figure 3). Loss of appetite and shortness of breath were the only symptoms among patients of this group for which fewer patients achieved an improvement than a deterioration (Figure 3).

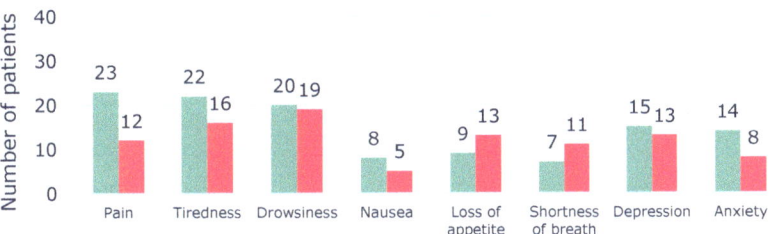

Figure 3. Number of Deprescribing Subgroup patients (n = 48) with improvements (green) and deteriorations (red), respectively, in each symptom after deprescribing.

The figure below shows the number of patients who exhibited the individual symptoms (Figure 4) to some degree before and after deprescribing, respectively. The majority of patients suffered from tiredness, drowsiness, and pain. These data show a general tendency that there were no more patients who developed symptoms after deprescribing, apart from symptoms regarding shortness of breath.

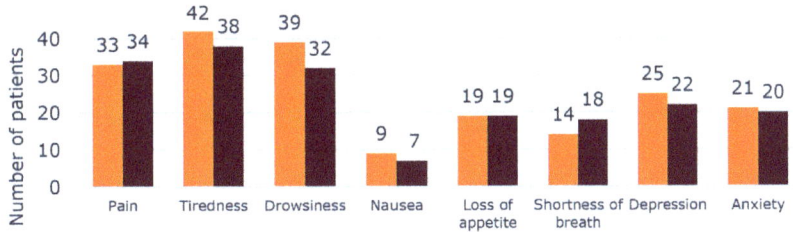

Figure 4. Number of Deprescribing Subgroup patients (n = 48) with any presentation of each symptom (answers higher than 0 on the Edmonton Symptom Assessment System (revised version) scale) before (orange) and after (brown) deprescribing. There was no significant difference for any symptoms.

One of the purposes of this work was to consider whether symptom assessment could contribute to additional knowledge about the patient-relevant effects of MRs. Hence, we tried to elucidate whether deprescribing of a medication related to a symptom, e.g., pain, had an influence on the symptom score for pain. Overall, we found no tendency for a deterioration of symptoms caused by deprescribing a drug. However, we found a tendency towards improvement for some symptoms. As an example, deprescribing of pain relievers (NSAIDs, paracetamol, opioids, or muscle relaxants) was performed for 12 patients. Of these, seven patients obtained a better pain score, four patients revealed unchanged pain scores, and only one patient experienced an increase in pain at follow-up.

2.4. Quality of Life

Overall, only a small change in the EQ-5D index and VAS score was observed during the study period, as shown in Table 2.

For both the Follow-Up Group and the Deprescribing Subgroup, small insignificant changes in the EQ-5D index were found. The overall Follow-Up Group revealed a small insignificant deterioration, whereas the Deprescribing Subgroup revealed a small insignificant improvement. Both groups showed a small insignificant improvement in the VAS score. The improvement was largest in the Deprescribing Subgroup, though it was smaller than the minimal clinically relevant difference of eight [19].

Table 2. The mean difference in quality of life (QoL), the EQ-5D index, and VAS score, respectively, from baseline (before the medication review (MR)) to follow-up (3 months after the MR). The mean difference is shown for patients in the Follow-Up Group (n = 86), who completed the QoL questionnaire at baseline and follow-up, and for the Deprescribing Subgroup (n = 48), respectively. For the EQ-5D index and VAS score, a higher score indicates a better QoL.

Patient Group	EQ-5D Index Mean Change Higher Better (CI 95%)	VAS Score Mean Change Higher Better (CI 95%)
Follow-Up Group (n = 86)	−0.002 (−0.036: 0.176)	1.5 (−3.8: 6.8)
Deprescribed Subgroup (n = 48)	0.019 (−0.034: 0.073)	6.4 (−0.7: 13.5)

3. Discussion

We explored the feasibility of using symptom assessment as an outcome of MRs among nursing home residents with polypharmacy using the ESAS-r [20] in comparison with a QoL assessment, i.e., EQ-5D [21]. One hundred and twenty-six patients met our inclusion criteria, were included in the study, and received MR (the Medication Review Group). However, only 86 patients completed the ESAS-r and EQ-5D (the Follow-Up Group). The primary barriers in the workflow, which prevented a full-sized Follow-Up Group, were related partly to the physical and mental health of the patients and to lack of resources among the nursing staff to support the patients in answering the questionnaires. The allocation of additional support to healthcare providers in nursing homes would probably improve the follow-up rate significantly.

The patient characteristics (Table 1) revealed a patient group which was comparable to other polypharmacy patient groups in nursing homes, although the prevalence of polypharmacy among the residents in this study was higher [22]. It was observed that the patients from the Deprescribing Subgroup on average used two drugs more than patients in the overall Follow-Up Group, i.e., 14 vs. 12 medications per patient. Similarly, the patients from the Deprescribing Subgroup were recommended one more medication change on average compared to the patients in the overall Follow-Up Group, indicating a higher degree of overmedication among the subgroup that had at least one drug deprescribed.

During the MR, deprescribing was by far the most frequent recommendation. The GPs thus agreed that 23% of all medications should be deprescribed. This was consistent with other MR studies for elderly polypharmacy patients, in which deprescribing made up around 15–32% of all recommended changes [23–28]. In a previous study, we found that GPs agreed to deprescribe 18% of all medications [29]. Likewise, a Dutch study showed that 13% of all medications had been deprescribed 1 week after an MR [30].

In the present study, the GPs accepted the majority (94%) of the recommendations suggested by the medication team. Of all the accepted recommendations, 45% were implemented at follow-up. This was the case for 35% of the deprescribing recommendations. Thus, the implementation rate was low compared to similar MR projects performed in collaboration with GPs, in which 77–93% of the recommendations were found to be implemented [26,31]. Hence, one can question why the implementation rate was so low considering that the GPs accepted the medication changes at the MR meeting. Thus, it could be interesting to clarify reasons for the lack of implementation.

In order to evaluate the potential of the use of symptom assessments as a future outcome of deprescribing interventions, we analyzed the change in symptoms between baseline and follow-up, i.e., before and after MRs, in three different ways: the mean change in symptom score; the number of patients with a deterioration or improvement of symptoms; and the identification of the total number of patients suffering from each symptom before and after the intervention. The changes in symptom scores were correlated with the changes in QoL.

Although not statistically significant, there was a clear trend towards an improvement of most symptom scores for the patients in the Deprescribing Subgroup between baseline and follow-up (Figure 2). This also applied to the overall Follow-Up Group, which, however, showed a weaker tendency for improvement than the Deprescribing Subgroup.

We deprescribed pain relievers for 12 patients, and 11 of these patients showed no deterioration in pain scores, indicating that they did not benefit from the pain relievers. This observation is in line with a recent Danish guideline, which does not recommend pain relievers (NSAID, paracetamol, opioids, and muscle relaxing drugs) for chronic use in non-cancer patients due to the lack of evidence of effects and the risk of increased adverse reactions for these patients [32,33]. Furthermore, seven of these twelve patients reported less pain after deprescribing pain relievers, which may indicate that the pain relievers might even have contributed to maintaining the pain, i.e., medication-induced pain [34–36].

The observed trends for symptom score assessments were supported by the QoL results of the Deprescribing Subgroup. Thus, in this group a tendency towards an improvement of QoL was found, which was not seen in the overall Follow-Up Group. For the Follow-Up Group, the EQ-5D index decreased after MR, but the VAS-score was improved (Table 2). Thus, the results for the change in QoL of the Follow-Up Group pointed in opposite directions, suggesting no overall change in QoL. Hence, the results of our study indicated a trend towards an overall improvement in both symptoms and QoL outcomes in the Deprescribing Subgroup (Figures 2–4). However, apparently due to the lack of a critical mass in the study, the results did not show significant differences between baseline and follow-up values.

In summary, based on these results, symptom assessment may in the future be considered as a potential sensitive and specific method to assess an effect of deprescribing, i.e., either benefit or harm.

Strengths and Limitations

This study secured a broad representation of nursing home residents and GPs, i.e., 3 different nursing homes and 18 GPs were included. In this study we had the advantage of direct access to the nursing home record. This made it possible to obtain an accurate picture of the patients' current medication and the conditions regarding the individual medication administrations (both at baseline and follow-up), as well as limiting the loss-to-follow-up. Only the patients who died did not have a follow-up on the implementation of recommendations. The medication team consisted of two different professions to ensure high-quality recommendations, which was confirmed by the GPs' high degree of acceptance of the suggested recommendations. For the symptom assessment and QoL, we ensured high quality and international applicability by using the validated, internationally recognized and ESAS-r and EQ-5D questionnaires, translated into Danish.

This study had some limitations worth noting, including the small number of patients, the low implementation rate and the failure to complete all questionnaires. A small number of patients and no control group is a consequence of being a descriptive study, and underline that the results of this study cannot be generalized but rather should be an inspiration for future work. The 3-month follow-up period was chosen to ensure that the patients' state of health could be considered comparable in relation to their baseline score, to ensure a low loss-to-follow-up and at the same time to be long enough to enable us to assess the possible effect of deprescribing. However, a three-month follow-up period might have reduced the impact seen by deprescribing and multiple later follow-ups might be useful. In this study we saw a loss-to-follow-up of 7% due to death, but a further 7% of the initially included patients died before the intervention. A low implementation rate and the lack of completion of questionnaires might lead to selection bias, e.g., if the GPs only implemented recommendations in some intentionally selected patients or if only the patients with few symptoms were able to complete the questionnaires. In addition, the incomplete degree of implementation and completion of questionnaires suggested division into three post-hoc groups instead of prospective definition of groups. This is a further limitation of the study, which unfortunately reflects real world difficulties in conducting studies that include the present study population, i.e., frail elderly nursing home residents with high morbidity, and which involves interdisciplinary collaboration between physicians and nursing homes.

4. Materials and Methods

4.1. Design

This study was performed as a feasibility study based on an experimental design aiming at building initial understandings about symptom assessment as outcomes of medication reviews. The project was performed in a collaboration between the Department of Clinical Pharmacology at Copenhagen University Hospital Bispebjerg, Hvidovre Municipality, and the GPs of the included patients. Nursing homes in Hvidovre Municipality, Capital Region, Denmark, were offered MRs for elderly patients with polypharmacy. Patients were recruited in 2019, the MRs were conducted between March 2019 and February 2020 and the last follow-up was in May 2020. All patients were screened.

The MRs were prepared by an interdisciplinary medication team from the Department of Clinical Pharmacology at Copenhagen University Hospital Bispebjerg, consisting of a pharmacist and a medical doctor. The medication team visited each patient's GP and together they conducted the MR with a duration per patient of 10 min. During the MR, the medication team recommended changes to the patient's medication, e.g., deprescribing. Symptoms and QoL were measured before the MR and at follow-up (3 months after MR). A follow-up was performed by lookup in the individual care giver records after 3 months to allow time for the GPs to implement recommendations and for recommendations to impact symptoms and QoL, while preventing an excessive decline in the health state of these frail patients. The implementation of recommendations that were agreed upon by the GPs was evaluated at follow-up. The study design adheres to the Pharmacist Patient Care Intervention Reporting checklist:PaCIR [37] and the CONSORT extension for randomized pilot and feasibility trials used for non-randomized trials as proposed by Lancaster and Thabane [38].

4.2. Settings and Patients

The patients were recruited from the three public nursing homes in Hvidovre Municipality. Written informed consent was requested from the patients or their legal guardians to participate. Because we wanted to examine MRs in elderly polypharmacy patients, we included patients aged 65 years and older, who were prescribed five or more regular medications, including calcium tablets and strong vitamins (strong vitamins as defined by the Danish Medicines Agency [39]).

4.3. Medication Review

Based on the caregiver record, the medication list and input from the caregiving staff, the medication team prepared the MR for each patient. During the MR preparation, the medication team assessed the drug substance, dose, dosage form, dosage time and potential interactions for each medication in relation to the stated medications, indications and diagnoses. To assess the appropriateness of each drug, we used several decision tools in addition to national and regional guidelines, e.g., List of first choice medications, Capital Region, Denmark [40], Danish Deprescribing List [41], List of anticholinergic medicines [42] and National Database on Drug Interactions [43]. Each drug was assessed for the individual patient, and the same drug could be considered appropriate for some patients and inappropriate for others.

The medication team met with the patient's GP and discussed the medication. On the basis of the medication team's MR preparation and the newly acquired information from the GP, the medication team on site recommended changes to the patient's medication with a specific focus on deprescribing. The GP could either accept or reject each recommendation. However, the final decision and implementation was a shared decision between the patient and their GP, which took place after the meeting with the GPs.

The recommendations were categorized into six types: Discontinuation; reduction of dose; increase of dose; change to another drug; change of dosage time; and reduce pill burden. Discontinuation included both abrupt discontinuation and tempering, depending on national/regional recommendations. In this article we focus especially on deprescribing, which covers both discontinuation and reduction of dose.

4.4. Outcomes

4.4.1. Symptoms and QoL

Symptoms were measured using the Edmonton Symptom Assessment System (revised version) (ESAS-r) Scale [20]. The ESAS-r is a patient-reported instrument for patients near the end of life and is mostly used for monitoring symptoms in palliative care and hospices, but has also been used for monitoring symptoms in long-term care facilities [44–47] and to guide changes in the treatment of frail elderly patients [48]. The ESAS-r is based on a short numerical symptom scoring framework to enable quantitative measurements of symptoms with minimal patient burden [45,49]. The ESAS-r measures the intensity of each of eight symptoms (pain, tiredness, loss of appetite, nausea, depression, drowsiness, anxiety, and shortness of breath) using a numerical scale from 0 (no symptoms) to 10 (worst intensity of symptoms). ESAS-r also measures wellbeing using a numerical scale from 0 (best wellbeing) to 10 (worst wellbeing). ESAS-r measures multiple different symptoms that are typical for patients in the end of life, and symptoms which might be improved or deteriorated by medication. Deprescribing via an MR is an intervention without a specific medication or symptom target, and it may impact several symptoms. Therefore, ESAS-r may be suitable to evaluate the impact of deprescribing different medications. For each of the symptoms, the numerical value of 1 was used as the minimally clinically relevant difference for both improvement and deterioration [50]. In addition, we considered using the Neuropsychiatric Inventory (NPI) to assess the neuropsychiatric symptoms of patients with dementia [51]. However, this measurement would only assess behavioral disturbances of dementia and not physical symptoms. In addition, it would increase the patient burden. Thus, we decided not to use it in this study.

QoL was measured using EQ-5D. EQ-5D is a validated [21] extensively used, generic, non-disease-specific health-related QoL instrument, which is often used in the elderly population [9,13,52–54]. We used the five-level version of the EQ-5D instrument (EQ-5D-5L) which consisted of two sections. The first section—the EQ-5D index—consisted of five questions about health, which each had five ratings: mobility; self-care; usual activities, pain/discomfort; and anxiety/depression. The answers were converted (using the crosswalk index value calculator [55]) to a single score with values ranging from 1 (perfect health) to -0.59 (the worst imaginable health state), with the value of 0 indicating death. Furthermore, the EQ-5D has a visual analogue scale (VAS) which captures the responders' self-ratings of their health from 100 (perfect health) to 0 (worst possible health). In this study, the minimum clinically important difference of 0.03 was used for the EQ-5D index and 8 for the VAS score [19,56].

We examined the following outcomes regarding symptoms and QoL: the mean change for each symptom between baseline and follow-up; the number of patients with a deterioration of each symptom; the number of patients with an improvement of each symptom; the number of patients with any representation (1–10) of each symptom; and the mean change in QoL. QoL was compared with the results of the symptom assessment to examine if the symptom assessment supported QoL measurements and/or contributed further relevant information.

4.4.2. Medications and Recommendations

We examined the percentage of recommendations accepted by the GPs and the percentage of medications the GPs agreed to deprescribe to evaluate the relevance of the recommendations according to the GP and the perceived overmedication at baseline, respectively.

In addition, the number and percentage of implemented deprescribing recommendations at follow-up were measured, to evaluate the MR's effect on the medications.

4.5. Ethics

This project was approved by the Danish Data Protection Agency (I-Suite no 05564). According to Danish law, approval by the Danish Council on Ethics was not required and could not be obtained for this study, as we only recommended changes to the medication. The GPs decided which changes to accept and implement as part of their normal care for the patients. Each included patient or their legal guardian provided written informed consent.

4.6. Analysis and Statistics

Data were analyzed using SAS Enterprise Guide software (version 7.15. Copyright © 2022 SAS Institute Inc.). The data were collected in REDCap (Research Electronic Data Capture), which is a secure database approved for that purpose by the Danish Data Protection Agency [57].

Not all patients had completed the symptom assessment and QoL questionaries both at baseline and follow-up. Thus, we formed an investigational group including those who did (the Follow-Up Group).

To elucidate the symptom assessment for patients who had medication deprescribed, we created a subgroup (the Deprescribing Subgroup) consisting of only the patients from the Follow-Up Group who had a deprescribing intervention implemented at the follow-up.

Due to the descriptive nature of the study, we only included the most basic statistics to describe the results. The characteristics of the patients, divided into the different investigational groups (Table 1), were summarized and standard deviations were included for symptoms and QoL. For the outcomes, we analyzed the change with a paired t-test. For outcomes presented in tables, we included 95% confidence intervals, as they are more descriptive than a p-value, and we did not intend to show a significant change. For other outcomes, any significant change was mentioned in the text.

5. Conclusions

In this study we used the ESAS-r for symptom assessment as an outcome of medication reviews, with a focus on deprescribing. To our knowledge, this is a new approach. We observed a non-significant tendency towards improvement in most symptoms after deprescribing medication. This correlated with the tendency observed in QoL for these patients. The ESAS-r can be analyzed in different ways. However, we did not observe any clinically relevant effect on symptoms in patients who received deprescribing. Based on our results, we can conclude that symptom assessment is feasible and has potential as a valid outcome measure of deprescribing when performing MRs of elderly patients in nursing homes. However, an effort must be made to optimize the completion of questionnaires, either by improving the inclusion of healthier patients (e.g., home-dwelling elderly patients), or by ensuring caregivers are committed to helping the patients. A special focus should be directed towards an increased degree of implementation of recommendations.

In conclusion, our results indicate that symptom assessment may be a valuable, clinical and patient-relevant outcome of deprescribing studies, that is considered suitable for study upscaling and for use in other settings, e.g., home-dwelling elderly patients. This should be further elucidated in a randomized clinical setting with sufficient statistical power.

Author Contributions: Conceptualization, D.A.D. and C.V.; methodology, C.V. and D.A.D.; software, D.A.D.; validation, D.A.D. and G.K.M.; formal analysis, D.A.D.; investigation, D.A.D. and G.K.M.; resources, C.V.; data curation, D.A.D.; writing—original draft preparation, D.A.D. and S.F.; writing—review and editing, D.A.D., C.V., G.K.M. and S.F.; visualization, D.A.D.; supervision, C.V.; project administration, D.A.D.; funding acquisition, C.V. All authors have read and agreed to the published version of the manuscript.

Funding: We thank the The Danish Ministry of Health for funding to conduct the present study.

Institutional Review Board Statement: Not applicable.

Informed Consent Statement: Informed consent was obtained from all subjects or their legal guardians involved in the study.

Data Availability Statement: Data is contained within the article.

Acknowledgments: We wish to thank the staff at the three nursing homes in Hvidovre municipality, Hvidovre municipality and the GPs who participated in this project.

Conflicts of Interest: The authors declare no conflict of interest.

References

1. Hvidberg, M.F.; Johnsen, S.P.; Davidsen, M.; Ehlers, L. A Nationwide Study of Prevalence Rates and Characteristics of 199 Chronic Conditions in Denmark. *Pharm. Econ. Open* **2020**, *4*, 361–380. [CrossRef] [PubMed]
2. Hovstadius, B.; Petersson, G. Factors leading to excessive polypharmacy. *Clin. Geriatr. Med.* **2012**, *28*, 159–172. [CrossRef]
3. Sirois, C.; Domingues, N.S.; Laroche, M.-L.; Zongo, A.; Lunghi, C.; Guénette, L.; Kroger, E.; Emond, V. Polypharmacy Definitions for Multimorbid Older Adults Need Stronger Foundations to Guide Research, Clinical Practice and Public Health. *Pharmacy* **2019**, *7*, 126. [CrossRef] [PubMed]
4. Thorell, K.; Midlöv, P.; Fastbom, J.; Halling, A. Importance of potentially inappropriate medications, number of chronic conditions and medications for the risk of hospitalisation in elderly in Sweden: A case-control study. *BMJ Open* **2019**, *9*, e029477. [CrossRef] [PubMed]
5. Rodrigues, M.C.S.; de Oliveira, C. Drug-drug interactions and adverse drug reactions in polypharmacy among older adults: An integrative review. *Rev. Lat. Am. Enferm.* **2016**, *24*, e2800. Available online: https://www.ncbi.nlm.nih.gov/pmc/articles/PMC5016009/ (accessed on 27 April 2021). [CrossRef]
6. Weeda, E.R.; AlDoughaim, M.; Criddle, S. Association between Potentially Inappropriate Medications and Hospital Encounters Among Older Adults: A Meta-Analysis. *Drugs Aging* **2020**, *37*, 529–537. [CrossRef]
7. Ahmed, B.; Nanji, K.; Mujeeb, R.; Patel, M.J. Effects of polypharmacy on adverse drug reactions among geriatric outpatients at a tertiary care hospital in Karachi: A prospective cohort study. *PLoS ONE* **2014**, *9*, e112133. [CrossRef]
8. Cardwell, K.; Kerse, N.; Hughes, C.M.; Teh, R.; Moyes, S.A.; Menzies, O.; Rolleston, A.; Broad, J.B.; Ryan, C. Does potentially inappropriate prescribing predict an increased risk of admission to hospital and mortality? A longitudinal study of the 'oldest old'. *BMC Geriatr.* **2020**, *20*, 28. [CrossRef]
9. Franic, D.M.; Jiang, J.Z. Potentially inappropriate drug use and health-related quality of life in the elderly. *Pharmacotherapy* **2006**, *26*, 768–778. [CrossRef]
10. Bain, K.T.; Holmes, H.M.; Beers, M.H.; Maio, V.; Handler, S.M.; Pauker, S.G. Discontinuing medications: A novel approach for revising the prescribing stage of the medication-use process. *J. Am. Geriatr. Soc.* **2008**, *56*, 1946–1952. [CrossRef]
11. Lee, S.J.; Kim, C.M. Individualizing Prevention for Older Adults. *J. Am. Geriatr. Soc.* **2018**, *66*, 229–234. [CrossRef] [PubMed]
12. Bhardwaj, S.; Selvarajah, S.; Schneider, E.B. Muscular effects of statins in the elderly female: A review. *Clin. Interv. Aging* **2013**, *8*, 47–59. [PubMed]
13. Wouters, H.; Scheper, J.; Koning, H.; Brouwer, C.; Twisk, J.W.; van der Meer, H.; Boersma, F.; Zuidema, S.U.; Taxis, K. Discontinuing Inappropriate Medication Use in Nursing Home Residents: A Cluster Randomized Controlled Trial. *Ann. Intern. Med.* **2017**, *167*, 609–617. [CrossRef] [PubMed]
14. Scott, I.A.; Hilmer, S.N.; Reeve, E.; Potter, K.; Le Couteur, D.; Rigby, D.; Gnjidic, D.; Del Mar, C.B.; Roughead, E.E.; Page, A.; et al. Reducing Inappropriate Polypharmacy: The Process of Deprescribing. *JAMA Intern. Med.* **2015**, *175*, 827–834. [CrossRef] [PubMed]
15. Beuscart, J.; Pont, L.G.; Thevelin, S.; Boland, B.; Dalleur, O.; Rutjes, A.W.S.; Westbrook, J.I.; Spinewine, A. A systematic review of the outcomes reported in trials of medication review in older patients: The need for a core outcome set. *Br. J. Clin. Pharmacol.* **2017**, *83*, 942–952. [CrossRef] [PubMed]
16. Christensen, M.; Lundh, A. Medication review in hospitalised patients to reduce morbidity and mortality. *Cochrane Database Syst. Rev.* **2016**, *20*, CD008986. [CrossRef]
17. Kjeldsen, L.J.; Olesen, C.; Hansen, M.K.; Nielsen, T.R.H. Clinical Outcomes Used in Clinical Pharmacy Intervention Studies in Secondary Care. *Pharmacy* **2017**, *5*, 28. [CrossRef]
18. Huiskes, V.J.B.; Burger, D.M.; van den Ende, C.H.M.; van den Bemt, B.J.F. Effectiveness of medication review: A systematic review and meta-analysis of randomized controlled trials. *BMC Fam. Pract.* **2017**, *18*, 5. [CrossRef]
19. Zanini, A.; Aiello, M.; Adamo, D.; Casale, S.; Cherubino, F.; Della Patrona, S.; Raimondi, E.; Zampogna, E.; Chetta, A.; Spanevello, A. Estimation of minimal clinically important difference in EQ-5D visual analog scale score after pulmonary rehabilitation in subjects with COPD. *Respir. Care* **2015**, *60*, 88–95. [CrossRef]
20. Boel, K.; Haaber, K.; Byskov, L. Dansk versione af ESAS—Symptomregistrering. *OMSORG* **2009**, *1*, 41–46.21.
21. Janssen, M.F.; Pickard, A.S.; Golicki, D.; Gudex, C.; Niewada, M.; Scalone, L.; Swinburn, P.; Busschbach, J. Measurement properties of the EQ-5D-5L compared to the EQ-5D-3L across eight patient groups: A multi-country study. *Qual. Life Res. Int. J. Qual. Life Asp. Treat Care Rehabil.* **2013**, *22*, 1717–1727. [CrossRef] [PubMed]

22. Onder, G.; Liperoti, R.; Fialova, D.; Topinkova, E.; Tosato, M.; Danese, P.; Gallo, P.F.; Carpenter, I.; Finne-Soveri, H.; Gindin, J.; et al. Polypharmacy in nursing home in Europe: Results from the SHELTER study. *J. Gerontol. A Biol. Sci. Med. Sci.* **2012**, *67*, 698–704. [CrossRef] [PubMed]
23. Rhalimi, M.; Rauss, A.; Housieaux, E. Drug-related problems identified during geriatric medication review in the community pharmacy. *Int. J. Clin. Pharm.* **2018**, *40*, 109–118. [CrossRef] [PubMed]
24. Castelino, R.L.; Bajorek, B.V.; Chen, T.F. Are interventions recommended by pharmacists during Home Medicines Review evidence-based? *J. Eval. Clin. Pract.* **2011**, *17*, 104–110. [CrossRef] [PubMed]
25. Doucette, W.R.; McDonough, R.P.; Klepser, D.; McCarthy, R. Comprehensive medication therapy management: Identifying and resolving drug-related issues in a community pharmacy. *Clin. Ther.* **2005**, *27*, 1104–1111. [CrossRef]
26. Brulhart, M.I.; Wermeille, J.P. Multidisciplinary medication review: Evaluation of a pharmaceutical care model for nursing homes. *Int. J. Clin. Pharm.* **2011**, *33*, 549–557. [CrossRef]
27. Bryant, L.J.M.; Coster, G.; Gamble, G.D.; McCormick, R.N. The General Practitioner-Pharmacist Collaboration (GPPC) study: A randomised controlled trial of clinical medication reviews in community pharmacy. *Int. J. Pharm. Pract.* **2011**, *19*, 94–105. [CrossRef]
28. Khera, S.; Abbasi, M.; Dabravolskaj, J.; Sadowski, C.A.; Yua, H.; Chevalier, B. Appropriateness of Medications in Older Adults Living With Frailty: Impact of a Pharmacist-Led Structured Medication Review Process in Primary Care. *J. Prim. Care Community Health* **2019**, *10*, 2150132719890227. [CrossRef]
29. Dalin, D.A.; Vermehren, C.; Jensen, A.K.; Unkerskov, J.; Andersen, J.T. Systematic Medication Review in General Practice by an Interdisciplinary Team: A thorough but Laborious Method to Address Polypharmacy among Elderly Patients. *Pharmacy* **2020**, *8*, 57. [CrossRef]
30. Hurmuz, M.Z.M.; Janus, S.I.M.; van Manen, J.G. Changes in medicine prescription following a medication review in older high-risk patients with polypharmacy. *Int. J. Clin. Pharm.* **2018**, *40*, 480–487. [CrossRef]
31. Soendergaard, B.; Kirkeby, B.; Dinsen, C.; Herborg, H.; Kjellberg, J.; Staehr, P. Drug-related problems in general practice: Results from a development project in Denmark. *Pharm. World Sci. PWS* **2006**, *28*, 61–64. [CrossRef] [PubMed]
32. Rothenberg, D.; Sædder, E.; Kasch, H.; Gram-Hansen, J.; Højsted, J.; Bjørnholdt, K.T.; Juul, L.; Tschemerinsky-Kirkeby, L.; Kamp-Jensen, M.; Jensen, M.P. The National list of Recommendations: Pharmacological Treatment of Chronic Nociceptive Pain] Den Nationale Rekommendationsliste: Farmakologisk Behandling af Kroniske Nociceptive Smerter. *Dan. Health Auth.* **2018**. Available online: https://www.sst.dk/da/viden/laegemidler/anbefalinger/den-nationale-rekommendationsliste-_nrl_/kroniske-nociceptive-smerter (accessed on 24 February 2021).
33. Rothenberg, D.; Sædder, E.; Kasch, H.; Gram-Hansen, J.; Højsted, J.; Bjørnholdt, K.T.; Juul, L.; Tschemerinsky-Kirkeby, L.; Kamp-Jensen, M.; Jensen, M.P. The National list of Recommendations: Pharmacological Treatment of Neuropathic Pain] Den Nationale Rekommendationsliste: Farmakologisk Behandling af Neuropatiske Smerter. *Dan. Health Auth.* **2018**. Available online: https://www.sst.dk/da/viden/laegemidler/anbefalinger/den-nationale-rekommendationsliste-_nrl_/farmakologisk-behandling-af-neuropatiske-smerter (accessed on 24 February 2021).
34. Lee, M.; Silverman, S.M.; Hansen, H.; Patel, V.B.; Manchikanti, L. A comprehensive review of opioid-induced hyperalgesia. *Pain Physician* **2011**, *14*, 145–161. [CrossRef] [PubMed]
35. Higgins, C.; Smith, B.H.; Matthews, K. Evidence of opioid-induced hyperalgesia in clinical populations after chronic opioid exposure: A systematic review and meta-analysis. *Br. J. Anaesth.* **2019**, *122*, e114–e126. [CrossRef] [PubMed]
36. Russell, M.B. Epidemiology and management of medication-overuse headache in the general population. *Neurol. Sci.* **2019**, *40*, 23–26. [CrossRef]
37. Pg, C.; Al, B.; Bj, I.; Jd, H.; Ma, K.; Lg, P. PaCIR: A tool to enhance pharmacist patient care intervention reporting. *J. Am. Pharm. Assoc. JAPhA* **2019**, *59*, 615–623. Available online: https://pubmed.ncbi.nlm.nih.gov/31400991/ (accessed on 11 April 2022).
38. Lancaster, G.A.; Thabane, L. Guidelines for reporting non-randomised pilot and feasibility studies. *Pilot Feasibility Stud.* **2019**, *5*, 114. [CrossRef]
39. The Danish Medicines Agency. [Vitamine and Mineral Preparations]. Available online: https://laegemiddelstyrelsen.dk/da/special/naturlaegemidler-og-vitamin-og-mineralpraeparater/vitamin-og-mineralpraeparater/ (accessed on 7 June 2021).
40. Basislisten. Available online: https://www.sundhed.dk/sundhedsfaglig/information-til-praksis/hovedstaden/almen-praksis/laegemidler/basislisten-hovedstaden/ (accessed on 10 February 2021).
41. Danish Health Authority. The Deprescribing List. Available online: https://www.sst.dk/da/viden/laegemidler/medicingennemgang/seponeringslisten (accessed on 1 January 2019).
42. Danish Health Authority. Anticholinergic Medicines. Available online: https://www.sst.dk/da/viden/laegemidler/medicingennemgang/antikolinerge-laegemidler (accessed on 10 February 2021).
43. Interaktionsdatabasen.dk. Available online: http://interaktionsdatabasen.dk/ (accessed on 10 February 2021).
44. Brechtl, J.R.; Murshed, S.; Homel, P.; Bookbinder, M. Monitoring Symptoms in Patients with Advanced Illness in Long-Term Care: A Pilot Study. *J. Pain Symptom Manag.* **2006**, *32*, 168–174. [CrossRef]
45. Beddard-Huber, E.; Jayaraman, J.; White, L.; Yeomans, W. Evaluation of the Utility of the Edmonton Symptom Assessment System (revised) Scale on a Tertiary Palliative Care Unit. *J. Palliat. Care* **2015**, *31*, 44–50. [CrossRef]

46. Sandvik, R.K.; Selbaek, G.; Bergh, S.; Aarsland, D.; Husebo, B.S. Signs of Imminent Dying and Change in Symptom Intensity During Pharmacological Treatment in Dying Nursing Home Patients: A Prospective Trajectory Study. *J. Am. Med. Dir. Assoc.* **2016**, *17*, 821–827. [CrossRef]
47. Lamppu, P.J.; Laakkonen, M.-L.; Finne-Soveri, H.; Kautiainen, H.; Laurila, J.V.; Pitkälä, K.H. Training Staff in Long-Term Care Facilities–Effects on Residents' Symptoms, Psychological Well-Being, and Proxy Satisfaction. *J. Pain Symptom Manag.* **2021**, *62*, e4–e12. [CrossRef] [PubMed]
48. Moorhouse, P.; Mallery, L.H. Palliative and therapeutic harmonization: A model for appropriate decision-making in frail older adults. *J. Am. Geriatr. Soc.* **2012**, *60*, 2326–2332. [CrossRef] [PubMed]
49. Nekolaichuk, C.; Watanabe, S.; Beaumont, C. The Edmonton Symptom Assessment System: A 15-year retrospective review of validation studies (1991–2006). *Palliat. Med.* **2008**, *22*, 111–122. [CrossRef] [PubMed]
50. Hui, D.; Shamieh, O.; Paiva, C.E.; Perez-Cruz, P.E.; Kwon, J.H.; Muckaden, M.A.; Park, M.; Yennu, S.; Hun Kang, J.; Bruera, E. Minimal clinically important differences in the Edmonton Symptom Assessment Scale in cancer patients: A prospective, multicenter study. *Cancer* **2015**, *121*, 3027–3035. [CrossRef]
51. Cummings, J.L.; Mega, M.; Gray, K.; Rosenberg-Thompson, S.; Carusi, D.A.; Gornbein, J. The Neuropsychiatric Inventory: Comprehensive assessment of psychopathology in dementia. *Neurology* **1994**, *44*, 2308–2314. [CrossRef]
52. Harrison, S.L.; Kouladjian O'Donnell, L.; Bradley, C.E.; Milte, R.; Dyer, S.M.; Gnanamanickam, E.S.; Liu, E.; Hilmer, S.N.; Crotty, M. Associations between the Drug Burden Index, Potentially Inappropriate Medications and Quality of Life in Residential Aged Care. *Drugs Aging* **2018**, *35*, 83–91. [CrossRef]
53. Polinder, S.; Boyé, N.D.A.; Mattace-Raso, F.U.S.; Van der Velde, N.; Hartholt, K.A.; De Vries, O.J.; Lips, P.; Van der Cammen, T.J.M.; Patka, P.; Van Beeck, F.; et al. Cost-utility of medication withdrawal in older fallers: Results from the improving medication prescribing to reduce risk of FALLs (IMPROveFALL) trial. *BMC Geriatr.* **2016**, *16*, 179. [CrossRef]
54. Olsson, I.N.; Runnamo, R.; Engfeldt, P. Medication quality and quality of life in the elderly, a cohort study. *Health Qual. Life Outcomes* **2011**, *9*, 95. [CrossRef]
55. Van Hout, B.; Janssen, M.F.; Feng, Y.S.; Kohlmann, T.; Busschbach, J.; Golicki, D.; Lloyd, A.; Scalone, L.; Kind, P.; Pickard, A.S. Interim scoring for the EQ-5D-5L: Mapping the EQ-5D-5L to EQ-5D-3L value sets. *Value Health J. Int. Soc. Pharm. Outcomes Res.* **2012**, *15*, 708–715. [CrossRef]
56. Coretti, S.; Ruggeri, M.; McNamee, P. The minimum clinically important difference for EQ-5D index: A critical review. *Expert Rev. Pharm. Outcomes Res.* **2014**, *14*, 221–233. [CrossRef]
57. Harris, P.A.; Taylor, R.; Thielke, R.; Payne, J.; Gonzalez, N.; Conde, J.G. Research electronic data capture (REDCap)—A metadata-driven methodology and workflow process for providing translational research informatics support. *J. Biomed. Inform.* **2009**, *42*, 377–381. [CrossRef] [PubMed]

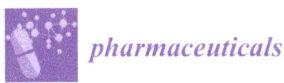

Article

Medicines Reconciliation in the Emergency Department: Important Prescribing Discrepancies between the Shared Medication Record and Patients' Actual Use of Medication

Tanja Stenholdt Andersen [1,2,†], Mia Nimb Gemmer [1,2,†], Hayley Rose Constance Sejberg [1,2], Lillian Mørch Jørgensen [2,3], Thomas Kallemose [3], Ove Andersen [2,3,4], Esben Iversen [3] and Morten Baltzer Houlind [1,3,5,*]

1 The Capital Region Pharmacy, 2730 Herlev, Denmark; tanja.stenholdt.andersen@regionh.dk (T.S.A.); mia.nimb.gemmer@regionh.dk (M.N.G.); hayley.rose.constance.sejberg@regionh.dk (H.R.C.S.)
2 Emergency Department, Copenhagen University Hospital Amager and Hvidovre, 2650 Hvidovre, Denmark; lillian.moerch.joergensen@regionh.dk (L.M.J.); ove.andersen@regionh.dk (O.A.)
3 Department of Clinical Research, Copenhagen University Hospital Amager and Hvidovre, 2650 Hvidovre, Denmark; thomas.kallemose@regionh.dk (T.K.); esben.iversen@regionh.dk (E.I.)
4 Department of Clinical Medicine, Faculty of Health and Medical Sciences, University of Copenhagen, 2200 Copenhagen, Denmark
5 Department of Drug Design and Pharmacology, University of Copenhagen, 2100 Copenhagen, Denmark
* Correspondence: morten.baltzer.houlind@regionh.dk; Tel.: +45-28-83-85-63
† These authors share first authorship.

Abstract: Medication reconciliation is crucial to prevent medication errors. In Denmark, primary and secondary care physicians can prescribe medication in the same electronic prescribing system known as the Shared Medication Record (SMR). However, the SMR is not always updated by physicians, which can lead to discrepancies between the SMR and patients' actual use of medication. These discrepancies may compromise patient safety upon admission to the emergency department (ED). Here, we investigated (a) the occurrence of discrepancies, (b) factors associated with discrepancies, and (c) the percentage of patients accessible to a clinical pharmacist during pharmacy working hours. The study included all patients age ≥ 18 years who were admitted to the Hvidovre Hospital ED on three consecutive days in June 2020. The clinical pharmacists performed medicines reconciliation to identify prescribing discrepancies. In total, 100 patients (52% male; median age 66.5 years) were included. The patients had a median of 10 [IQR 7–13] medications listed in the SMR and a median of two [IQR 1–3.25] discrepancies. Factors associated with increased rate of prescribing discrepancies were age < 65 years, time since last update of the SMR ≥ 115 days, and patients' self-dispensing their medications. Eighty-four percent of patients were available for medicines reconciliations during the normal working hours of the clinical pharmacist. In conclusion, we found that discrepancies between the SMR and patients' actual medication use upon admission to the ED are frequent, and we identified several risk factors associated with the increased rate of discrepancies.

Keywords: shared medication record; medication reconciliation; drug information service; hospital pharmacy service; electronic prescribing; electronic medical record; clinical pharmacist; emergency department

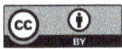

1. Introduction

Medicines reconciliation is an essential task for preventing medication errors in both primary and secondary care [1–4]. It ensures correct and updated information about patients' medication, which is especially important when patients transfer between sectors. Medicines reconciliation requires a detailed medication history, which includes examination of all recently dispensed prescriptions combined with patient interviews [5].

In Denmark, hospitals and primary care physicians (e.g., general practitioners, ophthalmologists, private dermatologists, etc.) have access to the Shared Medication Record (SMR), which is a central electronic database containing information about all medications prescribed and dispensed at a community pharmacy within the past two years for residents and citizens of Denmark [6,7]. The SMR provides an overview of the current medication status for all patients and gives the patient's healthcare team access to up-to-date prescribing information [6,7]. For example, the SMR indicates whether a patient has a dosette box from the community pharmacist or receives help with dispensing medication via home care, district nurses, or care assistants. Furthermore, sales records in the SMR for purchased medications can also indicate patient non-compliance. If a physician involved in the patient's treatment notices any obvious medication errors, they are required to fix the errors and update the SMR [8]. Altogether, the SMR aims to prevent medication errors by increasing accessibility to patients' current medication status [6,9].

Discrepancies between the SMR and patients' actual use of medicines can result in improper prescribing or medication errors, either during hospitalization or after discharge [10,11]. This is particularly relevant in acute settings where patients often cannot speak for themselves about their medication history [12]. In such cases, the SMR is a valuable resource for clinicians and pharmacists—but only if it is accurate. Therefore, it is always important to discuss and confirm a patient's current medication status directly with the patient or their caregiver [10,13]. Ideally, medicines reconciliation should be performed within the primary sector to keep the SMR up to date and improve its reliability during acute admissions.

It is important to note that the SMR categorizes the patient's medications into orders and prescriptions. When a patient is admitted to the hospital, any active orders in the SMR are automatically transferred to the hospital's local electronic prescribing system. This does not include active prescriptions that are no longer connected to an order. The admitting physician must review all active orders in the SMR and consider whether the patient should continue to receive these medications during hospitalization [14]. This becomes problematic if the general practitioner (GP) has not reviewed the patient's orders. For example, the SMR could contain an old order for a medication without a stop date or without an active prescription, which might indicate that the medication is no longer in use. If these orders are not corrected, they can be transferred to the hospital's prescribing system and ultimately lead to improper prescribing of a medication the patient does not need. Prior to discharge, the physician must again consider which orders should be continued after discharge. Each time a change is made in the SMR at discharge (e.g., new order/prescription, deprescription, or change in dose/frequency), the physician is required to indicate that the SMR has been updated [14].

Previous studies have shown that the SMR is not used as intended by physicians during medicines reconciliation [15–17], but it is unknown how often discrepancies occur in the emergency department (ED). Therefore, the purpose of this study is to investigate (a) the number and types of discrepancies, (b) the factors associated with discrepancies, and (c) the number of medicines reconciliations that could realistically be completed by a clinical pharmacist.

2. Results

2.1. Patient Characteristics

A total of 117 patients were admitted to the ED during the study period. Of these, 17 were excluded due to no active orders/prescriptions in the SMR (n = 11), patient isolation (n = 3), discharge against medical advice (n = 2), or death during admission (n = 1). Medicines reconciliation and a complete medication review was completed for 100 patients: 51 primary, 40 secondary, and nine retrospective. Patient characteristics for the final study population (n = 100) are shown in Table 1. Median age was 66.5 years, and 52% of patients were men. Patients used a median of six (IQR: 3–9) regular medications and two (IQR: 1–3) PRN medications. Fifty-five patients were referred by emergency services or an out-of-hours healthcare professional, 37 were referred by a GP or outpatient clinic, and eight were self-referrals.

Table 1. Patient characteristics of the included patients (n = 100).

Demographic Data	Median (IQR) or n (%)
Sex (men)	52 (52)
Age (years)	66.5 (53–80)
Admitted during normal working hours 8:00 a.m.–3:00 p.m.	48 (48)
Admitted outside normal working hours 3:01 p.m.–07:59 a.m.	52 (52)
Referred to the ED by a GP or Outpatient clinic	37 (37)
Referred to the ED by an emergency or out-of-hours service healthcare professional	55 (55)
Self-referral to the ED	8 (8)
Triage level ≥ 3	78 (78)
Length of hospital stay	2 (1–4)
Patients with a hospital interaction within 90 days before index admission	66 (66)
eGFR mL/min/1.73 m^2	83 (56–90)
<60 mL/min/1.73 m^2	29 (29)
Medication listed in the SMR	10 (7–13)
Medication used (regularly scheduled and PRN)	8 (5–11)
Medication used (regularly scheduled)	6 (3–9)
Patients using ≥ 1 regular medications	93 (93)
Patients using ≥ 5 regular medications	63 (63)
Days since the last SMR update *	59 (14–154)
<30 days since the last SMR update	35 (35)
<31–89 days since the last SMR update	16 (16)
≥ 90 days since the last SMR update	39 (39)
GP completed last update of the SMR *	24 (26)
Help with medication dispensing	29 (29)

* n = 92; ED, emergency department; eGFR, estimated glomerular filtration rate; GP, general practitioner; SMR, Shared Medication Record; PRN, Pro re nata.

2.2. Number of Prescribing Discrepancies

From a total of 852 prescriptions (648 regular medications and 204 PRN medications), the clinical pharmacists identified 240 discrepancies between the SMR and patients' actual use of medication during medicines reconciliation. Figure 1 shows the distribution of discrepancies per patient: 81% of patients had ≥ 1 discrepancy, while 14% had ≥ 5 discrepancies. The median number of discrepancies found per patients was two [IQR 1–3.25].

2.3. Types of Prescribing Discrepancies

Table 2 shows the most frequent types of discrepancies. The most common discrepancies were order no longer in use (65%), dosing frequency incorrect (15%), and order missing (12%). All discrepancies classified by anatomical therapeutic index (ATC) are shown in (Table A1). Discrepancies were most frequently observed for medications classified as A02 (antacids and certain laxatives) or N02 (analgesics such as opioids). Among the discrepancies involving opioids, four were orders no longer in use, and two were due to missing orders. Discrepancies involving medications classified as J01 (systemic antibiotics) included 14 cases where the indication for antibiotic treatment was no longer relevant.

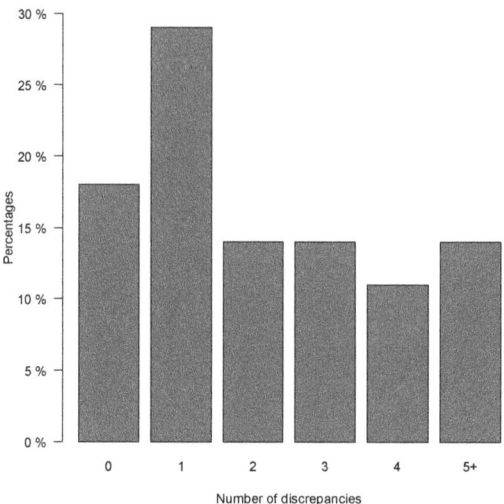

Figure 1. The percentage of patients with a specific number of discrepancies found between actual use of medication compared to the shared medication record (SMR).

Table 2. Types and number of discrepancies.

Types of Discrepancies	Discrepancies, n (%)	Patients, %
Order not in use	157 (65)	61
Incorrect dose frequency	37 (16)	24
Omission of order	29 (12)	15
Duplicate order	9 (4)	9
Incorrect dosage	8 (3)	6

2.4. Factors Associated with the Rate of Prescribing Discrepancies

Table 3 shows factors associated with the rate of discrepancies. Patients aged 65–80 and >80 both had reduced rates of discrepancies per medication listed in the SMR, 42% (CI: 29–52) and 51% (CI: 38–62), respectively, compared with patients aged <65 years. Adjusting for age and sex, patients with ≥115 days since the previous SMR update had a 53% (CI: 29–82) higher discrepancy rate per medication listed in the SMR compared with patients with ≤27 days since the previous SMR update. Patients who required assistance with medication dispensing also had a 72% (CI: 65–78) reduced rate of discrepancies per medication listed in the SMR compared with patients who dispensed medication themselves. Patients who required assistance dispensing their medications also had a 72% (CI: 65–78) reduced discrepancy rate per medication listed in the SMR compared with patients who dispensed medication themselves. The prescribing discrepancy rate was not associated with the type of physician who last updated the SMR, the time of admission to the ED, or triage level. Sensitivity analysis excluding discrepancies due to order not in use only showed additional association for patients admitted outside of normal working hours, with a 159% (CI: 84–263) increased rate of discrepancies per medication listed in the SMR compared to patients admitted during normal working hours (Table A2).

2.5. Medicines Reconciliations Completed during Normal Working Hours

Time of admission and discharge from the ED are shown in Table 4. Forty-nine patients (49%) were admitted during normal working hours (8.00 a.m.–3.00 p.m.), and 51 patients (51%) were admitted outside of normal working hours. Among patients admitted outside normal working hours, 35 patients were still in the ED the following morning.

Table 3. Factors associated with prescribing discrepancies between the Shared Medication Record (SMR) and patients actual use of medications.

Covariate (Number of Patients)	Incidence Rate Ratio	Confidence Interval	p-Value
Age, years			
<65 (44)	Ref	Ref	Ref
65–79 (30)	0.58	0.48–0.71	<0.001
≥80 (26)	0.49	0.38–0.92	<0.001
Female	Ref	Ref	Ref
Male 65–79 (52)	0.96	0.80–1.15	1.00
All models are adjusted for age and sex			
Days since the last SMR update *			
First tertile: 0–27 (33)	Ref	Ref	Ref
Second tertile: 28–114 (28)	1.16	0.96–1.40	1.00
Third tertile: ≥115 (29)	1.53	1.29–1.82	<0.001
Who updated the SMR last *			
Hospital (37)	Ref	Ref	Ref
Outpatients clinic (29)	1.02	0.84–1.23	1.00
GP (24)	1.19	0.98–1.43	0.836
Time of admission to the ED			
During normal working hours (48)	Ref	Ref	Ref
Outside normal working hours (52)	1.04	0.87–1.24	1.00
Help with medication dispensing			
No (71)	Ref	Ref	Ref
Yes (29)	0.31	0.24–0.39	<0.001
Triage level			
1 or 2 (23)	Ref	Ref	Ref
3 (51)	0.95	0.75–1.19	1.00
4 (26)	1.16	0.90–1.49	1.005

* n = 90, ED, emergency department; GP, general practitioner; SMR, Shared Medication Record. Note: The p-values are adjusted for multiple comparisons.

Table 4. Time intervals for admission and/or discharge in relation to the clinical pharmacists' normal working hours.

Time	Number of Patients	Patients with ≥1 Prescribing Discrepancy, n (%)
Admitted during normal working hours (8.00 a.m.–3.00 p.m.)	49	37 (76)
Admitted outside normal working hours (3.01 p.m.–7.59 a.m.), but still admitted the following morning (until at least 9.30 a.m.)	35	27 (77)
Admitted and discharged outside normal working hours (3.01 p.m.–7.59 a.m.)	16	15 (94)

Therefore, it was possible for the clinical pharmacists to complete medicines reconciliation for 84 patients (84%) during normal working hours. Of these, 64 patients (76%) had ≥1 discrepancy found during medicines reconciliation.

3. Discussion

3.1. Main Findings

This study investigated the number and types of discrepancies found between the SMR and patients actual medication use upon acute admission to the ED. Clinical pharmacists identified a total of 240 prescribing discrepancies among 100 patients. The median number of discrepancies per patient was two, and 81% of patients had ≥1 discrepancy. The most common types of discrepancy found were order no longer in use, dosing frequency incorrect, and order missing. Factors associated that increased discrepancy rates included age <65, and extended time since prior SMR update. The study also evaluated the percentage of medicines reconciliations that could be completed by a clinical pharmacist within working hours. Medicines reconciliation was possible for 84% of patients.

3.2. Results in Context of Other Studies

The frequency of discrepancies upon ED admission were lower than what has been observed in other Danish studies [15,16,18]. This may be explained by differences in clinical setting and inclusion criteria. For example, Buck et al. and Bülow et al. studied patients in the ED, geriatric ward, and the orthopedic surgery ward. Their inclusion criteria were age >50 years with ≥5 medications [15,18]. It has previously been demonstrated that increased medication use is associated with an increased risk of discrepancies [19–22], so the findings by Bülow et al. 2019 [16], Bülow et al. 2021 [15] and Buck et al. [18] may be related to the higher prevalence of polypharmacy. These studies did not find an association between age and the frequency of discrepancies found, which is likely due to the difference in clinical settings compared to our study. The study by Pippins et al. found that age <85 was associated with a higher risk of unintended medication discrepancies with potential for causing harm [23]. We found in our study that age <65 was associated with a higher frequency of discrepancies. However, in contrast to Pippins et al., we found that patients who required assistance with medication dispensing had a reduced rate of discrepancy compared to patients that dispensed medication themselves. This difference in findings between Pippins et al. and our study could be because of the Danish SMR system, where a similar tool was lacking in the Pippins et al. study. In Denmark, patients who receive help with dispensing their medication via home care, district nurses, or care assistants, get their medicines dispensed directly from orders in the SMR. The association between discrepancies and time since prior SMR update observed in our study is similar to findings from Bülow et al. 2021 [15]. Cornich et al. did not find a significantly higher discrepancy rate for admissions that took place outside of normal working hours [24]. Our study possibly indicates an increased discrepancy rate for patients admitted outside of normal working hours.

The types of discrepancies found in our study are comparable to other Danish studies [15,16,18,25]. We found that 65% of discrepancies were due to medication being no longer in use, which is similar to results from Bülow et al. 2019 [16] and Bülow et al. 2021 [15] but higher than results from Buck et al. [18]. We found that 15% of discrepancies were due to errors in dosing frequency. The two studies by Bülow [15,16] divide this category into two subcategories: PRN administration of regularly scheduled prescriptions, and regular scheduled administration of a PRN prescription. If these categories are merged, then the combined frequency of discrepancies found due to errors in dosing frequency from Bülow et al. 2019 [16] is similar to our study, but the frequency in Bülow et al. 2021 [15] is more than double what we observed. We found that 12% of discrepancies were due to an omission of order, which is similar to Bülow et al. 2019 [16] and Bülow et al. 2021 [15], but lower than what has been reported by Buck et al. [18] and Houlind et al. [25]. However, these studies use different terminology to describe the types of discrepancies, which makes direct comparison difficult. Finally, we found that antacids and analgesics were medication groups most frequently associated with prescribing discrepancies, which corresponds with the findings from Bülow et al. 2021 [15].

3.3. Updating the SMR: Possible Solutions and Reflections

The SMR can help healthcare professionals obtain an overview of a patient's medication use, detect noncompliance, and help prevent medication errors. However, our results indicate that dosing discrepancies are common regardless of how a patient is referred to the ED. This suggests that relying solely on the SMR for a patient's medication history is unsafe, which is supported by several other studies [26–29]. A valid medication history should include at least two information sources with different perspectives (i.e., prescribing and dispensing) [5,13]. Clinical pharmacists are essential for this purpose, as they have an opportunity to actively discuss medication use with the patient [2]. In addition, allowing clinical pharmacists to perform medicines reconciliation would enable physicians to focus on other aspects of patient care.

We found that 84% of patients were physically available for medicines reconciliation during normal working hours, meaning that medicines reconciliation combined with a medication review could in theory be performed for as many as 28 patients per day. However, previous studies have shown that medicines reconciliation takes approximately 30 min per patient (Buck et al.: 29 min, Urban et al.: 35.4 min, Cornich et al.: 24 min) [18,22,24], and a complete medication review would require even more time [30]. This suggests that a single person could perform no more than 14 medicines reconciliations per day. If the goal is to identify all discrepancies for all patients, then more staff resources must be dedicated. Alternatively, factors associated with prescribing discrepancies can be used to identify patients at highest risk for serious medication errors.

Accurate medicines reconciliation during admission increases the chances that the medication list will be updated at discharge. All physicians are expected to update the SMR any time they change a patient's medication [8], but this does not always occur. Despite best practice guidelines, primary care physicians are not legally required to update the SMR [8]. In secondary care, updating the SMR is required by regional standard operating procedures [14]. In practice, maintaining an accurate electronic medication list is time consuming [31,32], and correct use of the SMR is limited by factors such as motivation, technical problems, time constraints, and familiarity with the electronic system [17].

Since patients potentially interact with many physicians across healthcare sectors, it must be made clear who has this responsibility for ensuring that the patient's medication list is kept up to date [33]. Rose et al. suggest that a patient's GP should be responsible for ensuring the SMR is kept up to date [31]. Unfortunately, no national agreement has been made within the primary sector in Denmark. Another solution could be to utilize clinical pharmacists, either in the hospital or in outpatient clinics. Hospital-based pharmacists could update the SMR at discharge, thereby preventing inappropriate prescriptions from continuing until the patient sees their primary care physician. Dedicated pharmacists in primary care could assist with medicines reconciliation for patients who are in a stable phase of their treatment, thereby preventing medication errors during future hospitalization. This pharmacist-based concept is utilized in other countries but remains uncommon in Denmark, in part because pharmacists in Denmark are not considered authorized healthcare professionals and, therefore, have limited access to the SMR. A third solution could be to promote patient involvement. For example, patients could be prompted on a yearly basis to review their own medication list to identify any prescriptions no longer in use. Increased patient involvement in general may also encourage dialogue between the patient and their GP that could help resolve any issues regarding medication compliance or inappropriate use.

3.4. Strengths and Limitations

The main strength of this study is that it identifies a daily clinical challenge in the ED regarding discrepancies found between the SMR and patients' actual medication use. Furthermore, the study included patients on three consecutive days. This study also has some important limitations. First, the study was not designed to investigate the clinical significance or long-term consequences of prescribing discrepancies. Second, this was a single-center study and results are not necessarily generalizable to other healthcare settings. Third, we did not investigate how many discrepancies continued from admission to discharge, so we could not evaluate the effectiveness of a pharmacist-based intervention. The timing and duration of the study could also be considered a limitation, as there may be variation in the frequency of discrepancies found on different days of the week. Finally, our results rely on the accuracy of patients' reported use of medication.

4. Materials and Methods

4.1. Ethics Approval

Data collection was performed during standard patient care as part of a quality improvement project by MNG, TSO and HRCS. Quality improvement projects in Denmark do not require prior ethical approval. The study was approved by a local committee at Copenhagen University Hospital, Amager and Hvidovre (WZ20017637-2020-77). All data were stored in anonymized form.

4.2. Setting

The tax-funded Danish healthcare system provides free and equal healthcare to citizens and residents of Denmark. Copenhagen University Hospital Amager & Hvidovre, Hvidovre, Denmark (hereafter Hvidovre Hospital) covers 10 municipalities with a population of approximately 550,000. Each year, the hospital has approximately 16,500 medical admissions, of which 85% are acute admissions to the ED. The Hvidovre Hospital ED is always open and has an acute medical ward with a capacity of 29 beds. Patients are typically referred to the acute medical ward by their GP, outpatient clinic, medical helplines, on-call/out-of-hours services, or by calling the emergency services. Patients can also be referred to the acute medical unit internally from other ED units. Patients can stay in the ED for up to three days before they are discharged or transferred to a specialized medical ward in the hospital.

The ED has permanent affiliations with pharmacy technicians, clinical pharmacists, physiotherapists, and doctors from a variety of medical specialties. During weekdays, pharmacy technicians dispense and administer medications and prepare discharge prescriptions between 7 a.m. and 2 p.m. Pharmacy technicians are often the first to notice specific medication issues, which are then referred to a clinical pharmacist. There is typically only one clinical pharmacist available between 8 a.m. and 3 p.m. The clinical pharmacist reviews and resolves any medication issues noted by the pharmacy technician. They also complete medicines reconciliation for as many patients as possible, prioritizing newly admitted geriatric patients and patients from particular medical specialties.

4.3. Design and Patients

The study included all patients age $\geq$18 years who were admitted to the Hvidovre Hospital ED on three consecutive days in June 2020. Exclusion criteria were: (i) no active orders/prescriptions in the SMR or no dispensed medication within the previous two years in the SMR, (ii) patient isolation, (iii) discharge against medical advice prior to interview with the clinical pharmacist, and (iv) death during admission.

4.4. Data Collection and the Best Possible Medication History

Three senior clinical pharmacists ($\geq$5 years of experience) performed medicines reconciliation in the ED during the three-day period. For each patient, the clinical pharmacist recorded the patient's sex, age, number of regular medications, and number of PRN medications. The SMR and electronic patient record were used to determine the time of admission, type of referral, triage level, time of discharge, and details about the most recent update of the SMR prior to admission. The clinical pharmacist then obtained a medication history for all prescribed and over-the-counter (OTC) medications as well as any vitamins and dietary supplements, noting whether the patient dispensed their own medication or received assistance. The medication history was collected from at least one prescribing source and one dispensing source. Prescribing sources included the SMR, dose dispensing card, or the patient's GP. Dispensing sources included purchasing records from the SMR, patient interview, examination of medicine labels, or telephone contact with the patient's relative, nursing facility, or district nurse. The purpose of locating the dispensing source was to identify any discrepancies between how a medication was prescribed and how it was used by the patient.

The medication history was categorized as primary, secondary, or retrospective: primary if the pharmacist completed medicines reconciliation before a physician transferred information from the SMR into the electronic prescribing system, secondary if the pharmacist completed medicines reconciliation after this transfer occurred, and retrospective if the pharmacist completed medicines reconciliation after patient discharge. Retrospective medication histories were obtained by contacting the patient by telephone.

4.5. Outcomes

The primary outcome was the number and types of discrepancies between the SMR and patients' actual use of medication. A discrepancy was defined as any inconsistency between the SMR and the medication history obtained by the clinical pharmacist. Discrepancies were classified as: (a) order not in use, (b) incorrect dose frequency, (c) omission of order, (d) duplicate order, or (e) dosage incorrect. Discrepancies for vitamins and dietary supplements were only recorded if the SMR indicated they had been prescribed by a physician. Secondary outcomes were: (i) factors associated with discrepancies, and (ii) the percentage of patients available for medicines reconciliation by a clinical pharmacist during normal working hours.

4.6. Statistics

All patient characteristics are presented as medians with interquartile range (IQR) or frequency with percentages. The discrepancy rate was calculated as the number of discrepancies, divided by the number of medications listed in the SMR. To investigate the association of different factors for the rate of discrepancies, Quasi-Poisson regression models were fitted. Quasi-Poisson was used to account for underdispersion in the models (all dispersion estimates were between 0.16 and 0.30). Factors included in the models were sex, age (<65 years, 65–79 years, or $\geq$80 years), time since last update of the SMR (tertiles), source of last SMR update (hospital, outpatient clinic, or GP), time of admission (during or outside normal working hours), assistance with medication dispensing (yes or no), and triage level (level 1–2, level 3, or level 4). Models were fitted for each factor including the specific factor with age and sex to adjust for confounding. However, age and sex models were not adjusted if they only included their specific factor. Results from the models are presented as incidence rate ratios (IRR) with confidence intervals (CI). Additionally, models were repeated with excluding discrepancies due to order not in use in the rate calculation. Bonferroni correction was used to account for multiple testing by upscaling p-values with number of tests, all upscaled p-values larger than 1 are set to 1. Data were processed using Microsoft Excel XLSTAT. All calculations and statistical analyses were performed in R 3.6.1 [34]. For all statistical tests, $p < 0.05$ was considered statistically significant.

5. Conclusions

In a cohort of 100 patients consecutively admitted to the ED, we found that 81% of patients had $\geq$1 discrepancy between the SMR and patients' actual use of medication. Age < 65, longer time since prior SMR update, and patient self-dispensing were associated with a higher frequency of discrepancies. During the study, 84% of the patients were available for medication reconciliation by a clinical pharmacist within normal working hours. The high frequency of discrepancies serves as a caution to clinicians who rely on the SMR when obtaining a medication history in daily practice. Future studies should utilize risk stratification models to identify patients with the highest risk of serious discrepancies leading to adverse clinical outcomes.

Author Contributions: T.S.A., M.N.G., H.R.C.S., L.M.J., O.A., T.K. and M.B.H. contributed to conception of the study design. M.N.G., T.S.A., H.R.C.S. and L.M.J., collected the data. T.S.A., M.N.G., H.R.C.S., E.I., M.B.H. and T.K. analyzed data. All others interpreted the data. M.N.G., T.S.A., H.R.C.S., E.I. and M.B.H. drafted the manuscript. All others revised the manuscript. All authors have read and agreed to the published version of the manuscript.

Funding: M.B.H. was supported by a postdoctoral fellowship from The Capital Region's Research Foundation for Health Research, Denmark (grant-A6882).

Institutional Review Board Statement: The study was approved by a local committee at Copenhagen University Hospital, Amager and Hvidovre (WZ20017637-2020-77).

Informed Consent Statement: Not applicable.

Data Availability Statement: The data presented in this study are not publicly available due to Danish legislation.

Acknowledgments: This study was performed as part of the Clinical Academic Group (ACUTE-CAG) for Recovery Capacity nominated by the Greater Copenhagen Health Science Partners (GCHSP).

Conflicts of Interest: The authors declare no conflict of interest.

Appendix A

Table A1. Distribution of discrepancies categorized by Anatomic Therapeutic Index (ATC).

ATC-Drug Group (Level 2)	Description	Number of Discrepancies, n (%)
A02	Drugs for acid related disorders	25 (22.7)
N02	Analgesics	13 (11.8)
C09	Agents acting on the renin-angiotensin system	11 (10.0)
A06	Drugs for constipation	5 (4.5)
B01	Antithrombotic agents	5 (4.5)
A12	Mineral supplements	5 (4.5)
C10	Lipid modifying agents	5 (4.5)
C01	Cardiac therapy	5 (4.5)
R03	Drugs for obstructive airway diseases	4 (3.6)
B03	Antianemic preparations	4 (3.6)
J01	Antibacterials for systemic use	4 (3.6)
N03	Antiepileptics	4 (3.6)
N05	Psycholeptics	3 (2.7)
A11	Vitamins	3 (2.7)
N06	Psychoanaleptics	2 (1.8)
A10	Drugs used in diabetes	2 (1.8)
M01	Anti-inflammatory and antirheumatic products	2 (1.8)
H02	Corticosteroids for systemic use	2 (1.8)
R01	Nasal preparations	1 (0.9)
C03	Diuretics	1 (0.9)
M03	Muscle relaxants	1 (0.9)
S01	Ophthalmologicals	1 (0.9)
L01	Antineoplastic agents	1 (0.9)
D01	Antifungals for dermatological use	1 (0.9)

Table A2. Factors associated with prescribing discrepancies between actual use of medication compared to dispensed medication in the shared medication record (SMR).

Covariate (Number of Patients)	Incidence Rate Ratio	Confidence Interval	p-Value
Age, years			
<65 (44)	Ref	Ref	Ref
65–79 (years) (30)	0.67	0.45–0.99	0.514
≥80 (years) (26)	0.53	0.33–0.86	0.119
Female	Ref	Ref	Ref
Male 65–79 (52)	0.98	0.68–1.43	1.00
All models are adjusted for age and sex			
Days since the last SMR update *			
First tertile: 0–27 (33)	Ref	Ref	Ref
Second tertile: 28–114 (28)	1.27	0.85–1.89	1.00
Third tertile: ≥115 (29)	1.14	0.76–1.73	1.00
Who updated the SMR last *			
Hospital (37)	Ref	Ref	Ref
Outpatients clinic (29)	1.03	0.69–1.54	1.00
GP (24)	1.22	0.82–1.81	1.00
Time of admission to the ED			
During normal working hours (48)	Ref	Ref	Ref
Outside normal working hours (52)	2.59	1.84–3.63	<0.001
Help with medication dispensing			
No (71)	Ref	Ref	Ref
Yes (29)	0.18	0.10–0.33	<0.001
Triage level			
1 or 2 (23)	Ref	Ref	Ref
3 (51)	0.97	0.62–1.53	1.00
4 (26)	0.79	0.45–1.37	1.00

* n = 90, ED, emergency department; GP, general practitioner; SMR, Shared Medication Record. Note: The p-values are adjusted for multiple comparisons.

References

1. Lau, H.S.; Florax, C.; Porsius, A.J.; De Boer, A. The Completeness of Medication Histories in Hospital Medical Records of Patients Admitted to General Internal Medicine Wards. *Br. J. Clin. Pharmacol.* **2000**, *49*, 597–603. [CrossRef] [PubMed]
2. Andersen, S.E.; Pedersen, A.B.; Bach, K.F. Medication History on Internal Medicine Wards: Assessment of Extra Information Collected from Second Drug Interviews and GP Lists. *Pharmacoepidemiol. Drug Saf.* **2003**, *12*, 491–498. [CrossRef] [PubMed]
3. Knez, L.; Suskovic, S.; Rezonja, R.; Laaksonen, R.; Mrhar, A. The Need for Medication Reconciliation: A Cross-Sectional Observational Study in Adult Patients. *Respir. Med.* **2011**, *105* (Suppl. 1), S60–S66. [CrossRef]
4. Beers, M.H.; Munekata, M.; Storrie, M. The Accuracy of Medication Histories in the Hospital Medical Records of Elderly Persons. *J. Am. Geriatr. Soc.* **1990**, *38*, 1183–1187. [CrossRef] [PubMed]
5. Shaw, J.; Seal, R.; Pilling, M. *Room for Review a Guide to Medication Review: The Agenda for Patients, Practitioners and Managers*; Medicines Partnership: London, UK, 2002.
6. Ministry of Health. Fælles Medicinkort (FMK)—Sundhedsdatastyrelsen. Available online: https://sundhedsdatastyrelsen.dk/da/registre-og-services/om-faelles-medicinkort (accessed on 28 November 2021). (In Danish)
7. The Danish Health Data Authority. Shared Medicine Card. Available online: https://www.danishhealthdata.com/find-health-data/,-w- (accessed on 28 November 2021).
8. The Danish Health Data Authority. Best Practice på FMK. Available online: https://sundhedsdatastyrelsen.dk/-/media/sds/filer/registre-og-services/faelles-medicinkort/fmk-sundhedsprofesionelle/best_practice_fmk.pdf (accessed on 30 November 2021). (In Danish)
9. Munck, L.K.; Hansen, K.R.; Mølbak, A.G.; Balle, H.; Kongsgren, S. The Use of Shared Medication Record as Part of Medication Reconciliation at Hospital Admission Is Feasible. *Dan. Med. J.* **2014**, *61*, A4817.

10. Mueller, S.K.; Sponsler, K.C.; Kripalani, S.; Schnipper, J.L. Hospital-Based Medication Reconciliation Practices: A Systematic Review. *Arch. Intern. Med.* **2012**, *172*, 1057–1069. [CrossRef]
11. Cornu, P.; Steurbaut, S.; Leysen, T.; De Baere, E.; Ligneel, C.; Mets, T.; Dupont, A.G. Effect of Medication Reconciliation at Hospital Admission on Medication Discrepancies during Hospitalization and at Discharge for Geriatric Patients. *Ann. Pharmacother.* **2012**, *46*, 484–494. [CrossRef]
12. DeAntonio, J.H.; Leichtle, S.W.; Hobgood, S.; Boomer, L.; Aboutanos, M.; Mangino, M.J.; Wijesinghe, D.S.; Jayaraman, S. Medication Reconciliation and Patient Safety in Trauma: Applicability of Existing Strategies. *J. Surg. Res.* **2020**, *246*, 482–489. [CrossRef]
13. Moore, P.; Armitage, G.; Wright, J.; Dobrzanski, S.; Ansari, N.; Hammond, I.; Scally, A. Medicines Reconciliation Using a Shared Electronic Health Care Record. *J. Patient Saf.* **2011**, *7*, 148–154. [CrossRef]
14. Region Hovedstaden. Lægemiddelkomitéer i Region Hovedstaden og Region Sjælland Lægemiddelordination. Available online: https://vip.regionh.dk/VIP/Admin/GUI.nsf/Desktop.html?open&openlink=https://vip.regionh.dk/VIP/Slutbruger/Portal.nsf/Main.html?open&unid=XDCFC8C0A263E4AB3C12578AA002C8412&level=159716&dbpath=/VIP/Redaktoer/RH.nsf/&windowwidth=1100&windowheight=600&windowtitle=S%F8g (accessed on 24 January 2022). (In Danish)
15. Bülow, C.; Noergaard, J.D.S.V.; Faerch, K.U.; Pontoppidan, C.; Unkerskov, J.; Johansson, K.S.; Kornholt, J.; Christensen, M.B. Causes of Discrepancies between Medications Listed in the National Electronic Prescribing System and Patients' Actual Use of Medications. *Basic Clin. Pharmacol. Toxicol.* **2021**, *129*, 221–231. [CrossRef]
16. Bülow, C.; Flagstad Bech, C.; Ullitz Faerch, K.; Trærup Andersen, J.; Byg Armandi, H.; Treldal, C. Discrepancies Between the Medication List in Electronic Prescribing Systems and Patients' Actual Use of Medicines. *Sr. Care Pharm.* **2019**, *34*, 317–324. [CrossRef] [PubMed]
17. Christensen, S.; Jensen, L.D.; Kaae, S.; Vinding, K.L.; Petersen, J. Implementation of the shared medication record is difficult. *Ugeskr. Laeg.* **2014**, *176*, 1389–1391. [PubMed]
18. Buck, T.C.; Gronkjaer, L.S.; Duckert, M.-L.; Rosholm, J.-U.; Aagaard, L. Medication Reconciliation and Prescribing Reviews by Pharmacy Technicians in a Geriatric Ward. *J. Res. Pharm. Pract.* **2013**, *2*, 145–150. [CrossRef] [PubMed]
19. Michaelsen, M.H.; McCague, P.; Bradley, C.P.; Sahm, L.J. Medication Reconciliation at Discharge from Hospital: A Systematic Review of the Quantitative Literature. *Pharmacy* **2015**, *3*, 53–71. [CrossRef] [PubMed]
20. Belda-Rustarazo, S.; Cantero-Hinojosa, J.; Salmeron-García, A.; González-García, L.; Cabeza-Barrera, J.; Galvez, J. Medication Reconciliation at Admission and Discharge: An Analysis of Prevalence and Associated Risk Factors. *Int. J. Clin. Pract.* **2015**, *69*, 1268–1274. [CrossRef]
21. Bjeldbak-Olesen, M.; Danielsen, A.G.; Tomsen, D.V.; Jakobsen, T.J. Medication Reconciliation Is a Prerequisite for Obtaining a Valid Medication Review. *Dan. Med. J.* **2013**, *60*, A4605.
22. Urban, R.; Armitage, G.; Morgan, J.; Marshall, K.; Blenkinsopp, A.; Scally, A. Custom and Practice: A Multi-Center Study of Medicines Reconciliation Following Admission in Four Acute Hospitals in the UK. *Res. Soc. Adm. Pharm. RSAP* **2014**, *10*, 355–368. [CrossRef]
23. Pippins, J.R.; Gandhi, T.K.; Hamann, C.; Ndumele, C.D.; Labonville, S.A.; Diedrichsen, E.K.; Carty, M.G.; Karson, A.S.; Bhan, I.; Coley, C.M.; et al. Classifying and Predicting Errors of Inpatient Medication Reconciliation. *J. Gen. Intern. Med.* **2008**, *23*, 1414–1422. [CrossRef]
24. Cornish, P.L.; Knowles, S.R.; Marchesano, R.; Tam, V.; Shadowitz, S.; Juurlink, D.N.; Etchells, E.E. Unintended Medication Discrepancies at the Time of Hospital Admission. *Arch. Intern. Med.* **2005**, *165*, 424–429. [CrossRef]
25. Houlind, M.B.; Andersen, A.L.; Treldal, C.; Jørgensen, L.M.; Kannegaard, P.N.; Castillo, L.S.; Christensen, L.D.; Tavenier, J.; Rasmussen, L.J.H.; Ankarfeldt, M.Z.; et al. A Collaborative Medication Review Including Deprescribing for Older Patients in an Emergency Department: A Longitudinal Feasibility Study. *J. Clin. Med.* **2020**, *9*, 348. [CrossRef]
26. Schytte-Hansen, S.; Karkov, L.L.; Balslev-Clausen, A.P. The personal electronic medicine profile contributes to the avoidance of wrong medication at transfer from primary to secondary sector. *Ugeskr. Laeg.* **2011**, *173*, 2793–2797. [PubMed]
27. Tamblyn, R.; Abrahamowicz, M.; Buckeridge, D.L.; Bustillo, M.; Forster, A.J.; Girard, N.; Habib, B.; Hanley, J.; Huang, A.; Kurteva, S.; et al. Effect of an Electronic Medication Reconciliation Intervention on Adverse Drug Events: A Cluster Randomized Trial. *JAMA Netw. Open* **2019**, *2*, e1910756. [CrossRef] [PubMed]
28. Jurado, C.; Calmels, V.; Lobinet, E.; Divol, E.; Hanaire, H.; Metsu, D.; Sallerin, B. The Electronic Pharmaceutical Record: A New Method for Medication Reconciliation. *J. Eval. Clin. Pract.* **2018**, *24*, 681–687. [CrossRef] [PubMed]
29. Meguerditchian, A.N.; Krotneva, S.; Reidel, K.; Huang, A.; Tamblyn, R. Medication Reconciliation at Admission and Discharge: A Time and Motion Study. *BMC Health Serv. Res.* **2013**, *13*, 485. [CrossRef]
30. Bracey, G.; Miller, G.; Franklin, B.D.; Jacklin, A.; Gaskin, G. The Contribution of a Pharmacy Admissions Service to Patient Care. *Clin. Med.* **2008**, *8*, 53–57. [CrossRef]
31. Rose, A.J.; Fischer, S.H.; Paasche-Orlow, M.K. Beyond Medication Reconciliation: The Correct Medication List. *JAMA* **2017**, *317*, 2057–2058. [CrossRef]
32. Mekonnen, A.B.; Abebe, T.B.; McLachlan, A.J.; Brien, J.-A.E. Impact of Electronic Medication Reconciliation Interventions on Medication Discrepancies at Hospital Transitions: A Systematic Review and Meta-Analysis. *BMC Med. Inform. Decis. Mak.* **2016**, *16*, 112. [CrossRef]

33. World Health Organization. *Medication Safety in Transitions of Care: Technical Report*; World Health Organization: Geneva, Switzerland, 2019.
34. R: A Language and Environment for Statistical Computing. R Foundation for Statistical Computing, Vienna, Austria. Available online: https://www.r-project.org/ (accessed on 30 November 2021).

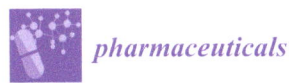

Article

Individualized versus Standardized Risk Assessment in Patients at High Risk for Adverse Drug Reactions (The IDrug Randomized Controlled Trial)–Never Change a Running System?

Katja S. Just [1], Catharina Scholl [2], Miriam Boehme [2], Kathrin Kastenmüller [3], Johannes M. Just [4], Markus Bleckwenn [5], Stefan Holdenrieder [6,7], Florian Meier [8], Klaus Weckbecker [4] and Julia C. Stingl [1,*]

1. Institute of Clinical Pharmacology, University Hospital RWTH Aachen, 52074 Aachen, Germany; kjust@ukaachen.de
2. Research Department, Federal Institute for Drugs and Medical Devices, 53175 Bonn, Germany; catharina.scholl@bfarm-research.de (C.S.); miriam.boehme@bfarm-research.de (M.B.)
3. Max-Planck Research Group, Würzburg Institute of Systems Immunology, University of Würzburg, 97078 Würzburg, Germany; kathrin.kastenmueller@uni-wuerzburg.de
4. Department of General Practice and Interprofessional Care, Medical Faculty of the University of Witten/Herdecke, 58448 Witten, Germany; johannes.just@uni-wh.de (J.M.J.); klaus.weckbecker@uni-wh.de (K.W.)
5. Department of General Practice, Medical Faculty, Leipzig University, 04103 Leipzig, Germany; markus.bleckwenn@medizin.uni-leipzig.de
6. Institute of Clinical Chemistry and Clinical Pharmacology, University Hospital Bonn, 53127 Bonn, Germany; stefan.holdenrieder@uni-bonn.de
7. Institute of Laboratory Medicine, German Heart Centre Munich, Technical University Munich, 80636 Munich, Germany
8. Wilhelm Loehe University of Applied Sciences (WLH), 90763 Fürth, Germany; florian.meier@wlh-fuerth.de
* Correspondence: jstingl@ukaachen.de; Tel.: +49-241-8089131

Citation: Just, K.S.; Scholl, C.; Boehme, M.; Kastenmüller, K.; Just, J.M.; Bleckwenn, M.; Holdenrieder, S.; Meier, F.; Weckbecker, K.; Stingl, J.C. Individualized versus Standardized Risk Assessment in Patients at High Risk for Adverse Drug Reactions (The IDrug Randomized Controlled Trial)–Never Change a Running System? *Pharmaceuticals* **2021**, *14*, 1056. https://doi.org/10.3390/ph14101056

Academic Editors: Charlotte Vermehren and Niels Westergaard

Received: 23 September 2021
Accepted: 11 October 2021
Published: 18 October 2021

Publisher's Note: MDPI stays neutral with regard to jurisdictional claims in published maps and institutional affiliations.

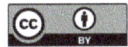

Copyright: © 2021 by the authors. Licensee MDPI, Basel, Switzerland. This article is an open access article distributed under the terms and conditions of the Creative Commons Attribution (CC BY) license (https://creativecommons.org/licenses/by/4.0/).

Abstract: The aim of this study was to compare effects of an individualized with a standardized risk assessment for adverse drug reactions to improve drug treatment with antithrombotic drugs in older adults. A randomized controlled trial was conducted in general practitioner (GP) offices. Patients aged 60 years and older, multi-morbid, taking antithrombotic drugs and at least one additional drug continuously were randomized to individualized and standardized risk assessment groups. Patients were followed up for nine months. A composite endpoint defined as at least one bleeding, thromboembolic event or death reported via a trigger list was used. Odds ratios (OR) and 95% confidence intervals (CI) were calculated. In total, $N = 340$ patients were enrolled from 43 GP offices. Patients in the individualized risk assessment group met the composite endpoint more often than in the standardized group (OR 1.63 [95%CI 1.02–2.63]) with multiple adjustments. The OR was higher in patients on phenprocoumon treatment (OR 1.99 [95%CI 1.05–3.76]), and not significant on DOAC treatment (OR 1.52 [95%CI 0.63–3.69]). Pharmacogenenetic variants of CYP2C9, 2C19 and VKORC1 were not observed to be associated with the composite endpoint. The results of this study may indicate that the time point for implementing individualized risk assessments is of importance.

Keywords: adverse drug reactions; pharmacogenetics; pharmacogenomics; personalized medicine; phenprocoumon; DOACs; older adults; bleeding; thromboembolism

1. Introduction

Personalized medicine is meant to improve efficacy and safety of drug treatment. However, strategies to modify drug treatment based on individual treatment risks are sparse. Older adults are often affected by adverse drug reactions (ADR) potentially leading to health emergencies [1,2]. It is estimated that around 6.5% of all admissions to the emergency department are caused by ADRs, mostly concerning older, multi-medicated adults [3]. Focusing only on older adults, even 8.7% of hospital admissions could be attributed to ADRs [4]. The prevalence might be even higher with rising age and drug intake [5]. While the role of potentially inappropriate medication for those admissions is not fully clear, ADRs are in general considered to be preventable [4]. Thereby, older adults often present bleeding ADR events due to antithrombotic drug treatment, with increasing risk at higher age [6]. Balancing the individual bleeding risk might be a fragile, challenging process in older adults. Therefore, older adults would probably benefit mostly from respecting the individual risk for ADRs.

While different antithrombotic drug treatments are available, the benefit–risk ratio in general needs to be balanced between preventing thromboembolic events without substantially increasing the risk for major bleedings. In the case of vitamin-K-antagonists (VKA), precise treatment goals are defined using international normalized ratios (INR), as the risk of bleeding increases not only with age, but also with the achieved intensity of coagulation [7]. However, also directly acting oral anticoagulants (DOAC), acetylsalicylic acid (ASA) and P2Y12-inhibitors such as clopidogrel, alone or in combination expose patients to a risk of bleeding [8,9].

Pharmacogenetics (PGx) is considered to smoothen the way to personalized medicine by improving drug efficacy as well as drug safety [10]. While around 80% of ADRs are considered to be dose-related, the individual drug metabolism affecting effective dose exposures might be in particular of importance for drug safety [11]. Heritable genetic variants can individually modify VKA drug effects through its target vitamin K epoxide reductase (VKORC1) and the metabolizing enzyme cytochrome P450 (CYP) 2C9. While PGx variability clearly impacts on drug effects of the VKA warfarin and dosing-guidelines exist [12], phenprocoumon is the VKA most commonly prescribed in Germany and other European countries [13]. However, using INR measurements the phenprocoumon treatment often gets empirically adjusted to the pharmacogenetic profile [14]. Beside the PGx variability, also other individual factors such as age, co-morbidities or co-medication via CYP3A4 interaction need to be considered to improve drug treatment and prevent ADRs due to anticoagulation [15,16].

The aim of the IDrug study was to compare effects of an individualized risk assessment for ADRs with a standardized risk assessment to improve safety of drug treatment in patients that are at high risk for bleeding and thromboembolic ADRs, thereby focusing on older, multi-morbid and multi-medicated patients with the intake of antithrombotic drugs.

2. Results

In total, $N = 365$ patients were enrolled in the IDrug study and randomized into the individualized or the standardized risk assessment group. Of those, $N = 340$ patients received the respective individualized or standardized risk assessment during visit one, which formed the intention to treat (ITT) cohort. Of those patients, $n = 273$ were followed-up according to the study plan (per protocol (PP) cohort). Within the individualized risk assessment group 80.2% ($n = 134$) and in the standardized risk assessment group 80.3% ($n = 139$) completed the whole follow-up according to the study plan. Supplement 1 lists reasons for dropping out of the ITT cohort (Table S1). Table 1 shows characteristics of the total ITT cohort and stratified to standardized and individualized risk assessment groups.

Table 1. Characteristics of the total population and stratified according to individualized and standardized risk assessment groups (N = 340).

Parameter	Missing, n (%)	Total Population, N = 340	Individualized Risk Assessment Group, n = 167	Standardized Risk Assessment Group, n = 173	p-Value
Age (years), median (IQR)	-	75 (71; 80)	75 (70; 78)	77 (72; 81)	**0.002**
Sex (female), n (%)	-	138 (40.6)	65 (38.9)	73 (42.2)	0.539
Number of drugs, median (IQR)	-	13 (8; 18)	13 (8; 18)	13 (8; 19)	0.955
HAS BLED (score), median (IQR)	-	2 (1; 3)	2 (1; 3)	2 (1; 3)	0.653
CHA2DS2 VASc (score), median (IQR)	-	4 (3; 5)	4 (3; 5)	4 (3; 5)	0.432
SF-36 score, median (IQR)					
Vitality	4 (1.2)	65 (50; 75)	65 (50; 80)	63 (45; 75)	0.212
Physical functioning	4 (1.2)	75 (55; 90)	80 (60; 91)	70 (50; 90)	**0.017**
Bodily pain	4 (1.2)	80 (52; 100)	84 (52; 100)	74 (52; 100)	0.672
General health perception	5 (1.5)	65 (50; 67)	65 (52; 77)	62 (49; 77)	0.531
Physical role functioning	5 (1.5)	100 (50; 100)	100 (50; 100)	100 (50; 100)	0.320
Emotional role functioning	5 (1.5)	100 (100; 100)	100 (100; 100)	100 (100; 100)	0.679
Social role functioning	4 (1.2)	100 (88; 100)	100 (97; 100)	100 (88; 100)	0.670
Mental health	4 (1.2)	84 (68; 92)	84 (71; 92)	84 (68; 92)	0.532
Time in study (days), median (IQR)	-	277 (259; 300)	279 (261; 302)	273 (254; 294)	0.062
GFR (mL/min/1.73m^2)	4 (1.2)	66.2 (51.7; 81.3)	67.4 (52.6; 81.5)	66.2 (51.3; 82.3)	0.424
Renal function, n (%)	-				0.240
GFR $\geq$ 90		32 (9.5)	14 (8.5)	18 (10.5)	
GFR 60–<90		178 (53.0)	91 (55.2)	87 (50.9)	
GFR 30–<60		119 (35.4)	59 (35.8)	60 (35.1)	
GFR 15–<30		5 (1.5)	0 (0)	5 (2.9)	
GFR < 15		2 (0.6)	1 (0.6)	1 (0.6)	
Highest educational degree, n (%)	19 (5.6)				0.925
Major school diploma		180 (56.1)	89 (56.3)	91 (55.8)	
Secondary school diploma		60 (18.7)	30 (19.0)	30 (18.4)	
Technical college diploma		16 (5.0)	8 (5.1)	8 (4.9)	
High school diploma		21 (6.5)	9 (5.7)	12 (7.4)	
College degree		43 (13.4)	22 (13.9)	21 (12.9)	
No diploma		1 (0.3)	0 (0)	1 (0.6)	
Number of antithrombotic drugs used, median (IQR)	-	1 (1; 1)	1 (1; 1)	1 (1; 1)	0.883
Antithrombotic drug use, n (%)	-				
VKA		209 (61.5)	103 (61.7)	106 (61.3)	0.997
DOAC		101 (29.7)	49 (29.3)	52 (30.1)	0.976
ASA		22 (6.5)	11 (6.6)	11 (6.5)	0.995
P2Y$_{12}$-inhibitor		53 (15.6)	28 (16.8)	25 (14.5)	0.831
PPI use, n (%)	-	168 (49.4)	78 (46.7)	90 (52.0)	0.327
Statin use, n (%)	-	187 (55.0)	92 (55.1)	95 (54.9)	0.974
CYP2C19 phenotype, n (%)	-				0.911
NM		241 (70.9)	120 (71.9)	121 (69.9)	
IM		87 (25.6)	41 (24.6)	46 (26.6)	
PM		12 (3.5)	6 (3.6)	6 (3.5)	
CYP2C9 phenotype, n (%)	-				0.488
NM		223 (65.6)	108 (64.7)	115 (66.5)	
IM		110 (32.4)	54 (32.3)	56 (32.4)	
PM		7 (2.1)	5 (3.0)	2 (1.2)	
VKORC1 phenotype, n (%)	-				0.724
Normal		295 (86.8)	146 (87.4)	149 (86.1)	
Poor		45 (13.2)	21 (12.6)	24 (13.9)	

IQR: interquartile range, GFR: glomerular filtration rate, VKA: vitamin-K-antagonist, DOAC: directly acting oral anticoagulants, ASA: acetylsalicylic acid, CKD: chronic kidney disease. Significant findings in bold text.

Patients in the standardized risk assessment group were of a median age of 77 years (IQR 72; 81) and, therefore, were older than those in the individualized risk assessment group (median 75 years (70; 78)) and accordingly scored with a median of 70 (50; 90) less concerning physical function based on the results of the SF-36 questionnaire (compared to 80 (60; 91)). All other parameters were equally distributed over both study groups. A high use of drugs was seen in both study groups with a median intake of 13 drugs (8; 18 in the individualized and 8; 19 in the standardized risk assessment group, respectively). Most patients in both groups received only one antithrombotic drug over the whole study time (median 1 (1; 1)), but in some patients a drug was switched or a treatment modified during follow-up. Therefore, results of antithrombotic drug use sums up to more than 100%. Characteristics of the PP cohort were comparable to the ITT cohort and can be found in Table S2.

Unadjusted results of the composite endpoint (at least one bleeding, thromboembolic event or death) and its single parameters are pictured in Table 2. The table gives the unadjusted ORs and 95% CI calculated using the Mantel–Haenszel common odds ratio estimate. For categorical parameters, in which the calculation of ORs was not possible due to rare occurrence, a p-value calculated using Chi-squared test is given.

Table 2. Frequencies and unadjusted odds of study endpoints ($N = 340$).

Endpoints	Total Population, $N = 340$	Individualized Risk Assessment Group, $n = 167$	Standardized Risk Assessment Group, $n = 173$	OR [95% CI]	p-Value
Composite endpoint, n (%)	195 (57.4)	102 (61.1)	93 (53.8)	1.35 [0.88–2.08]	
Death, n (%)	10 (2.9)	4 (2.4)	6 (3.5)	0.68 [0.19–2.47]	
Patients with bleeding event, n (%)	182 (53.5)	91 (54.5)	91 (52.6)	1.08 [0.70–1.65]	
Number of bleeding events, mean (SD)	0.68 (0.74)	0.67 (0.72)	0.68 (0.75)		0.887
Skin or mucosal bleeding, n (%)	160 (47.1)	76 (45.5)	84 (48.6)	0.89 [0.58–1.36]	
Hematochezia	15 (4.4)	10 (6.0)	5 (2.9)	2.14 [0.72–6.40]	
Hematuria	28 (8.2)	12 (7.2)	16 (9.2)	0.76 [0.35–1.66]	
Muscle or intra-articular bleeding, n (%)	6 (1.8)	2 (1.2)	4 (2.3)	0.51 [0.09–2.83]	
Intra-cranial bleeding, n (%)	1 (0.3)	1 (0.6)	0 (0)	-	0.308
Intra-ocular bleeding, n (%)	8 (2.4)	4 (2.4)	4 (2.3)	1.04 [0.26–4.22]	
Other bleeding, n (%)	12 (3.5)	7 (4.2)	5 (2.9)	1.47 [0.46–4.73]	
Patients with thromboembolic event, n (%)	25 (7.4)	16 (9.6)	9 (5.2)	1.93 [0.83–4.50]	
Number of thromboembolic events, mean (SD)	0.08 (0.30)	0.11 (0.37)	0.05 (0.22)		0.088
Superficial venous thrombosis, n (%)	3 (0.9)	2 (1.2)	1 (0.6)	2.09 [0.19–23.21]	
Deep venous thrombosis, n (%)	2 (0.6)	2 (1.2)	0 (0)	-	0.149
Pulmonary embolism, n (%)	1 (0.3)	0 (0)	1 (0.6)	-	0.325
Stroke/ TIA, n (%)	4 (1.2)	4 (2.4)	0 (0)	-	**0.041**
Myocardial infarction, n (%)	2 (0.6)	1 (0.6)	1 (0.6)	1.04 [0.06–16.70]	
Other thromboembolic event, n (%)	13 (3.8)	7 (4.2)	6 (3.5)		

Composite endpoint: any of the following death, bleeding event, or thromboembolic event. SD: standard deviation, TIA: transient ischemic attack. Significant findings in bold text.

In the unadjusted analysis, there was no significant difference between study groups concerning the composite endpoint, death, bleeding and thromboembolic events in general and most specific events. However, differences in frequencies can be seen. A stroke/transient ischemic attack was more common in the individualized risk assessment group ($p = 0.041$), but only in the ITT, not in the PP cohort (Table S3) and with a very small sample size (number of events: $n = 4$).

Table 3 shows the adjusted odds for the composite endpoint and separately for a bleeding event, a thromboembolic event, and death for the ITT cohort. Results for the PP cohort can be found in Table S4.

Table 3. Adjusted odds ratios for the individualized risk assessment group compared with the standardized risk assessment group for study endpoints (N = 340).

Endpoints	OR [95% CI] Model 1	OR [95% CI] Model 2	OR [95% CI] Model 3
Composite endpoint	**1.63 [1.03–2.60]**	**1.61 [1.00–2.58]**	**1.63 [1.02–2.63]**
Death	1.16 [0.22–6.08]	1.12 [0.20–6.27] *	1.06 [0.19–6.09] *
Bleeding event	1.33 [0.84–2.10]	1.30 [0.81–2.07]	1.31 [0.82–2.11]
Thromboembolic event	2.08 [0.84–5.11]	2.20 [0.87–5.57]	2.13 [0.83–5.44]

Composite endpoint: any of the following death, bleeding event, or thromboembolic event. Model 1: adjusted for age and sex. Model 2: adjusted for age, sex, educational degree, GFR, number of antithrombotic drugs taken, HAS BLED Score, CHA2DS2 VASc Score, number of patients enrolled per study center, and time in study. Model 3: adjusted for age, sex, educational degree, GFR, number of antithrombotic drugs taken, HAS BLED Score, CHA2DS2 VASc Score, number of patients enrolled per study center, time in study, CYP2C9, CYP2C19, and VKORC1 reduced activity phenotypes. * Time in study was not used as a parameter for the outcome death. Significant findings in bold text.

Patients that received an individualized risk assessment had higher odds for the composite endpoint (any of the following: bleeding, thromboembolic event, or death) than patients that received a standardized risk assessment (OR 1.63 [95% CI 1.02–2.63]) with multiple adjusting (Model 3). Being female was significantly associated with higher odds (2.17 [1.27–3.71]). None of the reduced activity phenotypes were associated with the composite endpoint (CYP2C9 OR 0.92 [0.56–1.51], CYP2C19 OR 1.11 [0.65–1.87], and VKORC1 OR 1.33 [0.67–2.65]). The single outcome parameters of the composite endpoint (bleeding event, thromboembolic event, or death) were not significantly more common in the individualized risk assessment group, but all ORs point towards an association with this group ranging from OR 1.06 [95% CI 0.19–6.09] for death to OR 2.13 [95% CI 0.83–5.44] for thromboembolic events.

There was no significant effect in the PP cohort, but ORs for the composite endpoint, bleeding, and thromboembolic event were all > 1 and CIs were large.

Secondary Analyses

Table 4 shows the adjusted models for the composite endpoint comparing patients in the individualized versus the standardized treatment group including only those patients taking VKA medication in the ITT cohort. Table S5 shows models for the PP cohort respectively.

The OR for the composite endpoint was even more pronounced in the models when including only patients on VKA treatment with an increase in the individualized treatment group (OR 1.99 [1.05–3.76]). Again, neither reduced CYP2C9, CYP2C19 nor VKORC1 activity were associated with the composite endpoint. Effect sizes of parameters were overall comparable in the PP cohort, even though not significant due to the small sample size. Including only patients with DOAC use revealed an OR of 1.52 [0.63–3.69] pointing to the same direction, but not reaching significance neither in the ITT nor the PP cohort (Table S6).

Figure 1 summarizes the adjusted ORs and 95% CI for patients in the individualized risk assessment group presenting with a certain outcome in the ITT cohort and in secondary analyses including only VKA and only DOAC users (Model 3).

Table 4. Secondary analyses for the composite endpoint comparing the individualized with the standardized risk assessment group including only patients with the intake of vitamin-K-antagonists (n = 209).

Parameters Included in Models	OR [95% CI] Model 1	OR [95% CI] Model 2	OR [95% CI] Model 3
Individualized risk assessment	**1.88 [1.02–3.44]**	**1.99 [1.06–3.74]**	**1.99 [1.05–3.76]**
Age (years)	**1.07 [1.02–1.12]**	1.05 [0.99–1.11]	1.05 [0.99–1.11]
Sex (female)	**1.90 [1.03–3.53]**	2.02 [0.99–4.13]	2.04 [0.98–4.26]
Educational degree	-	1.07 [0.87–1.32]	1.07 [0.86–1.32]
GFR (mL/min/1.73m^2)	-	0.99 [0.97–1.01]	0.99 [0.97–1.01]
Antithrombotic drugs taken (number)	-	1.20 [0.71–2.04]	1.25 [0.73–2.14]
HAS BLED (score)	-	0.97 [0.68–1.38]	0.94 [0.65–1.35]
CHA2DS2 VASc (score)	-	1.15 [0.87–1.52]	1.15 [0.86–1.52]
Amount of patients enrolled in study center	-	0.90 [0.75–1.07]	0.89 [0.75–1.07]
Time in study (days)	-	**1.01 [1.00–1.01]**	**1.01 [1.00–1.01]**
CYP2C9 phenotype (IM/ PM)	-	-	0.77 [0.39–1.52]
CYP2C19 phenotype (IM/ PM)	-	-	0.80 [0.39–1.66]
VKORC1 phenotype (reduced)	-	-	1.32 [0.51–3.41]

Composite endpoint: any of the following death, bleeding event, or thromboembolic event. Model 1: adjusted for age, and sex. Model 2: adjusted for age, sex, educational degree, GFR (glomerular filtration rate), number of antithrombotic drugs taken (excluding vitamin-K-antagonists), HAS BLED score, CHA2DS2 VASc score, number of patients enrolled per study center, and time in study. Model 3: adjusted for age, sex, educational degree, GFR (glomerular filtration rate), number of antithrombotic drugs taken (excluding vitamin-K-antagonists), HAS BLED score, CHA2DS2 VASc score, number of patients enrolled per study center, time in study, CYP2C9, CYP2C19, and VKORC1 phenotypes. Significant findings in bold text.

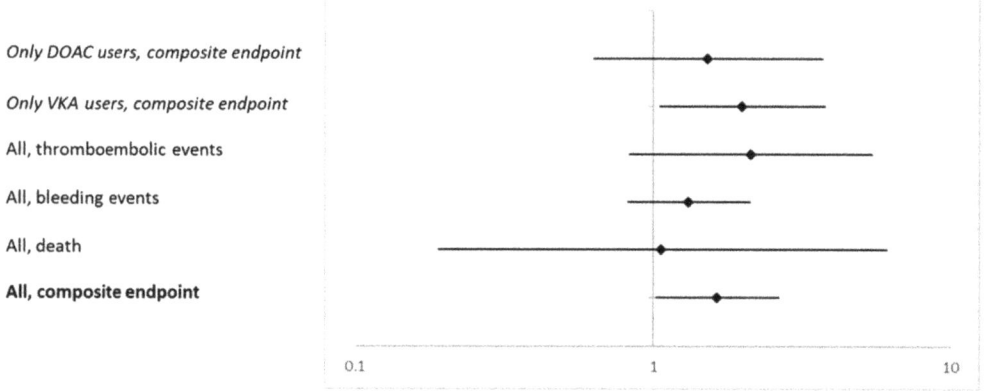

Figure 1. Adjusted ORs and corresponding 95% CI for the composite endpoint and the single items death, bleeding and thromboembolic events in the ITT cohort and for the composite endpoint including only VKA and DOAC users (all Model 3).

For around 40–45% of all patients, events were reported via the trigger list, but information was missing in the patient record. Using only the information documented in the patient record, no significant differences between the study groups were detected. A total of 35.3% (n = 61) of patients in the standardized risk assessment group and 34.1% (n = 57) of the patients in the individualized risk assessment group met the composite endpoint. This resulted in an unadjusted OR of 0.96 [0.61–1.50].

3. Discussion

In this analysis of the IDrug study, a pragmatic prospective multicenter randomized controlled trial, we compared effects of an individualized with a standardized risk assessment for preventing ADRs. As a main result of this analysis, patients in the individualized risk assessment group had poorer outcome and higher risk for the composite endpoint meaning experiencing a bleeding and/ or thromboembolic event or death than those in the standardized risk assessment group in adjusted analysis. This effect was even more pronounced in a subgroup analysis of patients on phenprocoumon treatment. However, this effect could not be seen when including only events documented in the patient record or in the unadjusted analysis. The PGx profile seemed to have no impact on the occurrence of ADRs.

An unadjusted increase in the event frequency of 7.3% and an adjusted OR of 1.63 for the composite endpoint in the group with individualized risk assessment are contrary to the study hypothesis that individualized risk information may help to adjust therapy and improve safety in situations with high risk for ADRs. Notably, we saw an association with the composite endpoint, while none of the single items reached statistical significance due to small sample sizes as pictured by large 95% CIs. The unadjusted analysis did not reveal significant differences between the two groups. The participating general practitioners (GP) and their staff reported different experiences with the trigger lists. It might be that women may have a tendency to be more communicative which may have led to a higher reporting rate of (possibly less severe) events [17].

Both the individualized and the standardized risk assessment leaflets contained general information on HAS-BLED and CHA2DS2-VASc scores, drug–drug interactions (DDIs), ageing, renal function, and pharmacogenetic factors, but the individualized risk assessment added extra individualized information per item [18]. In general, patients and GPs were blinded for the study group. However, most GP offices enrolled more than five patients in the study and therefore were confronted with both risk assessments. Therefore, we assume, that blinding became less effective for study group association when enrolling a higher number of patients, which could potentially have been prevented by cluster randomization. Ineffective blinding could have influenced alertness for outcome events in both study groups which may explain why the unadjusted analysis and the analysis using only the patient record data did not detect significant differences between the two groups. In addition, the individualized risk assessment may have led to an increase in doubts about the safety of the current pharmacological treatment both in GPs and patients, which may have resulted in changes in dosing, pharmacologic agent or medication compliance even though the current medication plan was maybe already well balanced.

In clinical practice, alerts integrated into electronic health records are frequently ignored [19,20]. In contrast, our study was a successful collaboration between GPs and clinical pharmacologist and most likely led to a high acceptance rate of recommendations. However, patients were not newly initiated with the drug and therefore, the timing of the risk assessment may have been inappropriate. Retrospectively, using an individualized risk assessment may have been more effective when used upon initiation of an antithrombotic therapy, when serious ADRs might even occur more often [21]. GPs have a high degree of experience with the indication and handling of antithrombotic agents and the benefit of an individualized risk assessment might be highest in patients initiating a new drug treatment such as that performed in the PREPARE trial within the U-PGx project and other PGx implementation projects [22,23].

With more than 50% of all patients meeting the composite endpoint the rate is quite high in our population. Based on other studies one might expect a rate of around 10–15% [21,24]. In general, with a median CHA2DS2-VASc score of four and a median HAS-BLED score of two, one would expect the benefit of the antithrombotic treatment outweighing its risk [25]. The high event rate in our population might be connected to a quite sensitive detection method. Over an observation period of nine months, patients were followed-up three times and a trigger list was used. However, in routine care patients would not have been visited that often, which might explain partly the high observed event rate. Furthermore, using a trigger list we were assessing all kinds of events including, i.e., minor nose bleeding. Bleeding ADRs were most commonly reported in our cohort, but most of the bleeding events were superficial skin or mucosal bleedings. Notably, including only events documented in the patient record, resulted in lower event rates. Meanwhile, the general rate of thromboembolic events seems in line with other studies [26], but was 4.4% higher in the individualized risk assessment group as compared to the standardized risk assessment group.

Associations were even more pronounced in patients taking phenprocoumon. This might be seen in line with a study showing adults aged 75 years and older spending more time out of the therapeutic range (time in therapeutic range, TTR) when genotype-based dosing was used [27]. TTR usually correlates negatively with hemorrhages and thromboembolic rates [26]. This might explain the higher risk for meeting the composite endpoint of bleeding and/or thromboembolic events or death in our cohort. In another analysis performed with this cohort, we concluded that the genotype had already been empirically respected with INR measurements [14]. Therefore, an added risk assessment might have irritated GPs' routine care and led to an increase in the composite endpoint. Nevertheless, the risk for adverse events might be even higher in patients without any anticoagulation where an anticoagulation is indicated [28]. Thus, an improved risk assessment might have the potential to initiate a better anticoagulation in older adults.

We did not find an association of a genotype-predicted phenotype with the composite endpoint. This might be seen in contrast to a recent analysis of emergency department admissions that showed a trend towards a combined PGx risk profile of low activity CYP2C9 and VKORC1 genotypes being associated with phenprocoumon-induced bleeding ADRs [29]. However, we included any type of bleeding and thromboembolic events, and a different result might be expected with only including serious ADRs. In addition, compared to the VKA warfarin, CYP3A4 next to CYP2C9 plays a major role in phenprocoumon metabolism. While frequencies of low activity metabolizer phenotypes were in general in line with reported frequencies in European populations [30,31], due to the small sample size absolute numbers of those phenotypes were low. Drug–drug interactions (DDI) might be even more relevant than the PGx profile per se [32]. This cohort was highly multi-medicated with a median intake of 13 drugs per person, although all medications including over the counter and dermatological products were counted. As this population was a cohort of multi-morbid, older adults, the prevalence of potential DDIs with more than 80% of patients was quite high and mostly involving antithrombotic drugs and non-steroidal anti-inflammatory drugs increasing the risk for bleeding [33]. Likewise, pharmacodynamic DDI, e.g., taking several antithrombotic drugs would obviously increase the risk for bleedings [34]. However, the median intake of antithrombotic drugs over the full study period was one and we adjusted the regression analyses for the number of antithrombotic drugs taken.

A strength of this study is the pragmatic design delivering real world data on drug safety in multi-morbid older adults on antithrombotic treatment and good characterization of individual risk factors such as PGx. However, the importance of PGx in age, in particular in the context of DDIs potentially leading to phenoconversion needs to be further studied [35,36]. While most studies enroll patients as older adults basing on the calendrical age (e.g., aged 65 years and older), we used a clinical estimate using multi-morbidity as inclusion criterion that correlated with multi-medication. Therefore, this cohort is formed by a group of clinically relevant older adults [37]. Even though the targeted sample size was not met, this is one of the bigger cohort studies in GP offices implemented in routine care, where the study setting is challenging [38,39] and therefore, delivers precious insight in clinical reality.

Still, the major limitations of this analysis accompany the use of trigger lists and that the calculated sample size of the study was not met [18]. The results need to be interpreted in this light. While the study design was oriented at clinical trial designs, the effort for enrollment and follow-up of the single patients and the single GP offices was high, in particular considering the multi-morbidity of the patients. Another limitation derives from the study design providing risk assessments in patients already on drug treatment. Thereby, the risk assessment especially in the individualized risk assessment group might have led to medication changes that would not have occurred without the risk assessment.

4. Materials and Methods

4.1. Study Design

Data of the individualized versus standardized risk assessment in patients at high risk for adverse drug reactions (IDrug; trial registration: German Clinical Trials Register: DRKS00006256) was analyzed. The IDrug study is a pragmatic prospective multicenter randomized controlled trial comparing the effect of an individualized versus a standardized risk assessment for reducing ADRs. Study design and information on enrollment is published elsewhere [18]. In brief, patients that were taking an antithrombotic drug together with at least one other regular medication were enrolled in general practitioner (GP) offices and randomized to receive either an individualized or a standardized risk assessment concerning their individual risk for an ADR respecting age, renal function, pharmacogenetics, drug–drug interactions, and bleeding- and thromboembolic risk factors. All patients were followed-up for nine months. The IDrug-study initially attempted to enroll $N = 960$ patients [18] with an assumed event rate of 10% and a potential reduction by 5%.

4.2. Study Population

Inclusion criteria of the IDrug study were patients aged 60 years and older, that had more than two concomitant diseases concerning at least two organ systems (multi-morbidity), took at least one antithrombotic drug and at least one additional drug continuously. While usually adults starting by the age of 65 years are considered as older, frailty of patients might differ largely in this age group. We chose a more clinically-relevant cohort with adding multi-morbidity as inclusion criterion. For study inclusion, the intake of a VKA (phenprocoumon or warfarin), of a DOAC (rivaroxaban, apixaban, or dabigatran), and of a P2Y12 inhibitor (clopidogrel or ticagrelor), was counted as antithrombotic drug. Patients were followed-up for nine months summing up to four visits in total.

All patients agreed to participate in the study and provided written informed consent. Patients were enrolled between September 2014 and March 2017 in GP offices in the area of Bonn, Cologne, and Rhine-Sieg-district, in Germany.

The IDrug study was approved by the Ethics Committees of the University of Bonn, of the Medical Association of North Rhine and of the Medical Association of Rhineland-Palatinate.

4.3. Study Centers

In total, $n = 43$ GP practices (here termed study centers) enrolled patients into the IDrug study. The number of patients enrolled per study center ranged between 1 and 50. Study centers were grouped according to the number of patients enrolled in the following way: overall, 17.4% of patients ($n = 59$) were enrolled in a study center enrolling between 1 and 5 patients, 20.0% of patients ($n = 68$) were enrolled in a study center enrolling between 6 and 10 patients, 17.6% of patients ($n = 60$) were enrolled in a study center enrolling between 11 and 15 patients, 14.7% of patients ($n = 50$) were enrolled in a study center enrolling between 16 and 20 patients, 6.5% of patients ($n = 22$) were enrolled in a study center enrolling between 21 and 25 patients, and 23.8% of patients ($n = 81$) were enrolled in a study center enrolling 26 patients and more.

4.4. Intervention

After enrollment patients were randomized to either receive an individualized or a standardized risk assessment. Age, renal function (creatinine-based glomerular filtration rate (GFR)), genotyping results for CYP2C9, CYP2C19, and VKORC1, potential drug–drug interactions (DDI), and results of the HAS-BLED and the CHA2DS-VASc-scores were used to create an individualized risk assessment by a medical doctor in clinical pharmacology training and supervised by a specialist in clinical pharmacology [18,33], therefore, offering a quality controlled and standardized assessment.

Leaflets were printed and sent to the GP offices. At the initial visit, patients gave their informed consent and all data (lab results, INR value, etc.) were documented. On the next visit, the GP handed out the leaflet with the risk assessment and gave a thorough explanation to the patient. The group with the standardized risk assessment received a look-a-like leaflet, in which single points were mentioned, but in a general and non-personalized way. This leaflet was also explained by the GP [18]. Therefore, the standardized risk assessment group received treatment with standard of care. This might also include DDI assessment or clinical scorings but may depend on clinical routine of the single GPs who tend to use their thorough knowledge of the patients history and habit as a basis of clinical decision making as much as scoring tools.

4.5. Data Collection

On study enrollment, age, renal function (GFR), genotyping results for CYP2C9, CYP2C19, and VKORC1, potential drug–drug interactions (DDI), and results of the HAS-BLED and the CHA2DS-VASc-scores were collected for all patients. The patient's medical history and current drug intake, including over-the-counter medication was documented. Further—sex, weight, height, blood test results, alcohol consumption, smoking status, highest educational degree, and antithrombotic treatment regimen were collected. All patients answered the SF-36 and a questionnaire about drug adherence. In addition, GPs usually had an overview over prescription frequency of single drugs in clinical routine.

4.6. Laboratory Methods

An EDTA-blood sample was drawn on enrollment visit from each patient and transferred to the central study laboratory for genotyping. DNA was extracted manually by the High Pure PCR Template Preparation Kit and amplified and detected using real-time-PCR with a LightCycler® 480 instrument (both Roche Diagnostics GmbH, Mannheim, Germany). Genotyping was performed for rs1799853 (CYP2C9*2), rs1057910 (CYP2C9*3) [31], rs4244285 (CYP2C19*2), rs12248560 (CYP2C19*3) [30], rs9934438 (VKORC1 1173C > T) [40] and rs9923231 (VKORC1 1639G > A) [41] using LightMix Kit human reagents (Cat-No 40-0298-32, 40-0304-32, 40-0302-64) from TIB Molbiol GmbH (Berlin, Germany). Melting curve analyses of fluorescent real-time-PCR amplification products were used for allelic identification. If no mutation for CYP2C9 and CYP2C19 was detected, wild type carrier status and extensive metabolism phenotype was assumed. Mutation in one allele was associated with intermediate, mutations in both alleles with slow (poor) metabolism phenotypes. Similarly, double mutations in VKORC1 were considered as slow (poor) metabolism phenotypes. DNA extraction and genotyping was performed by the Institute of Clinical Chemistry and Clinical Pharmacology of the University Bonn.

4.7. Phenotype Assessments

For all patients, phenotypes were extrapolated from genotypes. For CYP2C9 and CYP2C19 all patients carrying at least one reduced function allele (*2 or *3) were summarized as having a reduced activity phenotype (*2/*2, *3/*3, *2/*3, *1/*2, *1/*3) in this analysis. The absence of any *2 and the *3 allele was considered a wild-type leading to normal enzyme function. In case of VKORC1, patients carrying at least one C allele (VKORC1 1173C > T) were respected as having reduced clotting activity. The absence of a C allele was interpreted as wild-type carrier status and normal clotting activity.

4.8. Antithrombotic Treatment

Data on antithrombotic and drug treatment, and diagnoses were updated on each study visit. A patient was considered to take a specific drug in these analyses, if its use was reported in at least one study visit. To control the analyses for the summative risk of antithrombotic drug intake, a median number of antithrombotic drugs taken over the whole time of the study was calculated per patient. Therefore, the intake of a VKA (phenprocoumon or warfarin), of a DOAC (rivaroxaban, apixaban, or dabigatran), of ASA, of a P2Y12 inhibitor (clopidogrel or ticagrelor), and the administration of a heparin (heparin or low-molecular-weight heparin) was counted.

4.9. Study Outcome

On each study visit, patients were asked together with their GP about specific bleeding and thromboembolic events (yes, no) using a trigger list. Within this list, there was an option to report any other bleeding or thromboembolic event not specified in the list. If at least one point of the list was answered with yes, this was considered an event during follow-up. In a next analysis, only reported events documented in the patient record were included in the analysis in order to improve documentation quality. A composite endpoint was used, defined as the occurrence of at least one bleeding, or at least one thromboembolic event, or death during follow-up.

4.10. Randomization, Allocation to Study Arm, and Blinding

Randomization was conducted by the Biostatistics Unit of the Federal Institute for Drugs and Medical Devices in Germany. Participating GP offices sent lists of eligible patients. From these lists, patients were randomly selected for participation. Patients were enrolled by GP offices. Then, patients were randomized to receive an individualized or a standardized risk assessment. Randomization was stratified by GP office and sex [18]. According to the allocated study arm, the risk assessment was conducted in the Research Department of the Federal Institute for Drugs and Medical Devices in Germany. Risk assessments were sent out to the GP offices. GPs did not become informed about the study arm allocation of the patients. After finishing data plausibility checks and query management and closing the database, the allocation to study groups was implemented in the study database.

4.11. Statistical Analysis

The intention to treat (ITT) cohort was used for all analyses and, where applicable sensitivity analyses were conducted in the per protocol (PP) cohort (Supplement 1).

Descriptive analyses were conducted for the whole study sample and compared between the intervention and the control group. Continuous parameters were checked for normality using Kolmogorov-Smirnov test. Non-normally distributed continuous parameters are presented as median and interquartile ranges (IQR; Q1, Q3), while normally distributed variables are presented as means with standard deviation (SD). Categorical parameters are presented in absolute numbers and percentages. Continuous parameters were compared using a Mann-Whitney test and categorical parameters using a Chi-squared test.

According to the study plan, a composite endpoint was used. Subgroup analyses were performed for the single items of the composite endpoint (at least one bleeding event and specific bleeding events (yes, no), at least one thromboembolic event and specific thromboembolic events (yes, no), and death (yes, no)). The results of the individualized and the standardized risk assessment group for the composite endpoint were compared using Chi-squared test. The Mantel-Haenszel common odds ratio estimate was used to describe unadjusted odds ratios (OR) and 95% confidence intervals (CI). The distribution of number of events between groups was checked for normality using Kolmogorov–Smirnov. As these were normally distributed, groups were compared using a t-Test.

Logistic regression analyses were used for adjusting effects of the type of risk assessment (individualized vs. standardized) using different models. Model 1 included age (continuous) and sex (female: yes, no). Model 2 included age, sex, educational degree (categorical), GFR (continuous), number of antithrombotic drugs taken (continuous), HAS BLED score (continuous), CHA2DS2 VASc score (continuous), number of patients enrolled per study center (categorical), and time in study (continuous). Finally, Model 3 included age, sex, educational degree (categorical), GFR (continuous), number of antithrombotic drugs taken (continuous), HAS BLED score (continuous), CHA2DS2 VASc score (continuous), number of patients enrolled per study center (categorical), time in study (continuous), CYP2C9 phenotype (categorical reduced activity), CYP2C19 phenotype (categorical reduced activity), and VKORC1 phenotype (categorical reduced activity). The composite endpoint was used and sensitivity analyses were conducted on bleeding and thromboembolic events and deaths, separately. The time in study was not used as a parameter for analyzing the outcome death in Models 2 and 3 as death reduced the time in study.

Secondary analyses were conducted for the composite endpoint including first, only patients with reported VKA use and second reported DOAC use over study time. For adjustment, the number of antithrombotic drug intake in Models 2 and 3 was calculated without the respective drug class (e.g., number of antithrombotic drugs used excluding VKAs).

Another additional analysis compared the individualized vs. the standardized group using the Mantel–Haenszel common odds ratio estimate including only events from the patient record.

A p-value < 0.05 was considered significant. Statistical analyses were conducted with IBM® SPSS® Statistics (Version 25, IBM Inc., Armonk, NY, USA).

5. Conclusions

In conclusion, this study underlines the importance of risk assessments for altering safety of drug treatment. While GPs are open to risk assessments and modifying drug treatment in older adults in collaboration with clinical pharmacologists the effectiveness of this intervention and the appropriate time point for its implementation needs further investigations.

Supplementary Materials: The following are available online at https://www.mdpi.com/article/10.3390/ph14101056/s1, Table S1: reasons for dropping out of the intention to treat cohort ($N = 340$). Table S2: characteristics of the total per protocol population ($N = 273$) and stratified according to individualized and standardized risk assessment group. Table S3: unadjusted risk and frequencies of the composite primary study endpoint (any bleeding event, any thromboembolic event, or death) ($N = 273$). Table S4: adjusted odds ratios for the individualized risk assessment group compared with the standardized risk assessment group for study endpoints in the per protocol cohort ($N = 273$). Table S5: sensitivity analyses for the composite endpoint comparing individualized risk assessment group with the standardized risk assessment group including only patients with the intake of vitamin-K-antagonists in the per protocol cohort ($n = 167$).

Author Contributions: Conceptualization, K.S.J., J.M.J. and J.C.S.; supervision, J.C.S.; methodology, K.S.J. and J.M.J.; lab analysis, S.H. and C.S.; investigation, M.B. (Markus Bleckwenn), K.K., F.M. and K.W.; data curation, M.B. (Miriam Boehme); writing—original draft preparation, K.S.J.; funding acquisition, K.W. and J.C.S. All authors have read and agreed to the published version of the manuscript.

Funding: The IDrug study was financially supported by a research grant from the Federal Ministry of Education and Research (Grant Number 01GY1333A). This project has received funding from the European Union's Horizon 2020 research and innovation program under grant agreement No. 668353.

Institutional Review Board Statement: The study was conducted according to the guidelines of the Declaration of Helsinki, and approved by the responsible Ethics Committee of the University of Bonn (318/13).

Informed Consent Statement: Informed consent was obtained from all subjects involved in the study.

Data Availability Statement: Data is contained within the article and Supplementary Material.

Acknowledgments: The authors thank AK Leuchs and KL Schneider for their excellent previous work that supported the development of the present manuscript and research. In addition, thanks to the Biostatistics Unit of the Federal Institute for Drugs and Medical Devices in Germany led by N Benda for the support in carrying out the study and randomization of study groups.

Conflicts of Interest: The authors declare no conflict of interest.

References

1. Budnitz, D.S.; Lovegrove, M.C.; Shehab, N.; Richards, C.L. Emergency hospitalizations for adverse drug events in older Americans. *N. Engl. J. Med.* **2011**, *365*, 2002–2012. [CrossRef]
2. Budnitz, D.S.; Shehab, N.; Kegler, S.R.; Richards, C.L. Medication use leading to emergency department visits for adverse drug events in older adults. *Ann. Intern. Med.* **2007**, *147*, 755–765. [CrossRef]
3. Pirmohamed, M.; James, S.; Meakin, S.; Green, C.; Scott, A.K.; Walley, T.J.; Farrar, K.; Park, B.K.; Breckenridge, A.M. Adverse drug reactions as cause of admission to hospital: Prospective analysis of 18,820 patients. *BMJ* **2004**, *329*, 15–19. [CrossRef]
4. Oscanoa, T.J.; Lizaraso, F.; Carvajal, A. Hospital admissions due to adverse drug reactions in the elderly. A meta-analysis. *Eur. J. Clin. Pharmacol.* **2017**, *73*, 759–770. [CrossRef] [PubMed]
5. Chan, M.; Nicklason, F.; Vial, J.H. Adverse drug events as a cause of hospital admission in the elderly. *Intern. Med. J.* **2001**, *31*, 199–205. [CrossRef] [PubMed]
6. Just, K.S.; Dormann, H.; Schurig, M.; Böhme, M.; Steffens, M.; Plank-Kiegele, B.; Ettrich, K.; Seufferlein, T.; Gräff, I.; Igel, S.; et al. The phenotype of adverse drug effects: Do emergency visits due to adverse drug reactions look different in older people? Results from the ADRED study. *Br. J. Clin. Pharmacol.* **2020**, *86*, 2144–2154. [CrossRef] [PubMed]
7. Van der Meer, F.J.; Rosendaal, F.R.; Vandenbroucke, J.P.; Briët, E. Bleeding complications in oral anticoagulant therapy. An analysis of risk factors. *Arch. Intern. Med.* **1993**, *153*, 1557–1562. [CrossRef] [PubMed]
8. Ruff, C.T.; Giugliano, R.P.; Braunwald, E.; Hoffman, E.B.; Deenadayalu, N.; Ezekowitz, M.D.; Camm, A.J.; Weitz, J.I.; Lewis, B.S.; Parkhomenko, A.; et al. Comparison of the efficacy and safety of new oral anticoagulants with warfarin in patients with atrial fibrillation: A meta-analysis of randomised trials. *Lancet* **2014**, *383*, 955–962. [CrossRef]
9. García Rodríguez, L.A.; Lin, K.J.; Hernández-Díaz, S.; Johansson, S. Risk of upper gastrointestinal bleeding with low-dose acetylsalicylic acid alone and in combination with clopidogrel and other medications. *Circulation* **2011**, *123*, 1108–1115. [CrossRef] [PubMed]
10. Hamburg, M.A.; Collins, F.S. The path to personalized medicine. *N. Engl. J. Med.* **2010**, *363*, 301–304. [CrossRef]
11. Edwards, I.R.; Aronson, J.K. Adverse drug reactions: Definitions, diagnosis, and management. *Lancet* **2000**, *356*, 1255–1259. [CrossRef]
12. Johnson, J.A.; Caudle, K.E.; Gong, L.; Whirl-Carrillo, M.; Stein, C.M.; Scott, S.A.; Lee, M.T.; Gage, B.F.; Kimmel, S.E.; Perera, M.A.; et al. Clinical Pharmacogenetics Implementation Consortium (CPIC) Guideline for Pharmacogenetics-Guided Warfarin Dosing: 2017 Update. *Clin. Pharmacol. Ther.* **2017**, *102*, 397–404. [CrossRef]
13. Glaeske, G.; Schicktanz, C. *Barmer GEK Arzneimittelreport 2015*; Barmer GEK: St. Augustin, Germany, 2015.
14. Schneider, K.L.; Kunst, M.; Leuchs, A.K.; Bohme, M.; Weckbecker, K.; Kastenmuller, K.; Bleckwenn, M.; Holdenrieder, S.; Coch, C.; Hartmann, G.; et al. Phenprocoumon Dose Requirements, Dose Stability and Time in Therapeutic Range in Elderly Patients With CYP2C9 and VKORC1 Polymorphisms. *Front. Pharmacol.* **2019**, *10*, 1620. [CrossRef] [PubMed]
15. Sconce, E.A.; Kamali, F. Appraisal of current vitamin K dosing algorithms for the reversal of over-anticoagulation with warfarin: The need for a more tailored dosing regimen. *Eur. J. Haematol.* **2006**, *77*, 457–462. [CrossRef]
16. Dücker, C.M.; Brockmöller, J. Genomic Variation and Pharmacokinetics in Old Age: A Quantitative Review of Age- vs. Genotype-Related Differences. *Clin. Pharmacol. Ther.* **2019**, *105*, 625–640. [CrossRef] [PubMed]
17. Banovac, M.; Candore, G.; Slattery, J.; Houÿez, F.; Haerry, D.; Genov, G.; Arlett, P. Patient Reporting in the EU: Analysis of EudraVigilance Data. *Drug Saf.* **2017**, *40*, 629–645. [CrossRef]
18. Stingl, J.C.; Kaumanns, K.L.; Claus, K.; Lehmann, M.L.; Kastenmüller, K.; Bleckwenn, M.; Hartmann, G.; Steffens, M.; Wirtz, D.; Leuchs, A.K.; et al. Individualized versus standardized risk assessment in patients at high risk for adverse drug reactions (IDrug)—Study protocol for a pragmatic randomized controlled trial. *BMC Fam. Pr.* **2016**, *17*, 49. [CrossRef]
19. Van der Sijs, H.; Mulder, A.; van Gelder, T.; Aarts, J.; Berg, M.; Vulto, A. Drug safety alert generation and overriding in a large Dutch university medical centre. *Pharm. Drug Saf.* **2009**, *18*, 941–947. [CrossRef]
20. Phansalkar, S.; Zachariah, M.; Seidling, H.M.; Mendes, C.; Volk, L.; Bates, D.W. Evaluation of medication alerts in electronic health records for compliance with human factors principles. *J. Am. Med. Inform. Assoc.* **2014**, *21*, e332–e340. [CrossRef]
21. Hylek, E.M.; Evans-Molina, C.; Shea, C.; Henault, L.E.; Regan, S. Major hemorrhage and tolerability of warfarin in the first year of therapy among elderly patients with atrial fibrillation. *Circulation* **2007**, *115*, 2689–2696. [CrossRef]
22. Van der Wouden, C.H.; Bohringer, S.; Cecchin, E.; Cheung, K.C.; Davila-Fajardo, C.L.; Deneer, V.H.M.; Dolzan, V.; Ingelman-Sundberg, M.; Jonsson, S.; Karlsson, M.O.; et al. Generating evidence for precision medicine: Considerations made by the Ubiquitous Pharmacogenomics Consortium when designing and operationalizing the PREPARE study. *Pharmacogenet. Genom.* **2020**, *30*, 130. [CrossRef]

23. Dunnenberger, H.M.; Crews, K.R.; Hoffman, J.M.; Caudle, K.E.; Broeckel, U.; Howard, S.C.; Hunkler, R.J.; Klein, T.E.; Evans, W.E.; Relling, M.V. Preemptive Clinical Pharmacogenetics Implementation: Current Programs in Five US Medical Centers. *Annu. Rev. Pharmacol. Toxicol.* **2015**, *55*, 89–106. [CrossRef]
24. Chao, T.F.; Lip, G.Y.H.; Lin, Y.J.; Chang, S.L.; Lo, L.W.; Hu, Y.F.; Tuan, T.C.; Liao, J.N.; Chung, F.P.; Chen, T.J.; et al. Incident Risk Factors and Major Bleeding in Patients with Atrial Fibrillation Treated with Oral Anticoagulants: A Comparison of Baseline, Follow-up and Delta HAS-BLED Scores with an Approach Focused on Modifiable Bleeding Risk Factors. *Thromb. Haemost.* **2018**, *118*, 768–777. [CrossRef]
25. Hindricks, G.; Potpara, T.; Dagres, N.; Arbelo, E.; Bax, J.J.; Blomström-Lundqvist, C.; Boriani, G.; Castella, M.; Dan, G.A.; Dilaveris, P.E.; et al. 2020 ESC Guidelines for the diagnosis and management of atrial fibrillation developed in collaboration with the European Association for Cardio-Thoracic Surgery (EACTS). *Eur. Heart J.* **2021**, *42*, 373–498. [CrossRef]
26. Wan, Y.; Heneghan, C.; Perera, R.; Roberts, N.; Hollowell, J.; Glasziou, P.; Bankhead, C.; Xu, Y. Anticoagulation control and prediction of adverse events in patients with atrial fibrillation: A systematic review. *Circ. Cardiovasc. Qual. Outcomes* **2008**, *1*, 84–91. [CrossRef]
27. Zhang, Y.; de Boer, A.; Verhoef, T.I.; van der Meer, F.J.; Le Cessie, S.; Manolopoulos, V.G.; Maitland-van der Zee, A.H. Age-stratified outcome of a genotype-guided dosing algorithm for acenocoumarol and phenprocoumon. *J. Thromb. Haemost.* **2017**, *15*, 454–464. [CrossRef] [PubMed]
28. Ryan, F.; Byrne, S.; O'Shea, S. Managing oral anticoagulation therapy: Improving clinical outcomes. A review. *J. Clin. Pharm. Ther.* **2008**, *33*, 581–590. [CrossRef]
29. Just, K.S.; Dormann, H.; Schurig, M.; Böhme, M.; Fracowiak, J.; Steffens, M.; Scholl, C.; Seufferlein, T.; Gräff, I.; Schwab, M.; et al. Adverse Drug Reactions in the Emergency Department: Is There a Role for Pharmacogenomic Profiles at Risk?—Results from the ADRED Study. *J. Clin. Med.* **2020**, *9*, 1801. [CrossRef] [PubMed]
30. Scott, S.A.; Sangkuhl, K.; Gardner, E.E.; Stein, C.M.; Hulot, J.S.; Johnson, J.A.; Roden, D.M.; Klein, T.E.; Shuldiner, A.R. Clinical Pharmacogenetics Implementation Consortium guidelines for cytochrome P450-2C19 (CYP2C19) genotype and clopidogrel therapy. *Clin. Pharmacol. Ther.* **2011**, *90*, 328–332. [CrossRef] [PubMed]
31. Van Booven, D.; Marsh, S.; McLeod, H.; Carrillo, M.W.; Sangkuhl, K.; Klein, T.E.; Altman, R.B. Cytochrome P450 2C9-CYP2C9. *Pharmacogenet. Genom.* **2010**, *20*, 277–281. [CrossRef] [PubMed]
32. Annotation of DPWG Guideline for Phenprocoumon and CYP2C9. Available online: https://www.pharmgkb.org/guidelineAnnotation/PA166105004 (accessed on 20 September 2021).
33. Schneider, K.L.; Kastenmüller, K.; Weckbecker, K.; Bleckwenn, M.; Böhme, M.; Stingl, J.C. Potential Drug-Drug Interactions in a Cohort of Elderly, Polymedicated Primary Care Patients on Antithrombotic Treatment. *Drugs Aging* **2018**, *35*, 559–568. [CrossRef]
34. Lamberts, M.; Olesen, J.B.; Ruwald, M.H.; Hansen, C.M.; Karasoy, D.; Kristensen, S.L.; Køber, L.; Torp-Pedersen, C.; Gislason, G.H.; Hansen, M.L. Bleeding after initiation of multiple antithrombotic drugs, including triple therapy, in atrial fibrillation patients following myocardial infarction and coronary intervention: A nationwide cohort study. *Circulation* **2012**, *126*, 1185–1193. [CrossRef]
35. Klomp, S.D.; Manson, M.L.; Guchelaar, H.J.; Swen, J.J. Phenoconversion of Cytochrome P450 Metabolism: A Systematic Review. *J. Clin. Med.* **2020**, *9*, 2890. [CrossRef]
36. Shah, R.R.; Smith, R.L. Addressing phenoconversion: The Achilles' heel of personalized medicine. *Br. J. Clin. Pharmacol.* **2015**, *79*, 222–240. [CrossRef]
37. Coste, J.; Valderas, J.M.; Carcaillon-Bentata, L. Estimating and characterizing the burden of multimorbidity in the community: A comprehensive multistep analysis of two large nationwide representative surveys in France. *PLoS Med.* **2021**, *18*, e1003584. [CrossRef] [PubMed]
38. Kouladjian O'Donnell, L.; Gnjidic, D.; Sawan, M.; Reeve, E.; Kelly, P.J.; Chen, T.F.; Bell, J.S.; Hilmer, S.N. Impact of the Goal-directed Medication Review Electronic Decision Support System on Drug Burden Index: A cluster-randomised clinical trial in primary care. *Br. J. Clin. Pharmacol.* **2020**, *87*, 1499–1511. [CrossRef] [PubMed]
39. Godwin, M.; Ruhland, L.; Casson, I.; MacDonald, S.; Delva, D.; Birtwhistle, R.; Lam, M.; Seguin, R. Pragmatic controlled clinical trials in primary care: The struggle between external and internal validity. *BMC Med. Res. Methodol.* **2003**, *3*, 28. [CrossRef] [PubMed]
40. D'Andrea, G.; D'Ambrosio, R.L.; Di Perna, P.; Chetta, M.; Santacroce, R.; Brancaccio, V.; Grandone, E.; Margaglione, M. A polymorphism in the VKORC1 gene is associated with an interindividual variability in the dose-anticoagulant effect of warfarin. *Blood* **2005**, *105*, 645–649. [CrossRef] [PubMed]
41. Yuan, H.Y.; Chen, J.J.; Lee, M.T.; Wung, J.C.; Chen, Y.F.; Charng, M.J.; Lu, M.J.; Hung, C.R.; Wei, C.Y.; Chen, C.H.; et al. A novel functional VKORC1 promoter polymorphism is associated with inter-individual and inter-ethnic differences in warfarin sensitivity. *Hum. Mol. Genet.* **2005**, *14*, 1745–1751. [CrossRef] [PubMed]

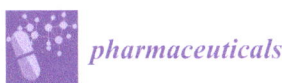 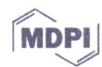

Article

Utility of suPAR and NGAL for AKI Risk Stratification and Early Optimization of Renal Risk Medications among Older Patients in the Emergency Department

Anne Byriel Walls [1,2], Anne Kathrine Bengaard [1,3,4], Esben Iversen [3], Camilla Ngoc Nguyen [1,2,3], Thomas Kallemose [3], Helle Gybel Juul-Larsen [3], Baker Nawfal Jawad [3,4,5], Mads Hornum [4,6], Ove Andersen [3,4,5], Jesper Eugen-Olsen [3] and Morten Baltzer Houlind [1,2,3,*]

1. Department of Drug Design and Pharmacology, University of Copenhagen, 2100 Copenhagen, Denmark; abw@sund.ku.dk (A.B.W.); anne.kathrine.pedersen.bengaard.02@regionh.dk (A.K.B.); camilla_ngoc@hotmail.com (C.N.N.)
2. The Capital Region Pharmacy, 2730 Herlev, Denmark
3. Department of Clinical Research, Copenhagen University Hospital—Amager and Hvidovre, 2650 Copenhagen, Denmark; esben.iversen1@hotmail.com (E.I.); thomas.kallemose@regionh.dk (T.K.); helle.gybel.jull-larsen@regioh.dk (H.G.J.-L.); baker.jawad@regionh.dk (B.N.J.); ove.andersen@regionh.dk (O.A.); jespereugenolsen@gmail.com (J.E.-O.)
4. Department of Clinical Medicine, University of Copenhagen, 2200 Copenhagen, Denmark; mads.hornum@regionh.dk
5. Emergency Department, Copenhagen University Hospital—Amager and Hvidovre, 2650 Hvidovre, Denmark
6. Department of Nephrology, Copenhagen University Hospital—Rigshospitalet, 2100 Copenhagen, Denmark
* Correspondence: morten.baltzer.houlind@regionh.dk; Tel.: +45-28-83-85-63

Abstract: Diagnosis of acute kidney injury (AKI) based on plasma creatinine often lags behind actual changes in renal function. Here, we investigated early detection of AKI using the plasma soluble urokinase plasminogen activator receptor (suPAR) and neutrophil gelatinase-sssociated lipocalin (NGAL) and observed the impact of early detection on prescribing recommendations for renally-eliminated medications. This study is a secondary analysis of data from the DISABLMENT cohort on acutely admitted older (≥65 years) medical patients (n = 339). Presence of AKI according to kidney disease: improving global outcomes (KDIGO) criteria was identified from inclusion to 48 h after inclusion. Discriminatory power of suPAR and NGAL was determined by receiver-operating characteristic (ROC). Selected medications that are contraindicated in AKI were identified in Renbase®. A total of 33 (9.7%) patients developed AKI. Discriminatory power for suPAR and NGAL was 0.69 and 0.78, respectively, at a cutoff of 4.26 ng/mL and 139.5 ng/mL, respectively. The interaction of suPAR and NGAL yielded a discriminatory power of 0.80, which was significantly higher than for suPAR alone ($p = 0.0059$). Among patients with AKI, 22 (60.6%) used at least one medication that should be avoided in AKI. Overall, suPAR and NGAL levels were independently associated with incident AKI and their combination yielded excellent discriminatory power for risk determination of AKI.

Keywords: acute kidney injury; early biomarker; plasma neutrophil gelatinase-associated lipocalin; soluble urokinase plasminogen activator receptor; medication optimization; older patients; emergency department

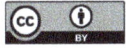

1. Introduction

Older people (≥65 years) represent a large and growing demographic worldwide [1,2]. In 2018 alone, approximately 465,000 older people in Denmark were admitted to an emergency department (ED) [3,4]. Acute kidney injury (AKI) occurs in 3–12% of hospitalized patients and is associated with an increased risk of medication-related toxicity, prolonged hospitalization and mortality [5–8]. The incidence of AKI is particularly high among older patients [9], who are characterized by multiple comorbid conditions that contribute to AKI development [10,11]. Increasing age is also associated with lower baseline glomerular filtration rate (GFR), which predisposes older patients to develop clinically relevant AKI [9,12]. Polypharmacy is common among older patients [13,14] and creates an additional risk in patients at risk for AKI because approximately 40% of all medications are nephrotoxic or require dose adjustment according to estimates of renal function [15]. Epidemiologic studies have identified medication toxicity as a contributing factor in 15–25% of patients with AKI [16,17]. Examples of common nephrotoxic medications that may contribute to AKI include non-steroidal anti-inflammatory drugs (NSAIDs) and renin–angiotensin–aldosterone system (RAAS) inhibitors [18,19]. The combination of age-related changes in kidney function, multiple comorbidities and exposure to polypharmacy with potential nephrotoxic medications is likely responsible for the high rate of AKI among older patients.

AKI involves complex pathophysiology and treatment is largely supportive [20]. AKI may develop prior to hospitalization and go undetected until routine blood samples including creatinine have been performed as a part of standard care [21]. However, increases in plasma creatinine due to AKI often lag 48–72 h behind the onset of injury, resulting in a delayed diagnosis [22,23]. Early detection of AKI at hospital admission may lead to earlier interventions to minimize risk factors or restrict medications that are contributing to AKI [24].

Previous studies have suggested the systemic inflammatory biomarker soluble urokinase plasminogen activator receptor (suPAR) as an early biomarker for detection of AKI [25–29]. suPAR is a signaling glycoprotein thought to be involved in kidney disease pathogenesis [27]. Hayek et al. recently showed that elevated suPAR is associated with increased risk of developing AKI in patients undergoing coronary angiography or cardiac surgery and in patients admitted to the intensive care unit [27]. Some have proposed that suPAR itself may cause kidney disease by damaging renal podocytes [30,31]. However, the applicability of suPAR in predicting AKI among older patients in the ED remains unclear. Another novel biomarker suggested for early detection of AKI is neutrophil gelatinase-associated lipocalin (NGAL) [32–34]. NGAL is a member of the lipocalin family of proteins, which is expressed and secreted from renal tubular cells at low concentrations. NGAL is produced in the kidney after ischemic or nephrotoxic injury [35–37], and various studies have demonstrated a rise in NGAL 24–36 h before an increase of creatinine is observed [24,38]. Although AKI is common among older patients, there is still a lack of knowledge of the predictive value of using suPAR, NGAL or the combination of suPAR and NGAL for early identification of AKI in older acutely hospitalized patients. The aims of this study are to assess the clinical utility of suPAR and NGAL as early markers of AKI and to quantify the number of renal risk medications that should be dose adjusted or paused in patients presenting with AKI.

2. Results

2.1. Patient Characteristics and Incidence of AKI

The original study included 369 patients. Due to the absence of pNGAL value at inclusion, 29 patients were excluded. Further, one patient was excluded due to chronic liver injury, resulting in a total of 339 patients for this study. Patient characteristics for the final study population ($n = 339$) are shown in Table 1. Among included patients, 63% were females, and the median age was 78 years. In median, patients used three renal risk medications. According to KDIGO criteria, 33 (9.7%) patients developing AKI were identified with AKI between inclusion and 48 h after, including 23 with creatinine increased to >1.5 times baseline and 10 patients with creatinine increased by >26.5 μmol/L. Of the 33 patients who developed AKI, 21 patients developed AKI stage 1, while 12 patients developed AKI stage ≥ 2. Compared to patients without AKI, patients who developed AKI had significantly higher Fi-OutRef, creatinine, cystatin C, CRP, IL6 and length of stay, as well as higher change in creatinine and eGFR from admission to discharge (all $p \leq 0.01$) (Table 1).

Table 1. Patient characteristics for all included patients, patients with and without AKI.

Variable	All Patients		Patients with AKI		Patients without AKI	
	N	Value	N	Value	N	Value
Demographics						
Age years, median (IQR)	339	77.6 (70.6; 84.4)	33	75.9 (72.3; 83.0)	306	77.9 (70.5; 84.5)
Female, n (%)	-	212 (62.5)	-	25 (75.8)	-	187 (61.1)
Body-mass index, median (IQR)	304	25.1 (22.3; 28.8)	26	24.8 (20.7; 28.9)	278	25.1 (22.5; 28.8)
Hospitalization-days, median (IQR)	339	2 (1; 6)	33	7 (4; 13)	306	2 (1; 5)
30-day morality, n (%)	339	12 (3.5)	33	3 (9.1)	306	9 (2.9)
Comorbidities						
Cardiovascular disease (%)	-	113 (33.3)	-	12 (36.4)	-	101 (33.0)
Diabetes (%)	-	57 (16.8)	-	5 (15.2)	-	52 (17.0)
Medication						
Total number of medications, median (IQR)	339	6 (3; 9)	33	8 (4; 12)	306	6 (3; 9)
Biomarkers *						
Creatinine µmol/L, median (IQR)	339	84.3 (66.2; 105.4)	33	120.8 (91.1; 169.5)	306	83.0 (65.4; 100.2)
Cystatin C mg/L, median (IQR)	339	1.21 (0.95; 1.60)	33	1.69 (1.26–2.56)	306	1.17 (0.94; 1.56)
eGFR mL/min/1.73 m^2, median (IQR)	339	65.6 (48.2; 81.9)	33	39.1 (26.7; 59.2)	306	67.4 (50.7; 82.3)
CRP-µg/mL, median (IQR)	314	15.5 (3.0; 63.7)	33	67.0 (22.3; 120.3)	281	14.0 (3.0; 53.4)
IL6-pg/mL, median (IQR)	336	4.6 (1.9; 13.3)	33	9.8 (3.6; 30.4)	303	4.3 (1.8; 11.1)
TNF-α–pg/mL, median (IQR)	336	7.4 (5.1; 107)	33	10.1 (6.7; 14.9)	303	7.3 (4.9; 10.5)
FI-OutRef, median (IQR)	314	5 (3; 7)	33	7 (6; 8)	282	5 (3; 7)
Change in creatinine and eGFR ***						
Δ$_{creatinine}$ inclusion to discharge	339	−1.0 (−9.0:7.0)	33	−33.0 (−57.0:−13.0)	306	0.0 (−7.0:7.0)
Δ$_{eGFR}$ inclusion to discharge	339	1.0 (−4.1:7.1)	33	20.4 (4.4:32.2)	306	0.0 (−4.7:4.9)

AKI, acute kidney injury; eGFR, estimated glomerular filtration rate calculated with chronic kidney disease epidemiology collaboration (CKD-EPI) equation based on creatinine; CRP, C-reactive protein; IL-6, interleukin 6; TNFα, tumor necrosis factor alpha. * p-values multiplied by seven. ** p-values multiplied by two.

2.2. Correlations of suPAR, NGAL and eGFR

There was significant correlation between eGFR and levels of suPAR and NGAL (r = −0.35 and −0.53, respectively, both $p < 0.001$) (Appendix A Figure A1a,b). There was also significant correlation between suPAR and NGAL (r = 0.36, $p < 0.001$) (Appendix A Figure A1c).

2.3. SuPAR and NGAL Levels in Patients Developing AKI

Compared to patients without AKI, those patients who developed AKI had a significantly higher median suPAR (5.8 ng/mL vs. 4.8 ng/mL, $p < 0.001$ (Figure 1a)) and higher median NGAL (229 ng/mL vs. 105 ng/mL, $p < 0.001$ (Figure 1b). Median suPAR was 5.8 (IQR 4.8–9.0) for patients with AKI stage 1 and 5.9 (IQR 4.5–8.7) for patients with AKI stage 2 ($p = 0.68$). Median NGAL was 157 (IQR 123–267) ng/mL for patients with AKI stage 1 and 389 (IQR 280–493) ng/mL for patients with AKI stage 2 ($p = 0.007$).

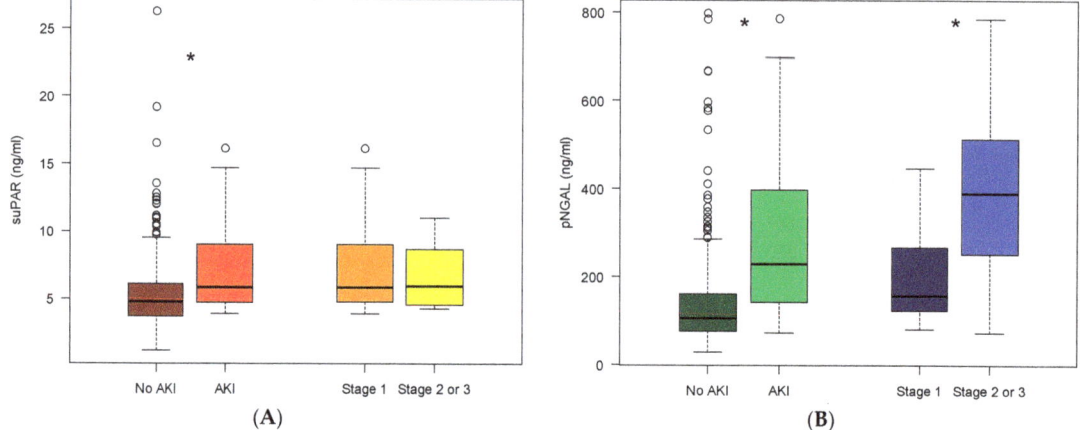

Figure 1. Plasma concentration of suPAR and NGAL at inclusion. (**A**) suPAR values in patients: without AKI (brown), developed AKI (red) within 48 h after inclusion, developed AKI stage 1 (orange), developed AKI stage ≥2 (yellow). (**B**) NGAL values in patients: without AKI (dark green), developed AKI (light green) within 48 h after inclusion, developed AKI stage 1 (dark blue), developed AKI stage ≥2 (light blue). The horizontal lines show minimum and maximum values of calculated non-outlier values; open circles indicate outlier values (* $p < 0.05$).

2.4. Risk Prediction for AKI by suPAR and NGAL

The discriminatory power of suPAR, NGAL or their combination for determining AKI are shown in Table 2 and Figure 2. As individual biomarkers for the detection of AKI, suPAR yielded an AUC of 0.69 with an optimal cut-off of 4.26 ng/mL, and NGAL yielded an AUC of 0.78 with an optimal cut-off of 139.5 ng/mL. No significant difference was found between AUC for suPAR and AUC for NGAL ($p = 0.117$). The interaction of suPAR and NGAL yielded an AUC of 0.80, which was significantly higher than AUC for suPAR alone ($p = 0.0059$) but not for NGAL alone ($p = 0.689$) (Figure 2). The addition of CRP or CRP + IL6 did not significantly improve AUC for any models ($p \geq 0.108$) (Appendix A Figure A2). However, the addition of CRP to suPAR improved the AUC to 0.76, which is considered to be acceptable discriminatory power.

Table 2. Diagnostic accuracy of suPAR, NGAL and the combination of both biomarkers, using optimal cut-off values, for predicting AKI.

	Cutoff	Sensitivity	Specificity	PPV	NPV	AUC (CI 95%)
suPAR (ng/mL)	4.26	0.94	0.40	0.15	0.98	0.69 (0.60–0.77)
NGAL (ng/mL)	139.5	0.76	0.67	0.20	0.96	0.78 (0.70–0.87)
Two-variable interaction	-	0.82	0.73	0.25	0.97	0.82 (0.73–0.90)

Two-variable interaction, includes interaction between suPAR and NGAL.

Cut-off values for combinations of suPAR and NGAL from the 2-variable interaction model show a dependency between the variables with lower values of NGAL requiring larger suPAR values (9.6 ng/mL suPAR at NGAL 2.6 ng/mL) and larger values of NGAL requiring smaller suPAR values (0.5 ng/mL suPAR at 205 ng/mL NGAL) (Figure 3). Further, the 3-variable interaction model show the dependency between suPAR and NGAL values at the cut-off was notably larger with eGFR < 60 mL/min/1.73 m^2 (Appendix A Figure A3).

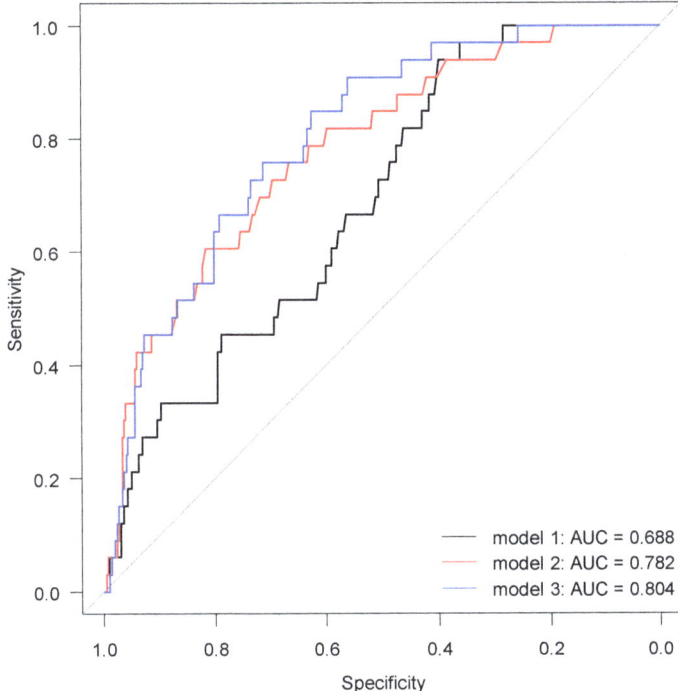

Figure 2. Receiver operating characteristic curve for predicting AKI. Model 1 includes suPAR; model 2 includes NGAL; and model 3 includes interaction between suPAR and NGAL (2-variable interaction).

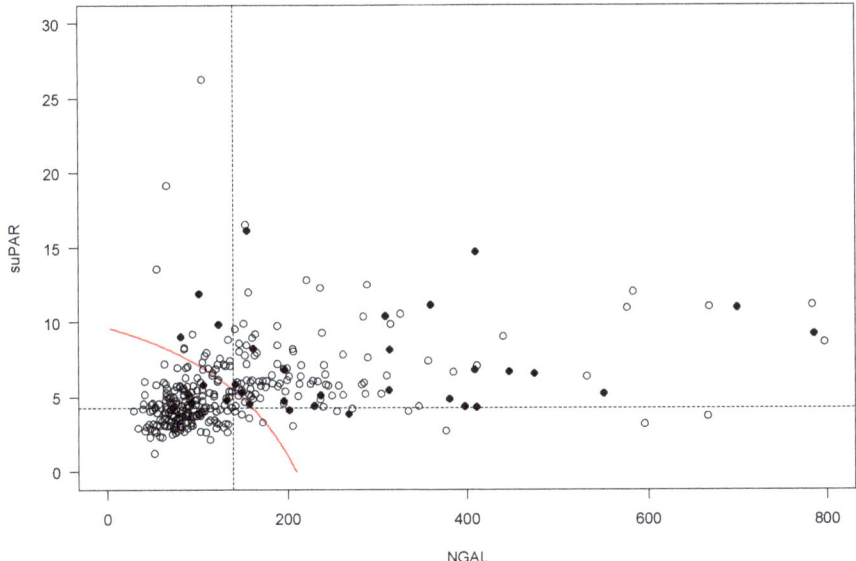

Figure 3. Two-biomarker cut-off approach with suPAR and NGAL (two-variable interaction). The dotted lines represent the cut-off values for NGAL and suPAR set to 139.5 ng/L and 4.26 ng/L, respectively. The red curve illustrates cut-off values for the combinations of suPAR and NGAL.

2.5. Renal Risk Medications in Patients Developing AKI

Among those with AKI, 20 (60.6%) patients used at least one medication that should be avoided in AKI, and 7 (21.2%) patients used two or more of these medications (Table 3).

Table 3. The table shows the frequency of patients with AKI using selected renal risk drugs that should be avoided.

	AKI (*n* = 33) (%)
Opioids	13 (39.4)
NSAIDs	4 (12.1)
Metformin	4 (12.1)
ACEIs/ARBs	10 (30.3)

AKI, acute kidney injury; NSAIDs, nonsteroidal anti-inflammatory drugs. ACEIs, angiotensin-converting enzyme inhibitors. ARBs, angiotensin II receptor blockers.

3. Discussion

3.1. Main Findings

In this study, we assess the applicability of suPAR and NGAL as early biomarkers of AKI in older acutely hospitalized patients. In total, 9.7% of the study group developed AKI within 48 h after study inclusion. Concentrations of suPAR and NGAL were correlated with AKI severity and reduced eGFR. ROC analysis for suPAR and NGAL yielded AUCs of 0.69 and 0.78 and cutoff values at 4.26 ng/mL and 139.5 ng/mL, respectively. The combination of suPAR and NGAL yielded an AUC of 0.80, which was significantly higher than for suPAR alone ($p = 0.032$). Among patients with AKI, 22 (60.6%) used at least one medication that should be avoided in patients with AKI.

3.2. AKI in Older Acutely Hospitalized Patients

Older patients are more susceptible to developing AKI due to multimorbidity [10,11], physiological reduction in GFR [9,12] and polypharmacy [13,14]. The prevalence of AKI in our study is 9.7%, which is slightly higher than what has been reported in similar studies [5,7,12]. This difference likely reflects the demographic composition of older medical patients predisposed to developing AKI [12]. Patients with AKI were hospitalized longer than those without AKI, which is in accordance with previous studies [7,8]. We also observed that the inflammatory biomarkers CRP, IL6 and *TNF-α* were higher among patients who developed AKI compared to those who did not, which highlights the role of severe infection in the pathogenesis of AKI [8,39]. Patients with AKI exhibited significantly higher median plasma levels of suPAR and NGAL compared to patients without AKI (Figure 1). Plasma suPAR and NGAL levels were also inversely correlated with baseline eGFR (Figure A1), which supports previous literature demonstrating the connection between these biomarkers and kidney function [25,27,29]. The associations with suPAR may indicate the role of suPAR in systemic inflammation, which is expected to be elevated in our study group. They may also indicate a value for suPAR in predicting AKI, which has previously been demonstrated in a variety of patient populations including those undergoing cardiac surgery, admitted to an intensive care unit or infected with COVID-19 [25–29,40]. However, suPAR appears to be unrelated to AKI severity, while plasma NGAL increased significantly with AKI severity, similar to findings by Soto et al. [32]. In future studies, more sophisticated prediction models may be developed using NGAL cutoff values for different degrees of AKI severity.

3.3. Plasma suPAR and NGAL

Several studies have suggested plasma suPAR as a biomarker for early detection of AKI. Our findings demonstrate that suPAR has a sensitivity of 94%, specificity of 40% and discriminative ability (AUC) of 0.69 for the development of AKI at a cutoff of 4.26 ng/mL. These findings are compatible with a similar study in patients undergoing cardiac surgery, which reported an AUC of 0.65 for the development of AKI at a suPAR cutoff value of 2.45 ng/mL [29]. Rasmussen et al. also investigated the discriminatory power of suPAR for AKI in patients undergoing cardiac surgery and reported an AUC of 0.60 [40]. The difference in cutoff values between these studies and our own may indicate a higher overall inflammatory state among patients in our study. In contrast, a study conducted in hospitalized patients with COVID-19 found an AUC of 0.75 at a cutoff value of 4.60 ng/mL [28], likely reflecting the high inflammatory burden of COVID-19.

Several previous studies also support the use of plasma NGAL for early AKI detection [34]. We found that NGAL has a sensitivity of 76%, specificity of 67% and discriminative ability of 0.78 for the development of AKI at a cutoff of 139.5 ng/mL. A multicenter study in the USA by Shapiro et al. assessed the predictive value of pNGAL in 1015 patients (average age 59) in the ED with suspected sepsis and found that pNGAL was 96% sensitive and 51% specific with an AUC of 0.78 for the development of AKI at a cutoff of 150 ng/mL [23]. Using the same pNGAL cutoff value, a study in Portugal by Soto et al. among 616 patients (average age 59) admitted to the ED reported an AUC between 0.77 and 0.82 for the development of AKI depending on when NGAL was measured [32]. Finally, a multicenter study in Italy by Di Somma et al. among 665 patients (average age 74) admitted to the ED reported an optimal pNGAL cutoff of 137 ng/mL, resulting in an AUC between 0.79 and 0.84, depending on AKI definition [41]. Overall, our reported AUC of 0.78 at a cutoff of 139.5 ng/mL is highly comparable to these other studies in similar patient populations. A recent meta-analysis reviewing NGAL as predictor for AKI reported an overall AUC of 0.74 at a cutoff of 165 ng/mL for all available studies [34], which is largely compatible with our findings. Results from the same meta-analysis highlighted that urinary NGAL measured in urine is also a robust biomarker for detecting AKI [34]. Measurement of urinary NGAL is non-invasive and should be considered in settings where measurement of plasma NGAL requires additional blood draws.

Since November 2013, suPAR but not NGAL has been routinely measured in all patients admitted to the ED at our hospital. We have previously shown that suPAR can be used for overall risk stratification and safe early discharge [25]. During weekdays, suPAR is measured once or twice per day, and results are available on average 16 h (range 2–74 h) after admission. Therefore, suPAR values are often not reported before clinical decisions are made for acute admissions. Quicker turnaround times are required if suPAR or NGAL should be used for early AKI risk stratification in the ED. One solution is to analyze both biomarkers using point-of-care or turbidimetric assays. It may also be useful for patients with elevated suPAR or NGAL during a previous admission to be flagged in the electronic patient record for future clinical encounters. A recent study by Mossanen et al. suggested that the combination of suPAR and NGAL may strengthen the prediction of AKI [29]. We found that plasma NGAL alone yielded an AUC of 0.78 for the development of AKI, while the addition of suPAR improved the AUC to 0.82. Such a change in discriminatory ability may not be clinically relevant, but results from Iversen et al. suggest that elevated suPAR at hospital admission reflects increased long-term risk of AKI after hospital discharge [25], maybe because suPAR in itself is involved in the pathogenesis of AKI [27]. Therefore, perhaps NGAL is more useful for predicting impending AKI in an acute setting whereas suPAR is more useful for predicting future AKI after discharge. In clinical settings where suPAR is already implemented as a standard biomarker, we suggest that suPAR in combination with CRP should be utilized for AKI risk stratification.

3.4. Optimization of Medication Prescribing

In total, 33 patients in our study developed AKI within 48 h of ED admission. These patients used a median of eight medications, approximately 40% of which are considered renal risk medications [15]. Among patients who developed AKI, 20 (60.6%) used ≥1 renal risk medication that should be avoided in patients with AKI, with opioids being the most common example. Given the known interactions between AKI and renal risk medications, early detection of AKI is essential for limiting the effects of nephrotoxic medications as well as reducing the dose of medications excreted by the kidneys. Results from this study indicate that plasma suPAR and NGAL can be used to screen patients for risk of developing AKI. A positive screen for high risk of AKI can prompt healthcare practitioners to perform a comprehensive medication review to identify renal risk medications that should be discontinued, dose-adjusted or monitored during hospitalization. We believe the use of routine biomarkers in combination with automated screening precautions would result in faster interventions to optimize medication prescribing among acutely hospitalized older patients at high risk for developing AKI.

3.5. Strengths and Limitations

The primary strength of this study is its applicability to a daily clinical challenge in the ED. Acutely hospitalized patients, and particularly those who are older with multimorbidity, are at elevated risk for developing AKI, yet there are currently no reliable tools for quickly identifying which patients are at the highest risk. Our study identifies screening tools that are both efficient and easily implemented given the time constraints of the ED. This study also has some limitations. First, we did not have access to creatinine values prior to admission. Second, our definition of AKI is limited to plasma creatinine and does not account for urine output. Third, both suPAR and NGAL can be affected by other clinical factors which may confound their association with thendevelopment of AKI. We attempted to account for these factors by excluding patients with chronic liver disease, but we could not account for subclinical conditions such as low-grade inflammation or asymptomatic infection. Fourth, we used Renbase® to determine prescribing recommendations for renal risk medications, but there may be discrepancies between Renbase® and other medication databases. Finally, the study is a single center study, and results should be confirmed in larger multicenter studies.

4. Materials and Methods

4.1. Setting

This study is a secondary analysis of data from the Disability in Older Medical Patients (DISABLMENT) cohort, which aimed to investigate the ability of physical performance measures and biomarkers to predict adverse health events in older patients after acute medical hospitalization and one year after discharge [42,43]. The study was performed in the Emergency Department (ED) at Hvidovre Hospital, University of Copenhagen, Denmark between July 2012 and September 2013.

4.2. Design and Participants

The original DISABLMENT [42,43] study included 369 older medical patients acutely admitted to the ED. The inclusion criteria were age ≥ 65 years and acutely admitted for a medical illness to the ED. The exclusion criteria were inability to cooperate, an inability to communicate in Danish, a cancer diagnosis or terminal disease, patient isolation, admission to an intensive care unit or imminent discharge hindering interview and physical testing. Using a computer-generated list, eligible patients were included using random sampling based on their social security number, as it was not possible to include all eligible patients due to assessment resources [42,43]. For the current study, patients were also excluded if the NGAL value was not measured or if they had a chronic liver injury (if prescribed in electronic patient record).

4.3. Ethical Statement

The original DISABLMENT cohort was conducted in accordance with the Declaration of Helsinki. Signed informed consent was obtained from all participants, and the study was approved by the Danish Data Protection Agency (0159 HVH-2012-005) and the Research Ethics Committees for the Capital Region (H-1-2011-167).

4.4. Patient Demographic, Length of Stay and Mortality

Patients' age and gender were recorded at admission. Patients were included in the study within 24 h after admission. Patient demographic information as physical parameters including weight and height were measured during this time. Data of cardiovascular disease and diabetes were identified by ICD-10 diagnosis codes or ATC medication codes in each patient's medical record within 10 years before inclusion in the study as described in Juul-Larsen et al. 2019 [44] Data regarding length of stay and 30-days mortality were obtained from the patient's electronic health records. Patients' frailty index (FI-OutRef) representing cumulative organ dysfunction, calculated as number of laboratory results outside of reference interval for 17 standard biomarkers, collected at admission: C-reactive protein (CRP), leucocytes, neutrophils, haemoglobin, mean corpuscular haemoglobin concentration (MCHC), mean corpuscular volume (MCV), thrombocytes, creatinine, blood urea nitrogen (BUN), sodium, potassium, albumin, alanine aminotransferase (ALAT), alkaline phosphatase, lactate dehydrogenase, (LDH), bilirubin and factors II, VII and X [45,46].

4.5. Timepoints for Measuring Biomarkers and Calculation of Baseline Plasma Creatinine

Patients' plasma creatinine, NGAL and suPAR value at inclusion (day 0) was obtained from the samples stored in a biobank. Creatinine values were measured repeatedly during hospitalization. Creatinine values at 24 h (day 1) and 48 h (day 2) after inclusion were obtained from the electronic patient record. The lowest measured creatinine value from admission to discharge, obtained from the electronic patient record or biobank, was defined as baseline (Appendix A Figure A4). Discharge creatinine was defined as the last measurement during admission.

4.6. Determination of Biomarkers

Blood samples were obtained at inclusion and stored at −80 °C in a Biobank at Copenhagen University Hospital in Hvidovre. Creatinine was measured by absorption photometry on a Roche Cobas® c 8000 701/702 with a module instrument using the Roche Creatinine Plus version 2 IDMS-traceable assay (coefficient of variation 1.5%). NGAL was measured on a Roche Cobas® c 8000 501/502 with the NGAL Test™ using particle-enhanced turbidimetric immunoassay (PETIA) (Bioporto®, Hellerup, Denmark) (coefficient of variation 3.7%). suPAR was measured using an enzyme-linked immunosorbent assay (suPARnostic® Auto Flex ELISA) (ViroGates A/S, Birkerød, Denmark) (coefficient of variation 3%) [43]. C-reactive protein (CRP) was measured by turbidimetric immunoassay on a Roche Cobas® 6000 platform in (Roche Diagnostic, Mannheim, Germany) [45]. Cystatin C was also measured on a Roche Cobas® c 8000 701/702 with a module instrument using the Roche Cystatin C Tina-quant generation 2 particle-enhanced immunonephelometric assay [45]. IL-6 and TNFα concentrations were measured on a Luminex® 200 platform (Luminex, Austin, TX, USA) using the Milliplex Human Cytokine/Chemokine Magnetic Bead Panel (Millipore, Billerica, MA, USA) as described in Klausen et al. 2017 [43].

4.7. Estimated Glomerular Filtration Rate

The chronic kidney disease epidemiology collaboration (CKD-EPI) equation based on creatinine (CKD-EPI$_{Cr}$) was used to estimate eGFR without adjustment for race [47]. Estimated GFR was calculated using the creatinine level at which suPAR and NGAL was measured at inclusion.

4.8. Medication

Patients' medication data were obtained from the Shared Medication Card Online, which records all prescriptions obtained by patients at a primary pharmacy [45]. This study only included medications for systemic use. Medication retrieved from a pharmacy within 4 months of hospital admission were included [45]. Prescriptions with end dates prior to admission or start dates after admission were excluded. Prescribed daily dose was calculated from dosing strength and frequency. The maximum daily dose was used if the medication was prescribed "as needed" [45].

According to Renbase®, renal risk drugs are defined as drugs that should either be avoided or dose-adjusted according to GFR [48]. Apart from the median value of renal risk drugs being used, this study is limited to a list of selected renal risk medications; metformin (A10BA02), NSAIDs (M01A (except of M01AX)), opioids which are further limited to tramadol (N02AX02), codeine (R05DA04) and morphine (N02AA01), whereas angiotensin-converting enzyme inhibitors (ACEIs) (C09AA) and angiotensin II receptor blockers (ARBs) (C09CA) were included for all drugs within the groups. These drugs should be avoided in the presence of AKI [49].

4.9. Outcomes

In this study, we have three outcomes to address the applicability of suPAR and NGAL as a prognostic kidney biomarker for AKI: (1) the accuracy of suPAR in predicting AKI between inclusion and 48 h after, (2) the accuracy of NGAL in predicting AKI between inclusion and 48 h after and (3) the accuracy of suPAR in combination with NGAL in predicting AKI between inclusion and 48 h after.

AKI is defined by the Kidney Disease: Improving Global Outcomes (KDIGO) Work Group criteria as an increase in creatinine to ≥ 1.5 times baseline or increase in creatinine by ≥ 0.3 mg/dL (≥ 26.5 µmol/L) within 48 h. The lowest measured creatinine value during hospitalization was defined as baseline creatinine. We identified patients with AKI from inclusion and within 48 h. Severity of AKI is classified according to the KDIGO criteria. Stage 1 is defined by an increase of 1.5–1.9 times baseline or an increase in creatinine by ≥ 26.5 µmol/L. An increase of 2.0–2.9 times baseline is defined as stage 2, and stage 3 is defined by an increase of 3.0 times baseline or more, or an increase in creatinine by (≥ 353.6 µmol/L) [50].

4.10. Statistical Analysis

Data were processed using Microsoft Excel XLSTAT. Continuous variables are given as median with interquartile range (IQR), and discrete variables are given as number with percent of patients. Continuous variables were compared by Mann–Whitney U test; tests for biomarkers, creatinine change and eGFR change were adjusted for multiple testing by Bonferroni correction by upscaling p-values with number of tests. Correlation between continues variables were estimated by Pearson correlation coefficient, and tested against a correlation of 0. The discriminatory value of NGAL and suPAR in relation to AKI was analyzed by receiver operating characteristic (ROC) analysis. Single-term models for suPAR (model 1) and NGAL (model 2), an interaction model with NGAL and suPAR included (2-variable interaction) (model 3) and an interaction model with NGAL, suPAR and eGFR (>60/<60 mL/min/1.73 m^2 at inclusion) included (3-variable interaction) were analyzed. Additionally, versions of model 1–3 with the addition of CRP and IL6 were also analyzed. Cut-off values from the ROC analysis were based on maximizing the Youden index. Models were fitted as logistic regression models and the linear predictor used as the continues predictor in the ROC analysis, cut-off values were calculated for the linear predictor and afterwards transformed back to specific suPAR and NGAL values. For interaction models, multiple cut-off values for suPAR are given dependent on the NGAL value and vice versa; because of this, the cut-off values are presented graphically. Area under the curve (AUC) is presented with 95% confidence interval (CI) and compared between the models. All analyses were performed using R 3.6.0 [30] with ROC analysis using the pROC r-package [51]. An AUC value of 0.7–0.8 is considered acceptable; 0.8–0.9 is considered excellent and a value more than 0.9 is considered outstanding [52]. A *p*-value of less than 0.05 was considered statistically significant.

5. Conclusions

AKI and use of renal risk medications are common among older patients in the ED. We found that suPAR and NGAL levels were independently associated with incident AKI, and the combination of suPAR and NGAL yielded excellent discriminatory power for risk of developing AKI. However, discriminatory power of suPAR and NGAL in combination was not statistically different from NGAL alone. The discriminatory power of suPAR and NGAL in older medical patients was similar to findings in the existing literature with other groups of patients.

Author Contributions: Concept, design and methodology, A.B.W., A.K.B., E.I., C.N.N., T.K., H.G.J.-L., B.N.J., M.H., O.A., J.E.-O. and M.B.H.; collection and assembly of data, A.B.W., E.I., C.N.N., H.G.J.-L. and M.B.H.; data analysis and interpretation, A.B.W., A.K.B., E.I., C.N.N., T.K., H.G.J.-L., B.N.J., M.H., O.A., J.E.-O. and M.B.H.; supervision, E.I., T.K. and M.B.H.; statistical analysis, C.N.N., T.K. and M.B.H.; funding, O.A.; writing—original draft preparation, A.B.W., A.K.B., E.I., C.N.N. and M.B.H.; writing—review and editing, A.B.W., A.K.B., E.I., C.N.N., T.K., H.G.J.-L., B.N.J., M.H., O.A., J.E.-O. and M.B.H. All authors have read and agreed to the published version of the manuscript.

Funding: The DISABLEMENT cohort was supported by The Danish Association of Physical Medicine and two grants from The Lundbeck Foundation: J. nr. FP 40/2012 and J. nr. FP 11/2013. The funders had no role in study design, data collection and analysis, decision to publish or preparation of the manuscript.

Institutional Review Board Statement: The original DISABLMENT cohort was conducted in accordance with the Declaration of Helsinki. The Danish Data Protection Agency (0159 HVH-2012-005), and the Research Ethics Committees for the Capital Region (H-1-2011-167) approved the study.

Informed Consent Statement: Informed consent was obtained from all subjects involved in the study.

Data Availability Statement: Data available on request due to restrictions. The data presented in this study are not publicly available due to Danish legislation. Request to access the dataset will require an individual inquiry to the Danish Data Protection agency for approval.

Acknowledgments: This study was performed as part of the Clinical Academic Group (ACUTE-CAG) for Recovery Capacity nominated by the Greater Copenhagen Health Science Partners (GCHSP). We would like to thank all patients and staff involved in the DISABLMENT study. A special thanks to Henrik Hedegaard Klausen, Ann Christine Bodilsen, Thomas Bandholm and Janne Petersen for their dedicated contribution to the DISABLMENT cohort. Finally, we would like to thank Maria Jahesh, Rubina Shirin, and Loise Hansen for collecting discharge creatinine data.

Conflicts of Interest: J.E.-O. is a cofounder, shareholder, and Chief Scientific Officer of ViroGates A/S. J.E.-O. and O.A. are named inventors on patents covering suPAR; the patents are owned by Copenhagen University Hospital Amager and Hvidovre, Hvidovre, Denmark and licensed to ViroGates A/S.

Appendix A

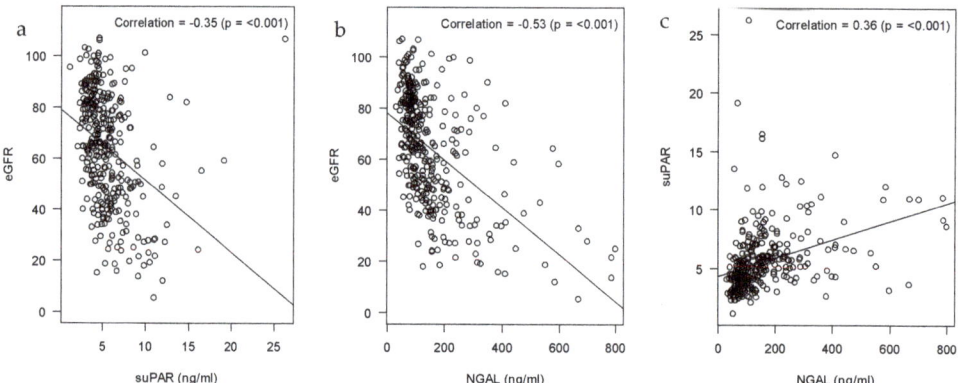

Figure A1. Correlation SuPAR vs. eGFR (**a**), correlation of NGAL vs. eGFR (**b**), correlation of NGAL vs. suPAR (**c**).

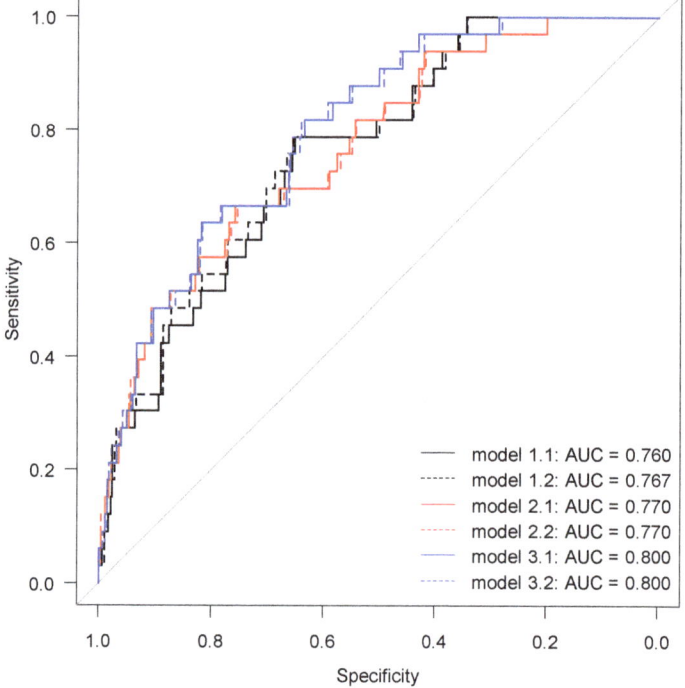

Figure A2. Receiver operating characteristic (ROC) curve for AKI prediction. Model 1.1 includes suPAR+CRP; model 1.2 includes model 1.1+IL6; model 2.1 includes NGAL+CRP; model 2.2 includes model 2.1+IL6; model 3.1 includes interaction between suPAR and NGAL (2-variable interaction) + CRP; and model 3.2 includes model 3.1+IL6.

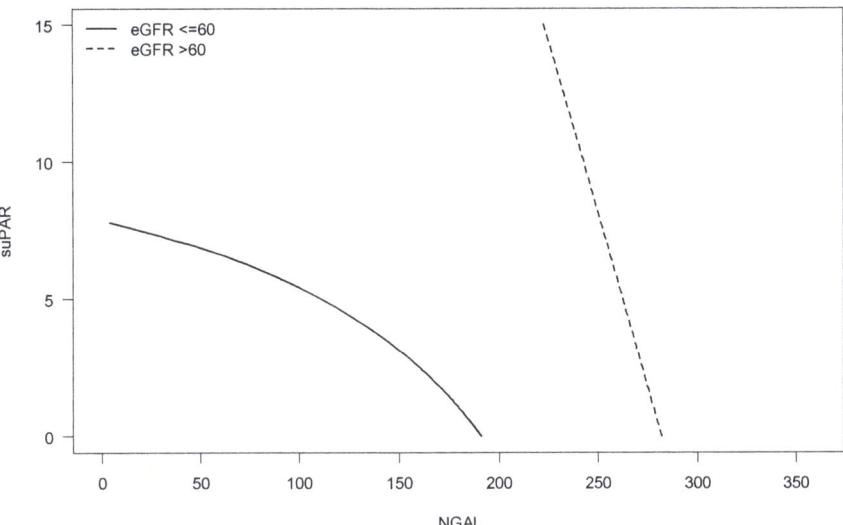

Figure A3. Three-biomarker cut-off approach with suPAR, NGAL and eGFR (3-variable interaction). The solid line represents cut-off values for the combinations of suPAR and NGAL when eGFR $\leq$ 60 and the dotted line represent cut-off values for the combinations of suPAR and NGAL when eGFR > 60.

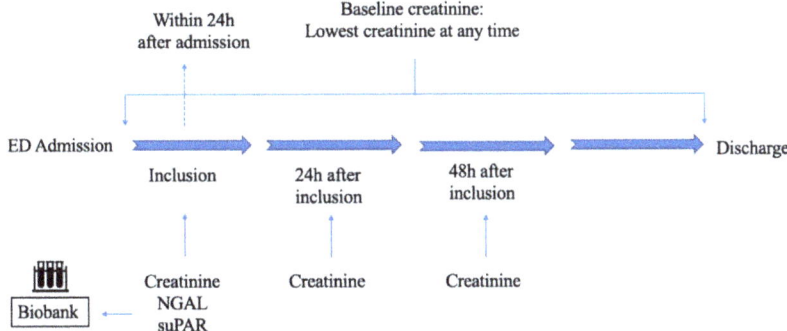

Figure A4. Flow diagram illustrating biomarker measurements during hospitalization. Creatinine was measured repeatedly during hospitalization, including admission, inclusion day (day 0), 24 h (day 1) and 48 h (day 2) after inclusion. Plasma neutrophil gelatinase-associated lipocalin (NGAL) and soluble urokinase plasminogen activator receptor (suPAR) were measured at inclusion, in addition to creatinine measured at inclusion, these markers were obtained from the samples stored in the Biobank. Patients were included within 24 h after admission. ED, emergency department.

References

1. World Health Organisation (WHO). Ageing and Health. 2018. Available online: http://www.who.int/news-room/fact-sheets/detail/ageing-and-health (accessed on 23 January 2020).
2. Christensen, K.; Doblhammer, G.; Rau, R.; Vaupel, J.W. Ageing Populations: The Challenges Ahead. *Lancet* **2009**, *374*, 1196–1208. [CrossRef]
3. Ministry of Health. Styrket Indsats for Den Ældre Medicisnke Patienter—National Handlingsplan. Available online: https://www.sum.dk/~{}/media/Filer%20-%20Publikationer_i_pdf/2016/Styrket-indsats-for-den-aeldre-medicinske-patient/National_Handlingsplan.pdf (accessed on 23 January 2020). (In Danish)
4. Statistics Denmark. StatBank Denmark. Available online: https://www.statistikbanken.dk/IND01 (accessed on 23 January 2020).

5. Foxwell, D.A.; Pradhan, S.; Zouwail, S.; Rainer, T.H.; Phillips, A.O. Epidemiology of Emergency Department Acute Kidney Injury. *Nephroloty* **2020**, *25*, 457–466. [CrossRef] [PubMed]
6. Wonnacott, A.; Meran, S.; Amphlett, B.; Talabani, B.; Phillips, A. Epidemiology and Outcomes in Community-Acquired versus Hospital-Acquired AKI. *Clin. J. Am. Soc. Nephrol.* **2014**, *9*, 1007–1014. [CrossRef] [PubMed]
7. Xu, X.; Nie, S.; Liu, Z.; Chen, C.; Xu, G.; Zha, Y.; Qian, J.; Liu, B.; Han, S.; Xu, A.; et al. Epidemiology and Clinical Correlates of AKI in Chinese Hospitalized Adults. *Clin. J. Am. Soc. Nephrol.* **2015**, *10*, 1510–1518. [CrossRef] [PubMed]
8. Porter, C.J.; Juurlink, I.; Bisset, L.H.; Bavakunji, R.; Mehta, R.L.; Devonald, M.A.J. A Real-Time Electronic Alert to Improve Detection of Acute Kidney Injury in a Large Teaching Hospital. *Nephrol. Dial. Transplant.* **2014**, *29*, 1888–1893. [CrossRef] [PubMed]
9. Coca, S.G. Acute Kidney Injury in Elderly Persons. *Am. J. Kidney Dis.* **2010**, *56*, 122–131. [CrossRef]
10. Cartin-Ceba, R.; Kashiouris, M.; Plataki, M.; Kor, D.J.; Gajic, O.; Casey, E.T. Risk Factors for Development of Acute Kidney Injury in Critically Ill Patients: A Systematic Review and Meta-Analysis of Observational Studies. *Crit. Care Res. Pract.* **2012**, *2012*, 691013. [CrossRef]
11. Pongsittisak, W.; Phonsawang, K.; Jaturapisanukul, S.; Prommool, S.; Kurathong, S. Acute Kidney Injury Outcomes of Elderly and Nonelderly Patients in the Medical Intensive Care Unit of a University Hospital in a Developing Country. *Crit. Care Res. Pract.* **2020**, *2020*, 2391683. [CrossRef]
12. Yokota, L.G.; Sampaio, B.M.; Rocha, E.P.; Balbi, A.L.; Sousa Prado, I.R.; Ponce, D. Acute Kidney Injury in Elderly Patients: Narrative Review on Incidence, Risk Factors, and Mortality. *Int. J. Nephrol. Renov. Dis.* **2018**, *11*, 217–224. [CrossRef]
13. Houlind, M.B.; Andersen, A.L.; Treldal, C.; Jørgensen, L.M.; Kannegaard, P.N.; Castillo, L.S.; Christensen, L.D.; Tavenier, J.; Rasmussen, L.J.H.; Ankarfeldt, M.Z.; et al. A Collaborative Medication Review Including Deprescribing for Older Patients in an Emergency Department: A Longitudinal Feasibility Study. *J. Clin. Med.* **2020**, *9*, 348. [CrossRef]
14. Christensen, L.D.; Reilev, M.; Juul-Larsen, H.G.; Jørgensen, L.M.; Kaae, S.; Andersen, O.; Pottegård, A.; Petersen, J. Use of Prescription Drugs in the Older Adult Population—A Nationwide Pharmacoepidemiological Study. *Eur. J. Clin. Pharmacol.* **2019**, *75*, 1125–1133. [CrossRef]
15. Wehling, M. (Ed.) *Drug Therapy for the Elderly*; Springer: Vienna, Austria, 2013; ISBN 978-3-7091-0911-3.
16. Ehrmann, S.; Helms, J.; Joret, A.; Martin-Lefevre, L.; Quenot, J.-P.; Herbrecht, J.-E.; Benzekri-Lefevre, D.; Robert, R.; Desachy, A.; Bellec, F.; et al. Nephrotoxic Drug Burden among 1001 Critically Ill Patients: Impact on Acute Kidney Injury. *Ann. Intensive Care* **2019**, *9*, 106. [CrossRef]
17. Joyce, E.L.; Kane-Gill, S.L.; Fuhrman, D.Y.; Kellum, J.A. Drug-Associated Acute Kidney Injury: Who's at Risk? *Pediatr. Nephrol.* **2017**, *32*, 59–69. [CrossRef]
18. Miano, T.A.; Shashaty, M.G.S.; Yang, W.; Brown, J.R.; Zuppa, A.; Hennessy, S. Effect of Renin-Angiotensin System Inhibitors on the Comparative Nephrotoxicity of NSAIDs and Opioids during Hospitalization. *Kidney360* **2020**, *1*, 604–613. [CrossRef] [PubMed]
19. Lucas, G.N.C.; Leitão, A.C.C.; Alencar, R.L.; Xavier, R.M.F.; Daher, E.D.F.; da Silva, G.B. Pathophysiological Aspects of Nephropathy Caused by Non-Steroidal Anti-Inflammatory Drugs. *J. Nephrol.* **2019**, *41*, 124–130. [CrossRef]
20. Murugan, R.; Kellum, J.A. Acute Kidney Injury: What's the Prognosis? *Nat. Rev. Nephrol.* **2011**, *7*, 209–217. [CrossRef] [PubMed]
21. Tollitt, J.; Bennett, N.; Darby, D.; Flanagan, E.; Chadwick, P.; Sinha, S.; Kalra, P.A.; Ritchie, J.; Poulikakos, D. The Importance of Acute Kidney Injury in Suspected Community Acquired Infection. *PLoS ONE* **2019**, *14*, e0216412. [CrossRef] [PubMed]
22. Ostermann, M.; Joannidis, M. Acute Kidney Injury 2016: Diagnosis and Diagnostic Workup. *Crit. Care* **2016**, *20*, 299. [CrossRef]
23. Shapiro, N.I.; Trzeciak, S.; Hollander, J.E.; Birkhahn, R.; Otero, R.; Osborn, T.M.; Moretti, E.; Nguyen, H.B.; Gunnerson, K.; Milzman, D.; et al. The Diagnostic Accuracy of Plasma Neutrophil Gelatinase—Associated Lipocalin in the Prediction of Acute Kidney Injury in Emergency Department Patients with Suspected Sepsis. *Ann. Emerg. Med.* **2010**, *56*, 52–59.e1. [CrossRef]
24. Buelow, M.W.; Dall, A.; Regner, K.; Weinberg, C.; Bartz, P.J.; Sowinski, J.; Rudd, N.; Katzmark, L.; Tweddell, J.S.; Earing, M.G. Urinary Interleukin-18 and Urinary Neutrophil Gelatinase-Associated Lipocalin Predict Acute Kidney Injury Following Pulmonary Valve Replacement Prior to Serum Creatinine. *Congenit. Heart Dis.* **2012**, *7*, 441–447. [CrossRef]
25. Iversen, E.; Houlind, M.B.; Kallemose, T.; Rasmussen, L.J.H.; Hornum, M.; Feldt-Rasmussen, B.; Hayek, S.S.; Andersen, O.; Eugen-Olsen, J. Elevated SuPAR Is an Independent Risk Marker for Incident Kidney Disease in Acute Medical Patients. *Front. Cell Dev. Biol.* **2020**, *8*, 339. [CrossRef] [PubMed]
26. Iversen, E.; Houlind, M.B.; Eugen-Olsen, J. Soluble Urokinase Receptor and Acute Kidney Injury—Letter to the editor. *N. Engl. J. Med.* **2020**, *382*, 2166–2167. [CrossRef] [PubMed]
27. Hayek, S.S.; Leaf, D.E.; Samman Tahhan, A.; Raad, M.; Sharma, S.; Waikar, S.S.; Sever, S.; Camacho, A.; Wang, X.; Dande, R.R.; et al. Soluble Urokinase Receptor and Acute Kidney Injury. *N. Engl. J. Med.* **2020**, *382*, 416–426. [CrossRef]
28. Azam, T.U.; Shadid, H.R.; Blakely, P.; O'Hayer, P.; Berlin, H.; Pan, M.; Zhao, P.; Zhao, L.; Pennathur, S.; Pop-Busui, R.; et al. Soluble Urokinase Receptor (SuPAR) in COVID-19-Related AKI. *J. Am. Soc. Nephrol.* **2020**, *31*, 2725–2735. [CrossRef] [PubMed]
29. Mossanen, J.C.; Pracht, J.; Jansen, T.U.; Buendgens, L.; Stoppe, C.; Goetzenich, A.; Struck, J.; Autschbach, R.; Marx, G.; Tacke, F. Elevated Soluble Urokinase Plasminogen Activator Receptor and Proenkephalin Serum Levels Predict the Development of Acute Kidney Injury after Cardiac Surgery. *Int. J. Mol. Sci.* **2017**, *18*, 1662. [CrossRef]
30. Wei, C.; El Hindi, S.; Li, J.; Fornoni, A.; Goes, N.; Sageshima, J.; Maiguel, D.; Karumanchi, S.A.; Yap, H.-K.; Saleem, M.; et al. Circulating Urokinase Receptor as a Cause of Focal Segmental Glomerulosclerosis. *Nat. Med.* **2011**, *17*, 952–960. [CrossRef]

31. Hayek, S.S.; Koh, K.H.; Grams, M.E.; Wei, C.; Ko, Y.-A.; Li, J.; Samelko, B.; Lee, H.; Dande, R.R.; Lee, H.W.; et al. A Tripartite Complex of SuPAR, APOL1 Risk Variants and Avβ3 Integrin on Podocytes Mediates Chronic Kidney Disease. *Nat. Med.* **2017**, *23*, 945–953. [CrossRef]
32. Soto, K.; Papoila, A.L.; Coelho, S.; Bennett, M.; Ma, Q.; Rodrigues, B.; Fidalgo, P.; Frade, F.; Devarajan, P. Plasma NGAL for the Diagnosis of AKI in Patients Admitted from the Emergency Department Setting. *Clin. J. Am. Soc. Nephrol.* **2013**, *8*, 2053–2063. [CrossRef]
33. Nickolas, T.L.; O'Rourke, M.J.; Yang, J.; Sise, M.E.; Canetta, P.A.; Barasch, N.; Buchen, C.; Khan, F.; Mori, K.; Giglio, J.; et al. Sensitivity and Specificity of a Single Emergency Department Measurement of Urinary Neutrophil Gelatinase-Associated Lipocalin for Diagnosing Acute Kidney Injury. *Ann. Intern. Med.* **2008**, *148*, 810–819. [CrossRef]
34. Albert, C.; Zapf, A.; Haase, M.; Röver, C.; Pickering, J.W.; Albert, A.; Bellomo, R.; Breidthardt, T.; Camou, F.; Chen, Z.; et al. Neutrophil Gelatinase-Associated Lipocalin Measured on Clinical Laboratory Platforms for the Prediction of Acute Kidney Injury and the Associated Need for Dialysis Therapy: A Systematic Review and Meta-Analysis. *Am. J. Kidney Dis.* **2020**, *76*, 826–841.e1. [CrossRef] [PubMed]
35. Mårtensson, J.; Bellomo, R. The Rise and Fall of NGAL in Acute Kidney Injury. *Blood Purif.* **2014**, *37*, 304–310. [CrossRef] [PubMed]
36. Mishra, J.; Ma, Q.; Prada, A.; Mitsnefes, M.; Zahedi, K.; Yang, J.; Barasch, J.; Devarajan, P. Identification of Neutrophil Gelatinase-Associated Lipocalin as a Novel Early Urinary Biomarker for Ischemic Renal Injury. *J. Am. Soc. Nephrol.* **2003**, *14*, 2534–2543. [CrossRef] [PubMed]
37. Mishra, J.; Mori, K.; Ma, Q.; Kelly, C.; Barasch, J.; Devarajan, P. Neutrophil Gelatinase-Associated Lipocalin: A Novel Early Urinary Biomarker for Cisplatin Nephrotoxicity. *Am. J. Nephrol.* **2004**, *24*, 307–315. [CrossRef] [PubMed]
38. Ronco, C. N-GAL: Diagnosing AKI as Soon as Possible. *Crit. Care* **2007**, *11*, 173. [CrossRef]
39. Patel, J.B.; Sapra, A. Nephrotoxic Medications. In *StatPearls*; StatPearls Publishing: Treasure Island, FL, USA, 2021.
40. Rasmussen, S.R.; Nielsen, R.V.; Møgelvang, R.; Ostrowski, S.R.; Ravn, H.B. Prognostic Value of SuPAR and HsCRP on Acute Kidney Injury after Cardiac Surgery. *BMC Nephrol.* **2021**, *22*, 120. [CrossRef] [PubMed]
41. Di Somma, S.; Magrini, L.; De Berardinis, B.; Marino, R.; Ferri, E.; Moscatelli, P.; Ballarino, P.; Carpinteri, G.; Noto, P.; Gliozzo, B.; et al. Additive Value of Blood Neutrophil Gelatinase-Associated Lipocalin to Clinical Judgement in Acute Kidney Injury Diagnosis and Mortality Prediction in Patients Hospitalized from the Emergency Department. *Crit. Care* **2013**, *17*, R29. [CrossRef]
42. Bodilsen, A.C.; Klausen, H.H.; Petersen, J.; Beyer, N.; Andersen, O.; Jørgensen, L.M.; Juul-Larsen, H.G.; Bandholm, T. Prediction of Mobility Limitations after Hospitalization in Older Medical Patients by Simple Measures of Physical Performance Obtained at Admission to the Emergency Department. *PLoS ONE* **2016**, *11*, e0154350. [CrossRef]
43. Klausen, H.H.; Bodilsen, A.C.; Petersen, J.; Bandholm, T.; Haupt, T.; Sivertsen, D.M.; Andersen, O. How Inflammation Underlies Physical and Organ Function in Acutely Admitted Older Medical Patients. *Mech. Ageing Dev.* **2017**, *164*, 67–75. [CrossRef]
44. Juul-Larsen, H.G.; Christensen, L.D.; Andersen, O.; Bandholm, T.; Kaae, S.; Petersen, J. Development of the "Chronic Condition Measurement Guide": A New Tool to Measure Chronic Conditions in Older People Based on ICD-10 and ATC-Codes. *Eur. Geriatr. Med.* **2019**, *10*, 431–444. [CrossRef]
45. Iversen, E.; Bodilsen, A.C.; Klausen, H.H.; Treldal, C.; Andersen, O.; Houlind, M.B.; Petersen, J. Kidney Function Estimates Using Cystatin C versus Creatinine: Impact on Medication Prescribing in Acutely Hospitalized Elderly Patients. *Basic Clin. Pharmacol. Toxicol.* **2019**, *124*, 466–478. [CrossRef]
46. Klausen, H.H.; Petersen, J.; Bandholm, T.; Juul-Larsen, H.G.; Tavenier, J.; Eugen-Olsen, J.; Andersen, O. Association between Routine Laboratory Tests and Long-Term Mortality among Acutely Admitted Older Medical Patients: A Cohort Study. *BMC Geriatr.* **2017**, *17*, 62. [CrossRef] [PubMed]
47. Levey, A.S.; Stevens, L.A.; Schmid, C.H.; Zhang, Y.L.; Castro, A.F.; Feldman, H.I.; Kusek, J.W.; Eggers, P.; Van Lente, F.; Greene, T.; et al. A New Equation to Estimate Glomerular Filtration Rate. *Ann. Intern. Med.* **2009**, *150*, 604–612. [CrossRef] [PubMed]
48. Nielsen, A.L.; Henriksen, D.P.; Marinakis, C.; Hellebek, A.; Birn, H.; Nybo, M.; Søndergaard, J.; Nymark, A.; Pedersen, C. Drug Dosing in Patients with Renal Insufficiency in a Hospital Setting Using Electronic Prescribing and Automated Reporting of Estimated Glomerular Filtration Rate. *Basic Clin. Pharmacol. Toxicol.* **2014**, *114*, 407–413. [CrossRef] [PubMed]
49. Harty, J. Prevention and Management of Acute Kidney Injury. *Ulst. Med. J.* **2014**, *83*, 149–157.
50. Khwaja, A. KDIGO Clinical Practice Guideline for Acute Kidney Injury. *Nephron Clin. Pract.* **2012**, *120*, c179–c184. [CrossRef]
51. Robin, X.; Turck, N.; Hainard, A.; Tiberti, N.; Lisacek, F.; Sanchez, J.-C.; Müller, M. PROC: An Open-Source Package for R and S+ to Analyze and Compare ROC Curves. *BMC Bioinform.* **2011**, *12*, 77. [CrossRef]
52. Mandrekar, J.N. Receiver Operating Characteristic Curve in Diagnostic Test Assessment. *J. Thorac. Oncol.* **2010**, *5*, 1315–1316. [CrossRef]

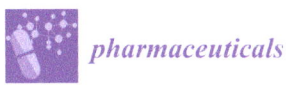

Article

Prevalence and Determinants of Multimorbidity, Polypharmacy, and Potentially Inappropriate Medication Use in the Older Outpatients: Findings from EuroAgeism H2020 ESR7 Project in Ethiopia

Akshaya Srikanth Bhagavathula [1,*], Mohammed Assen Seid [2], Aynishet Adane [3], Eyob Alemayehu Gebreyohannes [4], Jovana Brkic [1] and Daniela Fialová [1,5]

1. Department of Social and Clinical Pharmacy, Faculty of Pharmacy in Hradec Králové, Charles University, 500 05 Hradec Králové, Czech Republic; jovanabrkic37@gmail.com (J.B.); fialovad@faf.cuni.cz (D.F.)
2. Department of Clinical Pharmacy, School of Pharmacy, College of Medicine and Health Sciences, University of Gondar, Gondar P.O. Box 196, Ethiopia; hassenm100@gmail.com
3. Department of Internal Medicine, College of Medicine and Health Sciences, University of Gondar, Gondar P.O. Box 196, Ethiopia; ayne.2003@yahoo.com
4. Division of Pharmacy, School of Allied Health, University of Western Australia, Crawley, WA 6009, Australia; justeyob@gmail.com
5. Department of Geriatrics and Gerontology, 1st Faculty of Medicine, Charles University, 120 00 Prague, Czech Republic
* Correspondence: bhagavaa@faf.cuni.cz; Tel.: +420-776-444-393

Abstract: Few studies have been conducted on multimorbidity (two or more chronic diseases) and rational geriatric prescribing in Africa. This study examined the prevalence and determinants of multimorbidity, polypharmacy (five or more long-term medications), and potentially inappropriate medication (PIM) use according to the 2019 Beers criteria among the older adults attending chronic care clinics from a single institution in Ethiopia. A hospital-based cross-sectional study was conducted among 320 randomly selected older adults from 12 March 2020 to 30 August 2020. A multivariable logistic regression analysis was performed to identify the predictor variables. The prevalence of multimorbidity, polypharmacy, and PIM exposure was 59.1%, 24.1%, and 47.2%, respectively. Diuretics (10%), insulin sliding scale (8.8%), amitriptyline (7.8%), and aspirin (6.9%) were among the most frequently prescribed PIMs. Older patients experiencing pain flare-ups were more likely to have multimorbidity (adjusted odds ratio (AOR): 1.64, 95% confidence intervals: 1.13–2.39). Persistent anger (AOR: 3.33; 1.71–6.47) and use of mobility aids (AOR: 2.41, 1.35–4.28) were associated with polypharmacy. Moreover, cognitive impairment (AOR: 1.65, 1.15–2.34) and health deterioration (AOR: 1.61, 1.11–2.32) increased the likelihood of PIM exposure. High prevalence of multimorbidity and PIM use was observed in Ethiopia. Several important determinants that can be modified by applying PIM criteria in routine practice were also identified.

Keywords: multimorbidity; polypharmacy; potentially inappropriate medication use; older adults; prevalence; determinants; chronic; outpatient; 2019 Beers criteria; Ethiopia

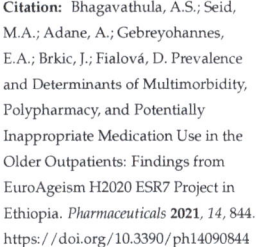

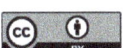

1. Introduction

The World Health Organization (WHO) defined multimorbidity as the coexistence of two or more chronic conditions in the same individual [1]. With a growing proportion of the older population, the health burden of multimorbidity is expected to increase more rapidly [2]. In general, multimorbidity among older people often leads to the use of multiple medications (also known as polypharmacy) and increases the risk of potentially inappropriate medication (PIM) use. Although there is no universal definition for polypharmacy, the most commonly used WHO definition is the concurrent use of five or more different medications [3]. In contrast, PIM use is defined as the use of "medication/medication class that should generally be avoided in people aged 65 years or older because they are either ineffective or pose unnecessary high-risk for such age group where a safer alternative is available" [4]. Moreover, multimorbidity simultaneously increases the use of multiple medications, and inappropriate use of multiple medications can lead to adverse drug events and increase morbidity and mortality in older patients [2,4]. Thus, optimizing pharmacotherapy and assessing the appropriateness of prescriptions in the older population have become global public health concerns.

Several studies have shown the effectiveness of comprehensive medication reviews in older people in reducing the number of medication-related problems and PIM use [5–9]. Over the past two decades, several evidence-based screening tools have been developed to avoid PIM use in older patients and prevent medication-related harms [10–12]. Mark Beers and associates developed the Beers Criteria in 1991, with several revisions made in 1997, 2003, 2012, 2015, and 2019 [13]. The American Geriatrics Society (AGS) approved and updated the Beers criteria in 2019 with several new modifications, clarifications of criteria, definitions, and explanations to ensure appropriate medication use among older adults and avoid adverse events associated with polypharmacy and PIM use [14]. However, the clinical use of AGS Beers criteria 2019 in improving medication appropriateness in older patients in African countries has not yet been determined.

Ethiopia is a sub-Saharan African (SSA) developing country located at the horn of Africa. The United Nations (UN) estimated that individuals aged 65 years and older accounted for 3.6% of the Ethiopian population in 2020 and is expected to reach 5.2% by 2050 [15]. Previous studies have investigated the extent of polypharmacy and PIM use using START/STOPP criteria and Beers criteria [16–21] and found poor medication-related quality of life among Ethiopian older patients [22]. Moreover, a recent meta-analysis from Ethiopia reported a high prevalence of PIM use (37%) among the older population [23]. However, the prevalence and determinants of multimorbidity, polypharmacy, and PIM use in the older population have not been previously evaluated. Thus, the objective of this study was to evaluate the prevalence and determinants of multimorbidity, polypharmacy, and PIM use, using the updated AGS Beers criteria 2019, in older patients attending chronic care outpatient clinics in Ethiopia.

2. Results

2.1. Demographic Characteristics of Study Participants

In this study, 320 older patients (aged 65 and above) participated with a response rate of 100%. The mean age of the study population was 71.9 (SD: 6.07) years. The majority of the subjects were men (59%), illiterate (65%), and married (70.3%). Table 1 shows the main sociodemographic and clinical characteristics of patients and the comprehensive geriatric assessment (CGA) variables. Among chronic conditions, the majority of patients had hypertension (66.6%), diabetes mellitus (36.8%), and other diseases (22.5%). The average CCI score was 2.53 (SD: 1.38), and the mean (SD) number of medications per patient was 3.4 (SD: 1.69). Around 40% of the participants had a history of hospitalization. Serum creatinine data were available for 188 patients (58.7%), and 13.1% of them had creatinine clearance (CrCl) levels of <30 mL/min.

The CGA results revealed that most participants were able to perform independently activities of daily living (85%) and understood verbal and non-verbal communications (72.8%). However, some had repeated health complaints (21.9%), experienced a fall in the past year (13.8%) and had cognitive deficiencies (17.5%) (Table 1).

Table 1. Characteristics of ambulatory older patients with multimorbidity, polypharmacy, and PIM use according to 2019 AGS Beers criteria (N = 320).

Variables	Overall	Multimorbidity (n = 189, 59.1%)	Polypharmacy (n = 77, 24.1%)	PIM [†] Use (n = 151, 47.2%)
Age (years)	71.9 (SD: 6.07)	71.6 (SD: 5.98)	71.5 (SD: 6.24)	72.8 (SD: 6.14)
65–74	209 (65.3)	124 (38.8)	49 (15.3)	93 (29.1)
≥75	111 (34.7)	65 (20.3)	28 (8.8)	58 (18.1)
Men	189 (59)	106 (33.1)	48 (15)	93 (29)
Women	131 (41)	83 (25.9)	29 (9)	58 (18.1)
Married	225 (70.3)	128 (40)	58 (18.1)	104 (32.5)
Illiterate	208 (65)	112 (35)	25 (7.8)	51 (15.9)
Overweight/Obese	14 (4.4)	9 (2.8)	5 (1.6)	6 (1.9)
Hospitalization previous year	126 (39.4)	80 (25)	35 (10.9)	64 (20)
Serum creatinine (micromol/L) (n = 188, 58.7%)	69.6 (SD: 27.6)	68.1 (SD: 28.2)	66.0 (SD: 27.4)	70.8 (SD: 28.8)
Creatine clearance < 30 mL/min	42 (13.1)	30 (9.4)	13 (4.1)	21 (6.6)
Charlson's comorbidity index (score)	2.53 (SD: 1.38)	3.1 (SD: 1.36)	2.54 (SD: 1.61)	2.25 (SD: 1.40)
Mild (1–2 points)	170 (53.1)	57 (17.8)	41 (12.8)	85 (26.6)
Moderate (3–4 points)	136 (42.5)	120 (37.5)	31 (9.7)	59 (18.4)
Severe (≥ 5 points)	14 (4.4)	12 (0.6)	5 (1.6)	7 (2.2)
Comorbidities				
Hypertension	213 (66.6)	157 (49.1)	54 (16.9)	100 (31.3)
Diabetes	118 (36.9)	103 (32.2)	27 (8.4)	52 (16.3)
Dyslipidemia	40 (12.5)	38 (11.9)	16 (5.0)	23 (7.2)
Coronary heart disease	31 (9.7)	28 (8.8)	5 (1.6)	16 (5.0)
Peptic ulcer disease	30 (9.4)	28 (8.8)	4 (1.3)	10 (3.1)
Congestive heart failure	11 (3.4)	9 (2.8)	2 (0.6)	5 (1.6)
Pneumonia	10 (3.1)	9 (2.8)	3 (0.9)	6 (1.9)
HIV	6 (1.9)	5 (1.6)	3 (0.9)	3 (0.9)
Other diseases	72 (22.5)	58 (18.1)	18 (5.6)	31 (9.7)
Number of medications	3.4 (SD: 1.69)	3.5 (SD: 1.66)	5.8 (SD: 1.24)	3.4 (SD: 1.72)
Comprehensive geriatric assessment *				
Understand verbal and non-verbal communication	233 (72.8)	145 (45.3)	63 (19.7)	92 (28.8)
Physical fitness	272 (85)	159 (49.7)	64 (20)	120 (37.5)
Using walking assistance devices	118 (36.9)	72 (22.5)	41 (12.8)	72 (22.5)
Lack of interest in activities	42 (13.1)	22 (6.9)	14 (4.4)	25 (7.8)
Persistent anger with self/others	51 (15.9)	30 (9.4)	22 (6.9)	24 (7.5)
Cognitive impairment	56 (17.5)	31 (9.7)	14 (4.4)	35 (10.9)
Had repeated health complaints	70 (21.9)	43 (13.4)	21 (6.6)	34 (10.6)
Experienced fall in the past year	44 (13.8)	21 (6.6)	11 (3.4)	21 (6.6)
Flare-ups of pain	56 (17.5)	36 (11.3)	20 (6.3)	26 (8.1)
Health fluctuation/deterioration	50 (15.6)	26 (8.1)	6 (1.9)	30 (9.4)

SD: standard deviation, [†] AGS Beers criteria 2019; HIV: human immunodeficiency virus. * selected area.

2.2. Prevalence of Multimorbidity, Polypharmacy, and PIM Use

The overall prevalence of multimorbidity was 59.1% (95% CI: 53.5–64.5), polypharmacy was 24.1% (95% CI: 19.4–29.3), and PIM exposure based on the AGS Beers criteria 2019 list was 47.2% (95% CI: 41.6–52.8). The majority of the patients, aged 65–70 years, had higher prevalence of multimorbidity (33.1%, 95% CI: 28–38.6), polypharmacy (10.3%, 95% CI: 7.2–14.2), and PIM use (22.8%, 95% CI: 18.3–27.8). The prevalence of multimorbidity, polypharmacy, and PIM use across different age groups is shown in Figure 1.

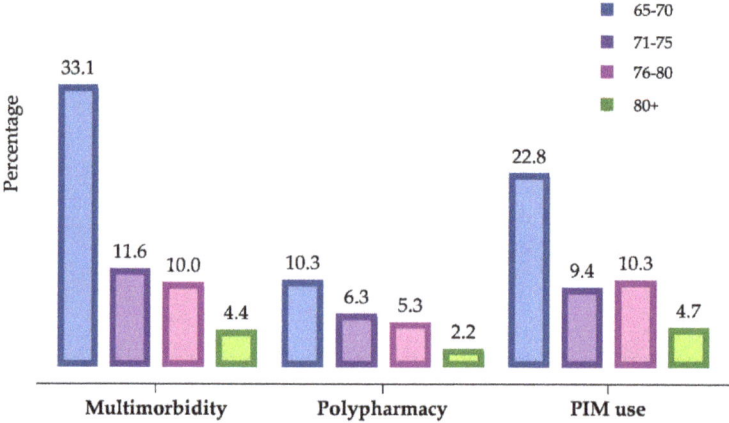

Figure 1. Distribution of multimorbidity, polypharmacy, and PIM use in older population.

A total of 203 PIMs were identified in 151 participants according to the AGS Beers Criteria 2019, and 34.1% of participants were prescribed at least one PIM, while 10.4% were prescribed two PIMs. However, prescribing three (2.6%) or four (0.3%) PIMs was uncommon. Figure 2 illustrates the proportion of individuals per age group who were prescribed a PIM.

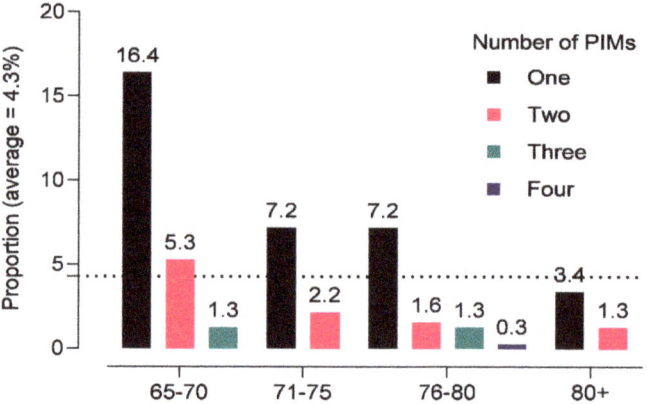

Figure 2. Proportion of older adults receiving potentially inappropriate medications according to 2019 AGS Beers criteria in an outpatient setting in Ethiopia.

The most commonly prescribed PIMs in the older patients were antidiabetic medications (13.5%), cardiovascular medications (9.7%), and antidepressants (7.8%). Potential drug–drug interactions were found in 2.8% of the cases. Moreover, most of the PIMs prescribed (24%) were medication classes to be used with caution among older adults aged ≥70 years (19.7%), particularly diuretics and aspirin for the primary prevention of cardiovascular events. Furthermore, 11.4% of the participants with reduced CrCl of <30 mL/min were exposed to PIMs (Table 2).

Table 2. Potentially inappropriate medication use among older outpatients according to 2019 AGS Beers criteria (total PIMs = 200).

Therapeutic Category	Drugs	Number of Patients (%)	Recommendation	Quality of Evidence	Strength of Recommendation
Antiparkinsonian agents	Trihexyphenidyl	1 (0.3)	Avoid	Moderate	Strong
Central alpha-agonists	Methyldopa	5 (1.6)	Avoid	Low	Strong
Antidepressants	Amitriptyline	25 (7.8)	Avoid	High	Strong
Cardiovascular agents	Diuretics	32 (10)	Use with caution	Moderate	Strong
	Aspirin	22 (6.9)	Use with caution in adults ≥ 70 years	Moderate	Strong
	RAS inhibitors or potassium-sparing diuretics	17 (5.3)	Avoid use in those with CrCl < 30 mL/min	Moderate	Strong
	Nifedipine	9 (2.8)	Avoid	High	Strong
	Chlorthalidone	9 (2.8)	Use with caution	Moderate	Strong
	Digoxin	5 (1.6)	Avoid dosages > 0.125 mg/day	Moderate	Strong
Endocrine agents	Insulin, sliding scale	28 (8.8)	Avoid	Moderate	Strong
	Glimepiride	15 (4.7)	Avoid	Moderate	Strong
Anti-infective agents	Ciprofloxacin	3 (0.9)	Avoid using when CrCl < 30 mL/min	Moderate	Strong
Gastrointestinal agents	Omeprazole	6 (1.9)	Avoid scheduled use for >8 weeks unless for high-risk patients	High	Strong
	Pantoprazole	3 (0.9)			
Drug–drug interactions	Trimethoprim-sulfamethoxazole + ACE inhibitors	11 (3.4)	Use with caution in patients on ACEI or ARB and decreased CrCl	Low	Strong
	Prazosin + Furosemide	9 (2.8)	Avoid in older women	Moderate	Strong

RAS: renin–angiotensin system; ACE: angiotensin-convertase enzyme; ARB: angiotensin-receptor blockers; CrCl: creatinine-clearance.

2.3. Determinants of Multimorbidity, Polypharmacy, and PIM Use

Bivariate and multivariate logistic regression analyses were performed to assess the factors that exhibit significant association with multimorbidity, polypharmacy, and PIM prescription. Although we found several significant factors associated with outcome variables in the crude analysis, these results slightly changed after adjusting for baseline variables (age, gender, education, marital status, and CCI score) (Table 3).

Table 3. Univariate and multivariable logistic regression analysis of determinants of multimorbidity, polypharmacy, and PIM exposure in older adults in Ethiopia.

Ageing Characteristics	Multimorbidity		Polypharmacy		PIM Use	
	Crude OR	*Adjusted OR*	*Crude OR*	*Adjusted OR*	*Crude OR*	*Adjusted OR*
Understand verbal and non-verbal communication	1.32 (1.02–1.71) *	1.37 (0.97–1.94)	2.04 (1.04–4.02) *	**2.06 (1.02–4.17) ***	0.47 (0.34–0.65) **	0.46 (0.33–0.65) **
Physical fitness †	0.87 (0.65–1.17)	0.95 (0.65–1.39)	0.85 (0.42–1.72)	0.82 (0.39–1.70)	0.68 (0.47–0.97) *	0.69 (0.47–1.00)
Using walking assistance devices	1.01 (0.80–1.27)	1.15 (0.84–1.58)	2.52 (1.47–4.32) **	**2.41 (1.35–4.28) ***	1.85 (1.36–2.51) **	**1.83 (1.32–2.53) ***
Lack of interest in activities	0.93 (0.67–1.28)	0.90 (0.60–1.34)	1.71 (0.84–3.47)	1.68 (0.81–3.47)	1.48 (1.02–2.15) *	**1.46 (1.00–2.14) ***
Persistent anger with self/others	1.08 (0.81–1.45)	1.03 (0.70–1.50)	2.91 (1.55–5.47) **	**3.33 (1.71–6.47) ***	1.18 (0.81–1.70)	1.21 (0.83–1.78)
Cognitive impairment	0.83 (0.46–1.48)	0.98 (0.67–1.43)	1.05 (0.53–2.09)	1.00 (0.49–2.05)	1.69 (1.21–2.37) **	**1.65 (1.15–2.34) ***
Had repeated health complaints	1.11 (0.86–1.44)	1.07 (0.76–1.50)	1.45 (0.80–2.63)	1.45 (0.78–2.69)	1.31 (0.95–1.80)	1.32 (0.95–1.84)
Experienced fall in the past year	0.71 (0.51–0.99) *	0.71 (0.46–1.08)	1.10 (0.52–2.31)	1.10 (0.51–2.35)	1.01 (0.67–1.51)	0.98 (0.65–1.48)
Flare-ups of pain	1.54 (1.16–2.04) **	**1.64 (1.13–2.39) ***	1.94 (1.03–3.67) *	**2.00 (1.03–3.89) ***	0.97 (0.66–1.42)	0.96 (0.65–1.43)
Health fluctuation/deterioration	0.89 (0.66–1.21)	0.79 (0.53–1.17)	0.37 (0.15–0.92) *	0.40 (0.16–1.01)	1.58 (1.11–2.24) *	**1.61 (1.11–2.32) ***

* $p < 0.05$; ** $p < 0.01$; OR: odds ratio, adjusted for: age, male gender, marital status—married, illiterate, and Charlson comorbidity index; † ability to perform daily activities normally; blue color: protective factor.

2.3.1. Multimorbidity

Older patients suffering from pain flare-ups were associated with multimorbidity (AOR: 1.64, 95% CI: 1.13–2.39).

2.3.2. Polypharmacy

Older patients who could understand verbal and non-verbal cues (AOR: 2.06, 95% CI: 1.02–4.17), used walking assistance devices (AOR: 2.41, 95% CI: 1.35–4.28), presented higher levels of anger (AOR: 3.33, 95% CI: 1.71–6.47), and experienced flare-up in pain (AOR: 2.00, 95% CI: 1.03–3.89) were more likely to have polypharmacy prescriptions.

2.3.3. PIM Use

PIM use was significantly associated with several factors, such as the use of walking assistance devices (AOR: 1.83, 95% CI: 1.32–2.53), cognitive impairments (AOR: 1.65, 95% CI: 1.15–2.34), poor health (AOR: 1.61, 95% CI: 1.11–2.32), and lack of interest in activities (AOR: 1.46, 95% CI: 1.00–2.14). Interestingly, older patients' abilities to understand verbal and non-verbal communications were associated with lower odds for PIM exposure (AOR: 0.17, 95% CI: 0.03–0.80). More details are given in Table 3.

3. Discussion

This study sought to assess the prevalence and determinants of multimorbidity, polypharmacy, and PIM use among older patients attending chronic care clinics in Ethiopia. Overall, the prevalence of multimorbidity and PIM use is becoming increasingly common in Ethiopia, and our findings are in concordance with other studies [18–20,23,24]. It was found that around 60% of the older adults had multimorbidity, a quarter of them experienced polypharmacy, and nearly half (47.1%) of them were being treated with at least one PIM during the study period. This highlights the need for multidisciplinary care in older patients and rational geriatric prescribing practices to minimize drug-related problems (DRPs).

To the best of our knowledge, this is the first study that applied the complete version of the 2019 Beers criteria to an SSA older population. None of the recent studies that have reported PIM use in the older population in West Africa [25], Nigeria [26,27], and South Africa [28] have used the 2019 AGS Beers criteria [10]. Furthermore, recently published studies from Ethiopia have used 2015 and 2019 criteria but have not reported the medications that are needed to avoid or to be used cautiously in the older population [29,30]. However, the current estimates of the prevalence of PIM use using the 2019 AGS Beers criteria were generally higher than those reported by previously published studies in Ethiopia using 2015 STOPP/START criteria and 2012 Beers criteria, reporting inappropriate medication use in 23% to 45% of the participants [20,31]. In addition, international studies using the 2019 AGS Beers criteria reported a high prevalence of PIM use in patients with heart failure in Lebanon (80%) [32], outpatients in Qatar (76%) [33], and patients with diabetes in India (74%) [34].

The most common classes of PIMs in our study were cardiovascular medications (27.8%), followed by endocrine agents (13.5%). In contrast, 84.2% of the PIMs were gastrointestinal medications in a Qatar study [33], and 44.6% were endocrine agents in India [34]. Other studies have reported different classes of PIMs, such as benzodiazepines [35], antidepressants and antipsychotics [36], and non-steroidal anti-inflammatory drugs [37]. The differences in PIM medication classes may be related to different study populations, study settings, availability of medications, and the criteria applied to identify PIMs. Based on our findings and in line with findings of other studies [33–37], it is crucial to reduce the overuse of unnecessary medications in older patients with multiple morbidities. Furthermore, our study revealed a considerable difference in the prevalence of multimorbidity and PIM use in different age groups and lower prevalence of polypharmacy across all age groups. This paradox in our study reflects the important differences between developed and developing countries, as most physicians in developing countries do not apply the principles of geriatric prescribing due to low awareness of explicit criteria.

Consistent with other studies, the multivariate logistic regression identified several age-specific factors associated with multimorbidity, polypharmacy, and PIM use [38–43]. As a rule of thumb, many body functions decline in old age, which is a frequent cause of multimorbidity [1,10,14,44,45]. The flare-up of nonspecific pain in older adults appears to be a principal component of multimorbidity and has higher odds of co-occurring with polypharmacy [37], this suggesting that pain flare-up predisposes one to polypharmacy. For example, 17.5% of participants in our study reportedly experienced pain most of the days, associated with higher odds of multimorbidity and polypharmacy. In addition, the study finds that an increase in the number of medications used in older patients was associated with persistent anger. A study documented that the increase in the number of depressive symptoms over time in older patients resulted from polypharmacy, social impairment, and behavioral agitation [46]. The study also found that medication review at baseline showed a moderated positive impact on social functioning and polypharmacy on depression was subsided over time [46]. However, the mechanism showing that polypharmacy causes anger was not clearly explored in the literature. The possible explanation could be that older people on polypharmacy may develop a sense of helplessness about their health status and stimulate more negative feelings, leading to behavioral agitation.

Furthermore, several factors related to geriatric syndrome, such as the use of mobility aids, functional limitations, distress, deterioration of health, and lack of interest in activities of daily living, are significant predictors of polypharmacy and PIM exposure in our study. Understanding oral and written communication was associated with > 50% lower odds of being prescribed PIMs. The reason for this may be that older patients can elicit and understand medication-related information and communicate information to their physicians. Thus, it has an advantage of perceived self-efficacy in obtaining information and attention to their medical concerns from physicians.

Polypharmacy is considered to be an important marker of multimorbidity and PIMs; it is like a double-edged sword. In our study, older patients experiencing flare-ups in pain in older population was associated with multimorbidity and polypharmacy. While it may be difficult to establish a causal relationship, our study's findings clearly show that polypharmacy is linked with chronic pain and inflammation that can result in morbidity and subsequently reduce the quality of life in older adults. However, developing a validated instrument or checklist to understand the cascade of multimorbidity, polypharmacy, and PIM use can subsequently help optimize medication use and improve rational drug prescribing in the older population.

Although RAS inhibitors and diuretics are deemed safe in the older population, the 2019 AGS Beers criteria recommended to avoid using them in older patients with reduced renal function [14]. In our study, around 16% of the PIMs are due to these medications. A Spanish study found an association of RAS inhibitors—with or without other drugs—with increased nephrotoxicity risk (17%) [47].

The present study also showed that 28 patients (8.8%) reported the insulin sliding scale as a PIM according to 2019 AGS explicit criteria. The insulin sliding scale is an agent approved for use in diabetic patients; however, in older patients, it may have a higher risk of hypoglycemia without an improvement in hyperglycemia management, and it is now recommended to avoid using it in older adults as per the 2019 AGS Beers criteria. In addition, a study from Oman using the 2015 Beers criteria identified amitriptyline (11%) among the top PIMs in the older patients [48], and a systematic review of Guaraldo et al. found that six out of seven studies (85.7%) mentioned amitriptyline among the most used PIMs in the older population [49]. The inappropriate medication use in Ethiopia could be due to low awareness of physicians about the risk of PIMs in older patients (disregarding the level of multimorbidity and polypharmacy) and lack of applicability of explicit criteria in their prescribing practice.

Limitations

This study has some limitations. First, this is a hospital-based cross-sectional study conducted in a single institution that did not show cause–effect relationships and cannot be generalized to other populations in Ethiopia. Second, some independent variables, such as patient characteristics, were self-reported and collected using a standardized tool. However, the accuracy of the information depends on subjects' abilities to recall events, and bias related to patients' forgetfulness or possible unwillingness to share information could not be ruled out. Low income and education levels limit the ability of self-report on certain health conditions and effort in clinical investigations, such as serum creatinine tests. Due to some missing data of some of the variables such as serum creatinine ($n = 188$) and history of hospitalization, we could include them in the logistic regression. Since the study was cross-sectional, a causal relationship could not be established. Moreover, inpatient facilities may have higher rates of multimorbidity, polypharmacy, and PIM use than outpatient settings [50]. Last, the appropriateness of the medication use was evaluated using the 2019 AGS Beers criteria, and the prevalence of certain PIMs, which were not included in the criteria list previously, might have been overestimated.

4. Materials and Methods

A cross-sectional study was conducted among older patients (≥ 65 years) attending the ambulatory care clinics from 12 March 2020, to 30 August 2020, in the University of Gondar (UOG) Teaching Hospital, Gondar, Northwest Ethiopia. The UOG Teaching Hospital, founded in 1954, is providing services to five million people living in and around Gondar. It is one of the biggest comprehensive specialized hospitals in the Amhara region and a major referral hospital for eight government healthcare centers. The UOG chronic care clinics provide services to patients with diabetes, cardiovascular diseases, hypertension, psychiatric issues, and other chronic diseases. It is estimated that around 10,000 patients with cardiovascular diseases and 8000 patients with diabetes have chronic illnesses follow-up every month.

This research was conducted as part of the EuroAgeism H2020 ESR7 project entitled "Inappropriate prescribing and availability of medication safety and medication management services in older patients in Europe and developing countries". The EuroAgeism ESR7 project, a multinational cross-sectional study, aimed to evaluate the rationality of drug prescribing in older patients in eight countries: the Czech Republic, Serbia, Estonia, Bulgaria, Croatia, Spain, Turkey, and Ethiopia.

4.1. Sample Size and Sampling Technique

The required sample size was calculated via Open Epi software using a single population proportion formula with the following assumptions of 27.7% prevalence of PIM use in older people in Gondar, Ethiopia [16], 95% confidence level, and 5% margin of error. Therefore, the total calculated sample size was 308. Older patients attending chronic care clinics who agreed to participate in a CGA during the study period and provided written informed consent were included in the study.

4.2. Data Collection

Research assistants conducted data collection and received intensive training on study tools, data collection methods, and ethical concerns. The data collection tools were pilot tested on 15 randomly selected patients before starting the actual data collection process. The data collection tools were translated to the local language (Amharic) with modifications and back-translated to English to conform to its original meanings. The research process was checked weekly, and data collection was performed under the supervision of the principal investigator and co-investigators. Eligible patients were approached for informed consent by research assistants during patients' visits to chronic care clinics. All patients who consented to participate completed a ESR7 study protocol (including CGA) administered by the research assistants, unaware of the study's aim and hypothesis. The data collection included (1) sociodemographic variables (age, gender, education, marital status, and living arrangements); (2) body mass index (BMI), history of medical problems, medications used, and information on recent hospitalizations were recorded and cross-checked with the patient medical records; (3) geriatric health assessment including diseases, symptoms, and other relevant information about health status, medication use, recent results of laboratory tests, adherence to medications, and questions related to the quality of life and satisfaction with provided care were also part of the study protocol. All assessments were completed in a separate room, and the collected data were de-identified by giving a unique code in database and paper forms.

Although a large number of data variables were collected following the EuroAgeism ESR7 study protocol, a set of other CGA variables related to i.e., the understanding of verbal and non-verbal communication, physical fitness, health and functional status, cognitive performance, barriers to physical and social activities, and dealing with pain flare-ups were considered also for this study. Several operational definitions were followed during the data collection and interpretation of the study findings.

- Multimorbidity is defined as the presence of two or more long-term conditions that cannot be cured but can be controlled through medications or other treatments [1].
- Polypharmacy is considered if the patient is taking at least five medications regularly [3].
- PIM use is defined as drug therapy whose potential risks outweigh potential benefits, and identified PIMs were classified according to the 2019 AGS Beers criteria [14].
- Charlson comorbidity index (CCI) score is used to measure the severity of the comorbidity for each patient quantitatively [43]. Patients were divided into three groups: mild, with a CCI score of 1–2; moderate, with a CCI score of 3–4; and severe, with a CCI score of ≥ 5.

4.3. Statistical Analysis

The collected data were visually checked for completeness and were coded and entered into MS Excel for Windows and exported to SPSS for analysis. Descriptive statistics, such as frequency, percentages, means, and standard deviations (SD), were conducted to describe the study population in relation to different variables. The prevalence rates of multimorbidity, polypharmacy, and PIM use in the older population were calculated for each age group. The number of PIMs identified in each age group was documented using the 2019 AGS Beers criteria. Univariate and multivariate regression analyses were conducted separately to identify the determinants (CGA variables) of multimorbidity, polypharmacy, and PIM exposure. Independent variables, such as age, gender, marital status, education, and CCI scores, were included in the adjusted multivariable regression model. An adjusted odds ratio (AOR) with a 95% confidence interval (CI) was used to measure the associations. A two-sided p-value of < 0.05 was considered statistically significant.

5. Conclusions

The study found that the prevalence of multimorbidity and PIM use among Ethiopian older adults was substantially high in an outpatient setting. The research identified several important determinants that could increase the risk of DRPs in the Ethiopian older population. These findings stress the need for multifaceted, interdisciplinary interventions to multiple chronic disease conditions; awareness of PIMs; and improvement of rational geriatric prescribing in Ethiopia.

Author Contributions: A.S.B.: conceptualization, methods, investigation, software, data analysis, visualization, writing, review and editing. M.A.S.: validation, data collection, validation, data curation, and project management. A.A.: validation, data collection, data curation, project management. E.A.G.: validation, data analysis, writing—original draft preparation. J.B.: methodology and funding acquisition; D.F.: investigation, funding acquisition, review and supervision. All authors have read and agreed to the published version of the manuscript.

Funding: This research received no external funding. Research works of D. Fialová and J. Brkič, have received funding from the European Union's Horizon 2020 research and innovation program under the Marie Skłodowska-Curie grant agreement No. 764632. Research work of D. Fialová has also been supported by the INOMED project NO.CZ.02.1.01/0.0/0.0/18_069/0010046 co-financed by the European Union, Progress Q42 at the Faculty of Pharmacy, Charles University (KSKF-research group 2, chaired by Assoc. Prof. D. Fialová), START/MED/093 CZ.02.2.69/0.0/0.0/19_073/0016935, SVV260 551 and I-CARE4OLD H2020 -965341.

Institutional Review Board Statement: The study was conducted according to the guidelines of the Declaration of Helsinki and approved by the Institutional Review Board (or Ethics Committee) of the University of Gondar—Vice President for Research and Community Services office (V/P/RCS/05/45/2019 and 24/10/2019).

Informed Consent Statement: Informed consent was obtained from all subjects involved in the study.

Data Availability Statement: Data is contained within the article.

Acknowledgments: The authors would like to thank the Research Assistants, University of Gondar and Gondar University Hospital, for their administrative and technical support in fulfilling the EuroAgeism H2020 ESR7 project data collection in Ethiopia.

Conflicts of Interest: The authors declare no conflict of interest.

References

1. Mercer, S.; Furler, J.; Moffat, K.; Fischbacher-Smith, D.; Sanci, L.; World Health Organization. Multimorbidity: Technical Series on Safer Primary Care. 2016. Available online: https://eprints.gla.ac.uk/133210/1/133210.pdf (accessed on 25 June 2021).
2. World Health Organization. *Global Age-Friendly Cities Project*; World Health Organization: Geneva, Switzerland, 2016.
3. World Health Organization. *Medication Safety in Polypharmacy: Technical Report*; World Health Organization: Geneva, Switzerland, 2019. Available online: http://apps.who.int/iris (accessed on 10 August 2021).

4. Beers, M.H.; Ouslander, J.G.; Rollingher, I.; Reuben, D.B.; Brooks, J.; Beck, J.C. Explicit criteria for determining inappropriate medication use in nursing home residents. UCLA Division of Geriatric Medicine. *Arch. Intern. Med.* **1991**, *151*, 1825–1832. [CrossRef] [PubMed]
5. Krause, O.; Wiese, B.; Doyle, I.M.; Kirsch, C.; Thürmann, P.; Wilm, S.; Sparenberg, L.; Stolz, R.; Freytag, A.; Bleidorn, J.; et al. Multidisciplinary intervention to improve medication safety in nursing home residents: Protocol of a cluster randomised controlled trial (HIOPP-3-iTBX study). *BMC Geriatr.* **2019**, *19*, 24. [CrossRef] [PubMed]
6. Dalton, K.; O'Mahony, D.; O'Sullivan, D.; O'Connor, M.N.; Byrne, S. Prescriber Implementation of STOPP/START Recommendations for Hospitalised Older Adults: A Comparison of a Pharmacist Approach and a Physician Approach. *Drugs Aging* **2019**, *36*, 279–288. [CrossRef] [PubMed]
7. McNicholl, I.R.; Gandhi, M.; Hare, C.B.; Greene, M.; Pierluissi, E. A Pharmacist-Led Program to Evaluate and Reduce Polypharmacy and Potentially Inappropriate Prescribing in Older HIV-Positive Patients. *Pharmacotherapy* **2017**, *37*, 1498–1506. [CrossRef] [PubMed]
8. Campins, L.; Serra-Prat, M.; Gózalo, I.; López, D.; Palomera, E.; Agustí, C.; Cabré, M.; REMEI Group. Randomized controlled trial of an intervention to improve drug appropriateness in community-dwelling polymedicated elderly people. *Fam. Pract.* **2017**, *34*, 36–42. [CrossRef] [PubMed]
9. Gillespie, U.; Alassaad, A.; Hammarlund-Udenaes, M.; Mörlin, C.; Henrohn, D.; Bertilsson, M.; Melhus, H. Effects of pharmacists' interventions on appropriateness of prescribing and evaluation of the instruments' (MAI, STOPP and STARTs') ability to predict hospitalization–analyses from a randomized controlled trial. *PLoS ONE* **2013**, *8*, e62401. [CrossRef] [PubMed]
10. American Geriatrics Society 2015 Beers Criteria Update Expert Panel. American Geriatrics Society 2015 updated Beers criteria for potentially inappropriate medication use in older adults. *J. Am. Geriatr. Soc.* **2015**, *63*, 2227–2246. [CrossRef] [PubMed]
11. Topinkova, E.; Madlova, P.; Fialova, D.; Klan, J. New evidence-based criteria for evaluating the appropriateness of drug regimen in seniors Criteria STOPP (Screening Tool of Older Person's Prescriptions) and START (Screening Tool to Alert Doctors to Right Treatment). *Vnitr. Lek.* **2008**, *54*, 1161–1169. (In Czech) [PubMed]
12. Renom-Guiteras, A.; Meyer, G.; Thürmann, P.A. The EU(7)-PIM list: A list of potentially inappropriate medications for older people consented by experts from seven European countries. *Eur. J. Clin. Pharmacol.* **2015**, *71*, 861–875. [CrossRef] [PubMed]
13. Inocian, E.P.; Reynaldo, R.F.; Dillon, D.; Ignacio, E.H. Using Beers Criteria to Avoid Inappropriate Prescribing for Older Adults. *Medsurg. Nurs.* **2021**, *30*, 113–117.
14. 2019 American Geriatrics Society Beers Criteria® Update Expert Panel. American Geriatrics Society 2019 updated AGS Beers Criteria® for potentially inappropriate medication use in older adults. *J. Am. Geriatr. Soc.* **2019**, *67*, 674–694. [CrossRef] [PubMed]
15. The United Nations Population Fund. 2021. Available online: https://www.unfpa.org/publications/state-world-population-2021 (accessed on 23 May 2021).
16. Mekonnen, A.B.; Bhagavathula, A.S. Inappropriate medication use in the elderly population attending Gondar University hospital: A preliminary assessment. *Int. J. Pharm. Pharm. Sci.* **2014**, *6*, 540–543.
17. Tefera, Y.G.; Alemayehu, M.; Mekonnen, G.B. Prevalence and determinants of polypharmacy in cardiovascular patients attending outpatient clinic in Ethiopia University Hospital. *PLoS ONE* **2020**, *15*, e0234000. [CrossRef] [PubMed]
18. Abegaz, T.M.; Birru, E.M.; Mekonnen, G.B. Potentially inappropriate prescribing in Ethiopian geriatric patients hospitalized with cardiovascular disorders using START/STOPP criteria. *PLoS ONE* **2018**, *13*, e0195949. [CrossRef] [PubMed]
19. Teka, F.; Teklay, G.; Ayalew, E.; Kassa, T.T. Prevalence of potentially inappropriate medications in Ayder referral hospital, Tigray region, Northern Ethiopia: Prospective study. *J. Drug Deliv. Ther.* **2016**, *6*, 16–21. [CrossRef]
20. Getachew, H.; Bhagavathula, A.S.; Abebe, T.B.; Belachew, S.A. Inappropriate prescribing of antithrombotic therapy in Ethiopian elderly population using updated 2015 STOPP/START criteria: A cross-sectional study. *Clin. Interv. Aging* **2016**, *11*, 819–827. [CrossRef] [PubMed]
21. Geresu, G.D.; Yadesa, T.M.; Abebe, B.A. Polypharmacy and the Contributing Factors Among Elderly Patients in Shashemene Referral Hospital, West Arsi, Oromia Region, Ethiopia. *J. Bioanal. Biomed.* **2017**, *9*, 277–282. [CrossRef]
22. Tegegn, H.G.; Erku, D.A.; Sebsibe, G.; Gizaw, B.; Seifu, D.; Tigabe, M.; Belachew, S.A.; Ayele, A.A. Medication-related quality of life among Ethiopian elderly patients with polypharmacy: A cross-sectional study in an Ethiopia university hospital. *PLoS ONE* **2019**, *14*, e0214191. [CrossRef] [PubMed]
23. Bhagavathula, A.S.; Gebreyohannes, E.A.; Fialova, D. Prevalence of polypharmacy and risks of potentially inappropriate medication use in the older population in a developing country: A systematic review and meta-analysis. *Gerontology* **2021**, 1–10. [CrossRef] [PubMed]
24. Jirón, M.; Pate, V.; Hanson, L.C.; Lund, J.L.; Jonsson, F.M.; Stürmer, T. Trends in prevalence and determinants of potentially inappropriate prescribing in the United States: 2007 to 2012. *J. Am. Geriatr. Soc.* **2016**, *64*, 788–797. [CrossRef] [PubMed]
25. Olusanya, A.; Ogunyemi, A.; Arikawe, A.; Megbuwawon, T.; Amao, O. Inappropriate drug use in the elderly outpatient population in a West-African metropolitan community. *Int. J. Clin. Pharmacol. Ther.* **2019**, *57*, 334–344. [CrossRef] [PubMed]
26. Akande-Sholabi, W.; Ajilore, O.C.; Showande, S.J.; Adebusoye, L.A. Potential inappropriate prescribing among ambulatory elderly patients in a geriatric centre in southwestern Nigeria: Beers criteria versus STOPP/START criteria. *Trop. J. Pharm. Res.* **2020**, *19*, 1105–1111. [CrossRef]

27. Abubakar, U.; Tangiisuran, B.; Kolo, M.; Yamma, A.I.; Hammad, M.A.; Sulaiman, S.A. Prevalence and predictors of potentially inappropriate medication use among ambulatory older adults in Northern Nigeria. *Drugs Ther. Perspect.* **2021**, *37*, 94–99. [CrossRef]
28. Saka, S.A.; Oosthuizen, F.; Nlooto, M. Potential inappropriate prescribing and associated factors among older persons in Nigeria and South Africa. *Int. J. Clin. Pharm.* **2019**, *41*, 207–214. [CrossRef] [PubMed]
29. Lemma, W.; Islam, M.; Loha, E.; Mahalwal, V.S. Drug prescribing patterns in geriatric patients in selected health facilities of Addis Ababa, Ethiopia. *J. Appl. Pharm. Sci.* **2020**, *10*, 103–109. [CrossRef]
30. Lemma, W.; Islam, M.; Loha, E. Potentially inappropriate medication prescribing patterns in geriatric patients in a health facility in Addis Ababa, Ethiopia. *Trop. J. Pharm. Res.* **2020**, *19*, 244–246. [CrossRef]
31. Sada, O. Irrational use of medications among elderly patients in an Ethiopian referral hospital. *Afr. J. Pharm. Pharmacol.* **2017**, *11*, 191–194. [CrossRef]
32. Zahwe, M.; Skouri, H.; Rachidi, S.; Khoury, M.; Noureddine, S.; Isma'eel, H.; Tamim, H.; Al-Hajje, A. Potentially inappropriate medications in elderly patients with heart failure: Beers Criteria-based study. *Int. J. Pharm. Pract.* **2020**, *28*, 652–659. [CrossRef] [PubMed]
33. Al-Dahshan, A.; Kehyayan, V. Prevalence and predictors of potentially inappropriate medication prescription among older adults: A cross-sectional study in the state of Qatar. *Drugs Real. World Outcomes* **2021**, *8*, 95–103. [CrossRef] [PubMed]
34. Sharma, R.; Chhabra, M.; Vidyasagar, K.; Rashid, M.; Fialova, D.; Bhagavathula, A.S. Potentially inappropriate medication use in older hospitalized patients with type 2 eiabetes: A cross-sectional study. *Pharmacy* **2020**, *8*, 219. [CrossRef] [PubMed]
35. He, D.; Zhu, H.; Zhou, H.; Dong, N.; Zhang, H. Potentially inappropriate medications in Chinese older adults: A comparison of two updated Beers criteria. *Int. J. Clin. Pharm.* **2021**, *43*, 229–235. [CrossRef] [PubMed]
36. Tian, F.; Li, H.; Chen, Z.; Xu, T. Potentially inappropriate medications in Chinese older outpatients in tertiary hospitals according to Beers criteria: A cross-sectional study. *Int. J. Clin. Pract.* **2021**, *75*, e14348. [CrossRef] [PubMed]
37. Nguyen, T.N.; Laetsch, D.C.; Chen, L.J.; Holleczek, B.; Meid, A.D.; Brenner, H.; Schöttker, B. Comparison of five lists to identify potentially inappropriate use of non-steroidal anti-inflammatory drugs in older adults. *Pain Med.* **2021**, pnaa480. [CrossRef] [PubMed]
38. Brockmöller, J.; Stingl, J.C. Multimorbidity, polypharmacy and pharmacogenomics in old age. *Pharmacogenomics* **2017**, *18*, 515–517. [CrossRef] [PubMed]
39. Muhlack, D.C.; Hoppe, L.K.; Stock, C.; Haefeli, W.E.; Brenner, H.; Schöttker, B. The associations of geriatric syndromes and other patient characteristics with the current and future use of potentially inappropriate medications in a large cohort study. *Eur. J. Clin. Pharmacol.* **2018**, *74*, 1633–1644. [CrossRef] [PubMed]
40. Manias, E.; Maier, A.; Krishnamurthy, G. Inappropriate medication use in hospitalised oldest old patients across transitions of care. *Aging Clin. Exp. Res.* **2019**, *31*, 1661–1673. [CrossRef] [PubMed]
41. Damoiseaux-Volman, B.A.; Medlock, S.; Raven, K.; Sent, D.; Romijn, J.A.; van der Velde, N.; Abu-Hanna, A. Potentially inappropriate prescribing in older hospitalized Dutch patients according to the STOPP/START criteria v2: A longitudinal study. *Eur. J. Clin. Pharmacol.* **2021**, *75*, 777–785. [CrossRef] [PubMed]
42. Yarnall, A.J.; Sayer, A.A.; Clegg, A.; Rockwood, K.; Parker, S.; Hindle, J.V. New horizons in multimorbidity in older adults. *Age Ageing* **2017**, *46*, 882–888. [CrossRef] [PubMed]
43. Charlson, M.E.; Pompei, P.; Ales, K.L.; MacKenzie, C.R. A new method of classifying prognostic comorbidity in longitudinal studies: Development and validation. *J. Chronic Dis.* **1987**, *40*, 373–383. [CrossRef] [PubMed]
44. Prithviraj, G.K.; Koroukian, S.; Margevicius, S.; Berger, N.A.; Bagai, R.; Owusu, C. Patient characteristics associated with polypharmacy and inappropriate prescribing of medications among older adults with cancer. *J. Geriatr. Oncol.* **2012**, *3*, 228–237. [CrossRef] [PubMed]
45. González-González, A.I.; Meid, A.D.; Dinh, T.S.; Blom, J.W.; van den Akker, M.; Elders, P.J.M.; Thiem, U.; De Gaudry, D.K.; Swart, K.M.A.; Rudolf, H.; et al. A prognostic model predicted deterioration in health-related quality of life in older patients with multimorbidity and polypharmacy. *J. Clin. Epidemiol.* **2021**, *130*, 1–12. [CrossRef] [PubMed]
46. Liu, C.P.B.; Leung, D.S.Y.; Chi, I. Social functioning, polypharmacy and depression in older Chinese primary care patients. *Aging Mental Health* **2011**, *15*, 732–741. [CrossRef] [PubMed]
47. Pedrós, C.; Formiga, F.; Corbella, X.; Arnau, J.M. Adverse drug reactions leading to urgent hospital admission in an elderly population: Prevalence and main features. *Eur. J. Clin. Pharmacol.* **2016**, *72*, 219–226. [CrossRef] [PubMed]
48. Al-Busaidi, S.; Al-Kharusi, A.; Al-Hinai, M.; Al-Zakwani, I.; Al-Ghafri, F.; Rizvi, S.; Al-Balushi, K. Potentially inappropriate prescribing among elderly patients at a primary care clinic in Oman. *J. Cross-Cult. Gerontol.* **2020**, *35*, 209–216. [CrossRef] [PubMed]
49. Guaraldo, L.; Cano, F.G.; Damasceno, G.S.; Rozenfeld, S. Inappropriate medication use among the elderly: A systematic review of administrative databases. *BMC Geriatr.* **2011**, *11*, 79. [CrossRef] [PubMed]
50. Jungo, K.T.; Streit, S.; Lauffenburger, J.C. Patient factors associated with new prescribing of potentially inappropriate medications in multimorbid US older adults using multiple medications. *BMC Geriatr.* **2021**, *21*, 163. [CrossRef] [PubMed]

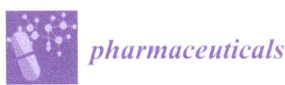 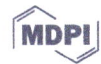

Article

Clinical Impact of Functional CYP2C19 and CYP2D6 Gene Variants on Treatment with Antidepressants in Young People with Depression: A Danish Cohort Study

Liv S. Thiele [1,†], Kazi Ishtiak-Ahmed [1,2,†], Janne P. Thirstrup [1,2,3], Esben Agerbo [4,5], Carin A. T. C. Lunenburg [1,2], Daniel J. Müller [6,7] and Christiane Gasse [1,2,8,*]

1. Department of Affective Disorders, Aarhus University Hospital Psychiatry, 8200 Aarhus, Denmark; 201409442@post.au.dk (L.S.T.); kazahm@rm.dk (K.I.-A.); janne.thirstrup@biomed.au.dk (J.P.T.); lunenburg.c@gmail.com (C.A.T.C.L.)
2. Department of Clinical Medicine, Aarhus University, 8200 Aarhus, Denmark
3. Department of Biomedicine, Aarhus University, 8000 Aarhus, Denmark
4. National Centre for Register-Based Research (NCRR), Aarhus BSS, Aarhus University, 8210 Aarhus, Denmark; ea@econ.au.dk
5. Centre for Integrated Register-Based Research Aarhus University (CIRRAU), 8210 Aarhus, Denmark
6. Pharmacogenetics Research Clinic, Campbell Family Mental Health Research Institute, Centre for Addiction and Mental Health, Toronto, ON M6J 1H4, Canada; daniel.mueller@camh.ca
7. Department of Psychiatry, University of Toronto, Toronto, ON M5S 1A1, Canada
8. Psychosis Research Unit, Aarhus University Hospital Psychiatry, 8200 Aarhus, Denmark
* Correspondence: chgass@rm.dk; Tel.: +45-51191476
† These authors contributed equally to this work.

Abstract: Background: The clinical impact of the functional CYP2C19 and CYP2D6 gene variants on antidepressant treatment in people with depression is not well studied. Here, we evaluate the utility of pharmacogenetic (PGx) testing in psychiatry by investigating the association between the phenotype status of the cytochrome P450 (CYP) 2C19/2D6 enzymes and the one-year risks of clinical outcomes in patients with depression with incident new-use of (es)citalopram, sertraline, or fluoxetine. Methods: This study is a population-based cohort study of 17,297 individuals who were born between 1981 and 2005 with a depression diagnosis between 1996 and 2012. Using array-based single-nucleotide-polymorphism genotype data, the individuals were categorized according to their metabolizing status of CYP2C19/CYP2D6 as normal (NM, reference group), ultra-rapid- (UM), rapid- (RM), intermediate- (IM), or poor-metabolizer (PM). The outcomes were treatment switching or discontinuation, psychiatric emergency department contacts, and suicide attempt/self-harm. By using Poisson regression analyses, we have estimated the incidence rate ratios (IRR) with 95% confidence intervals (95% CI) that were adjusted for covariates and potential confounders, by age groups (<18 (children and adolescents), 19–25 (young adults), and 26+ years (adults)), comparing the outcomes in individuals with NM status (reference) versus the mutant metabolizer status. For statistically significant outcomes, we have calculated the number needed to treat (NNT) and the number needed to genotype (NNG) in order to prevent one outcome. Results: The children and adolescents who were using (es)citalopram with CYP2C19 PM status had increased risks of switching (IRR = 1.64 [95% CI: 1.10–2.43]) and suicide attempt/self-harm (IRR = 2.67 [95% CI; 1.57–4.52]). The young adults with CYP2C19 PM status who were using sertraline had an increased risk of switching (IRR = 2.06 [95% CI; 1.03–4.11]). The young adults with CYP2D6 PM status who were using fluoxetine had an increased risk of emergency department contacts (IRR = 3.28 [95% CI; 1.11–9.63]). No significant associations were detected in the adults. The NNG for preventing one suicide attempt/suicide in the children who were using (es)citalopram was 463, and the NNT was 11. Conclusion: The CYP2C19 and CYP2D6 PM phenotype statuses were associated with outcomes in children, adolescents, and young adults with depression with incident new-use of (es)citalopram, sertraline, or fluoxetine, therefore indicating the utility of PGx testing, particularly in younger people, for PGx-guided antidepressant treatment.

Citation: Thiele, L.S.; Ishtiak-Ahmed, K.; Thirstrup, J.P.; Agerbo, E.; Lunenburg, C.A.T.C.; Müller, D.J.; Gasse, C. Clinical Impact of Functional CYP2C19 and CYP2D6 Gene Variants on Treatment with Antidepressants in Young People with Depression: A Danish Cohort Study. *Pharmaceuticals* 2022, 15, 870. https://doi.org/10.3390/ph15070870

Academic Editors: Charlotte Vermehren and Niels Westergaard

Received: 15 June 2022
Accepted: 11 July 2022
Published: 14 July 2022

Publisher's Note: MDPI stays neutral with regard to jurisdictional claims in published maps and institutional affiliations.

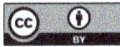

Copyright: © 2022 by the authors. Licensee MDPI, Basel, Switzerland. This article is an open access article distributed under the terms and conditions of the Creative Commons Attribution (CC BY) license (https://creativecommons.org/licenses/by/4.0/).

Keywords: pharmacogenetics; antidepressants; utility; population-based

1. Introduction

Antidepressants are essential of the pharmacological treatment of depression in youths and adults [1]. However, treatment with antidepressants is often not optimal, with about 30% of patients not recovering, even after several attempts of treatment with different antidepressants [2]. The insufficient treatment response and the adverse events may partly be attributed to the individual's capacity to metabolize the antidepressant (pharmacokinetics), which is affected by genetic variations of drug-metabolizing enzymes, e.g., the hepatic cytochrome P450 (CYP) system [3]. In particular, the highly polymorphic enzymes CYP2C19 and CYP2D6 play a central role in the metabolism of many antidepressants, including the selective serotonin-reuptake inhibitors (SSRIs) (es)citalopram, sertraline, and fluoxetine [3]. There is an increasing body of clinical evidence linking pharmacogenetic (PGx) variability of CYP2D6 and CYP2C19 to drug blood concentrations [4,5], the treatment response [4,6], and the remission rates [6] in patients with depression. Thus, by PGx testing of the genotypes of CYP2C19 and CYP2D6 metabolizer phenotypes according to the variable genotypes' activity can be classified into poor (PM), intermediate (IM), normal (NM), rapid (RM), or ultra-rapid metabolizer (UM) for the given enzyme. These phenotypes can guide the choice of drug and the dose adjustment in order to maximize the likelihood for treatment effectiveness and minimize the adverse events [7].

As a first-line treatment for depression, SSRIs are commonly used in the population worldwide, with more than 4% of the total Danish population using SSRIs in 2021 [8], 8% in UK in 2011 [9], and approximately 11% in the USA in 2021 [10]. The recommendations for PGx-guided dosing for PM and IM CYP2C19 phenotypes of the SSRIs (es)citalopram and sertraline have been published by the Dutch Pharmacogenetics Working Group (DPWG) and the Clinical Pharmacogenetics Implementation Consortium (CPIC) [11,12]. In addition, the drug labels of (es)citalopram and sertraline, by the national drug authorities in the USA, Switzerland, Canada, and Japan, consider PGx testing actionable, while the labelling for these drugs in the EU does not include any annotations for PGx testing [11]. Fluoxetine is the only approved SSRI for the treatment of depression in children in Denmark [13]. Fluoxetine is mainly metabolized by CYP2D6, but neither drug labels nor the DPWG or the CPIC offer dosing guidelines, due to insufficient relevant clinical evidence in children [11].

Despite the existing clinical evidence, drug labelling, actionable PGx recommendations for (es)citalopram and sertraline, and the frequent use of these first-line drugs in the population, the clinical utility of PGx testing is still broadly discussed nationally and internationally, particularly in youths [14], and the implementation of PGx testing remains low in psychiatry in Denmark [7,15], though it is increasing internationally [3]. The clinical utility of PGx can be defined as the ability of PGx-guided treatment and dosing to prevent the adverse effects expressed by the number needed to genotype (NNG) and number needed to treat (NNT) in order to avoid one adverse event [16]. Published PGx studies rarely report the clinical utility measures [17], which could support the communication of the evidence of PGx drugs with strong associations and/or frequent use in the population for the clinical implementation of PGx testing [16].

Here, we have examined the association of CYP2C19 and CYP2D6 gene variants translated into PGx phenotypes with treatment outcomes of switching or discontinuation, psychiatric emergency department contacts, and suicide attempt/self-harm in patients with depression with incident new-use of (es)citalopram, sertraline, or fluoxetine in children and adolescents ($\leq$18 years), young adults (19–25), and adults ($\geq$26 years).

2. Results
2.1. Characteristics of the Study Population

Of the 24,110 individuals with a hospital depression diagnosis given at any time between 1 January 1996 and 31 December 2012, 20,343 (84%) had redeemed at least one prescription for (es)citalopram, sertraline, or fluoxetine. Of the latter, 17,297 (85%) had valid genetic data and, therefore, formed the study population, of which 70% were females, 90% were younger than 26 years, and 90% were of Danish/European origin. Compared to the excluded individuals, the individuals of the study population were slightly younger, had filled their first prescription for the respective antidepressants in the more recent years in the study period, had their first prescription issued from the hospital, and had a diagnosis of autism more often, and a diagnosis of schizophrenia or bipolar disorder less often (Table S4).

Of the study population, the majority (62%) had redeemed at least one prescription for (es)citalopram during the study period (Table 1). According to the indicated use of fluoxetine in children, the mean age of the fluoxetine users was lower than in individuals initiating the other antidepressants. The differences in the baseline characteristics stratified by children and adolescents, young adults, and adults existed, but not regarding the frequency of CYP2C19 and CYP2D6 phenotypes (Tables S5 and 2).

Table 1. Baseline characteristics at the index date of the first-time prescription of sertraline, escitalopram, citalopram, and fluoxetine of the total study population (n = 17,297) of all individuals born between 1981 and 2005 with a depression diagnosis any time between 1996 and 2012.

	Antidepressants							
	Citalopram, n = 8281		Escitalopram, n = 2632		Sertraline, n = 4583		Fluoxetine, n = 1801	
	n	(%)	n	(%)	n	(%)	n	(%)
Sex								
Female	5896	(71.2)	1783	(67.7)	3164	(69.0)	1377	(76.5)
Male	2385	(28.8)	849	(32.3)	1419	(31.0)	424	(23.5)
Age in groups								
Children/adolescents (≤18 years)	3111	(37.6)	928	(35.3)	2513	(54.8)	1338	(74.3)
Young adults (19–25 years)	4263	(51.5)	1428	(54.3)	1567	(34.2)	403	(22.4)
Adults (26+ years)	907	(11.0)	276	(10.5)	503	(11.0)	60	(3.3)
Mean age in years, (SD)	20.3 (3.6)		20.5 (3.4)		19.2 (4.3)		17.5 (3.3)	
Region at index prescription								
Capital Region	2296	(27.7)	787	(29.9)	1068	(23.3)	514	(28.5)
Middle Jutland	2029	(24.5)	676	(25.7)	1161	(25.3)	323	(17.9)
North Jutland	887	(10.7)	227	(8.6)	574	(12.5)	148	(8.2)
Southern Denmark	1592	(19.2)	595	(22.6)	1073	(23.4)	374	(20.8)
Zealand	1477	(17.8)	347	(13.2)	707	(15.4)	442	(24.5)
Parents/adults SES *								
Missing	152	(1.8)	23	(0.9)	126	(2.7)	25	(1.4)
Employed	3670	(44.3)	1256	(47.7)	2292	(50.0)	1094	(60.7)
On social benefits	1839	(22.2)	465	(17.7)	1064	(23.2)	309	(17.2)
On study	1947	(23.5)	673	(25.6)	782	(17.1)	273	(15.2)
Others	673	(8.1)	215	(8.2)	319	(7.0)	100	(5.6)

Table 1. Cont.

	Antidepressants							
	Citalopram, n = 8281		Escitalopram, n = 2632		Sertraline, n = 4583		Fluoxetine, n = 1801	
	n	(%)	n	(%)	n	(%)	n	(%)
Within last year: No. of psychiatric hospital contacts								
0	4965	(60.0)	1450	(55.1)	2078	(45.3)	590	(32.8)
1	1220	(14.7)	408	(15.5)	844	(18.4)	371	(20.6)
2	445	(5.4)	143	(5.4)	311	(6.8)	193	(10.7)
3	213	(2.6)	80	(3.0)	143	(3.1)	68	(3.8)
4	107	(1.3)	36	(1.4)	100	(2.2)	42	(2.3)
>4	1331	(16.1)	515	(19.6)	1107	(24.2)	537	(29.8)
Past: No. of past mental diagnoses								
0	2757	(33.3)	798	(30.3)	952	(20.8)	241	(13.4)
1	2511	(30.3)	880	(33.4)	1217	(26.6)	566	(31.4)
2	1648	(19.9)	550	(20.9)	1169	(25.5)	603	(33.5)
3	845	(10.2)	268	(10.2)	779	(17.0)	253	(14.0)
4	361	(4.4)	105	(4.0)	296	(6.5)	96	(5.3)
>4	159	(1.9)	31	(1.2)	170	(3.7)	42	(2.3)
Past ever: history of self-harm/suicide attempt								
Yes	1312	(15.8)	431	(16.4)	651	(14.2)	321	(17.8)
Within last year: history of self-harm/suicide attempt								
Yes	586	(7.1)	206	(7.8)	346	(7.5)	197	(10.9)
Within last 90ds: strong CYP2D6 inhibitor use								
Yes	67	(0.8)	32	(1.2)	66	(1.4)	10	(0.6)
Within last 90ds: moderate CYP2D6 inhibitor use								
Yes	142	(1.7)	42	(1.6)	77	(1.7)	14	(0.8)
Within last 90ds: weak CYP2D6 inhibitor use								
Yes	One of the categories had <5 observations							
Within last 90ds: strong CYP2C19 inhibitor use								
Yes	216	(2.6)	73	(2.8)	109	(2.4)	39	(2.2)
Within last 90ds: moderate CYP2C19 inhibitor use								
No	8281	(100.0)	2632	(100.0)	4583	(100.0)	1801	(100.0)
Within last 90ds: weak CYP2C19 inhibitor use								
Yes	189	(2.3)	59	(2.2)	122	(2.7)	41	(2.3)

Table 1. *Cont.*

	Antidepressants							
	Citalopram, n = 8281		Escitalopram, n = 2632		Sertraline, n = 4583		Fluoxetine, n = 1801	
	n	(%)	n	(%)	n	(%)	n	(%)
Within last 90ds: CYP2C19 inducer use								
Yes	All categories had <5							
Within last 90ds: Antiepileptic drug use								
Yes	80	(1.0)	35	(1.3)	69	(1.5)	13	(0.7)
Year as category of first prescription								
1995–2001	237	(2.9)	0	0	185	(4.0)	44	(2.4)
2001–2005	2201	(26.6)	524	(19.9)	988	(21.6)	264	(14.7)
2006–2010	4447	(53.7)	1890	(71.8)	1931	(42.1)	828	(46.0)
2011–2016	1396	(16.9)	218	(8.3)	1479	(32.3)	665	(36.9)

* For those who had missing information on their own socioeconomic status (SES) we extracted SES from their parents. For a detailed description of all the variables see Supplement Table S3. Ds = days.

Table 2. Prevalence of CYP2C19 and CYP2D6 phenotypes of individuals born between 1981 and 2005, with a depression diagnosis any time between 1996 and 2012, with at least one prescription for escitalopram, citalopram, sertraline, or fluoxetine.

	Antidepressants									
	Total, n = 17,297		Escitalopram, n = 2632		Citalopram, n = 8281		Sertraline, n = 4583		Fluoxetine, n = 1801	
	n	(%)	n	(%)	n	(%)	n	(%)	n	(%)
CYP2D6 phenotype										
CYP2D6_NM	10,770	(62.3)	1629	(61.9)	5159	(62.3)	2855	(62.3)	1127	(62.6)
CYP2D6_IM	5781	(33.4)	873	(33.2)	2778	(33.5)	1533	(33.4)	597	(33.1)
CYP2D6_PM	746	(4.3)	130	(4.9)	344	(4.2)	195	(4.3)	77	(4.3)
CYP2C19 phenotype										
CYP2C19_UM	678	(3.9)	118	(4.5)	304	(3.7)	194	(4.2)	62	(3.4)
CYP2C19_RM	4483	(25.9)	687	(26.1)	2168	(26.2)	1143	(24.9)	485	(26.9)
CYP2C19_NM	7553	(43.7)	1122	(42.6)	3600	(43.5)	2042	(44.6)	789	(43.8)
CYP2C19_IM	4215	(24.4)	652	(24.8)	2024	(24.4)	1111	(24.2)	428	(23.8)
CYP2C19_PM	368	(2.1)	53	(2)	185	(2.2)	93	(2)	37	(2.1)

Abbreviations: NM: normal metabolizer, IM: intermediate metabolizer, PM: poor metabolizer, RM: rapid metabolizer, UM: ultrarapid metabolizer.

2.2. Associations between the CYP2C19 and CYP2D6 Phenotypes and Clinical Outcomes

Overall, irrespective of the outcomes, the study population of 17,297 individuals contributed to a total follow-up time of 17,237 person-years (PYs) since the treatment initiation with the respective drugs, with a mean follow-up period of 364 days. During the study period, 793 individuals emigrated and 124 died.

The incidence rates (IR) per 100 person-years with 95% CI of outcomes, according to the index drug use, are reported in Table S6. Figure 1 and Table S7 describe the association between the CYP2C19 and CYP2D6 phenotypes and the clinical outcomes in the individuals with depression who were using (es)citalopram, sertraline, or fluoxetine by the age groups.

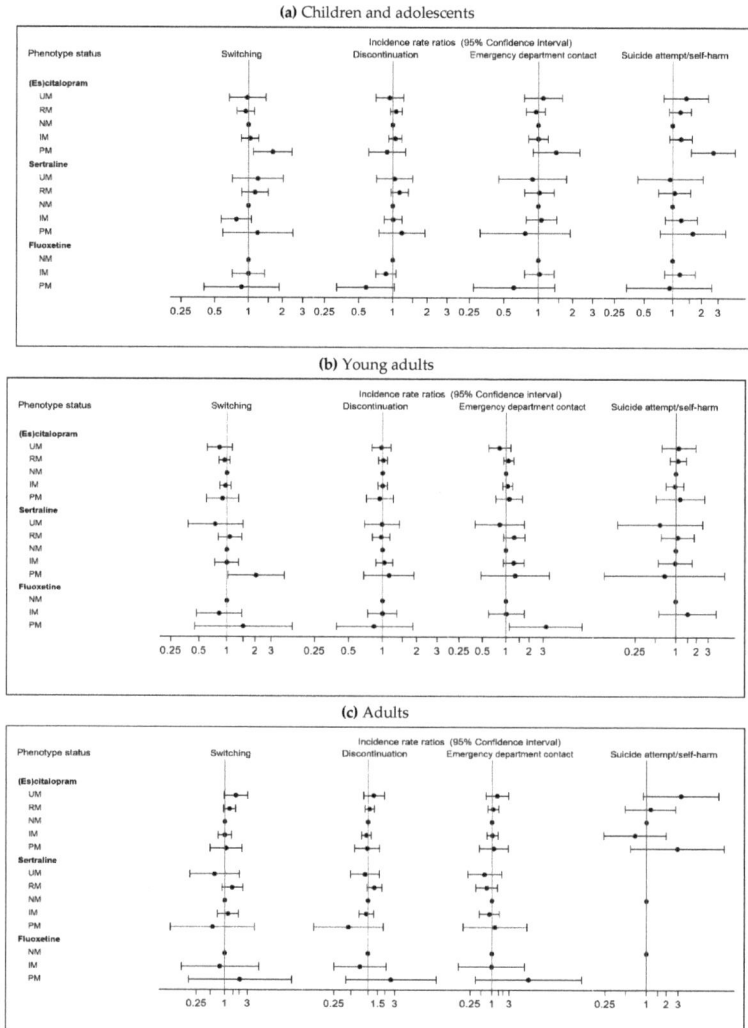

Figure 1. Adjusted incidence rate ratios (IRR) and 95% confidence intervals of the associations between the CYP2C19 and CYP2D6 phenotypes and clinical outcomes in people with a hospital depression diagnosis between 1 January 1996 and 31 December 2012 and a first-time prescription for (es)citalopram, sertraline, or fluoxetine between 1 January 1996 and 31 December 2016, stratified by age groups (≤18, 19–25, 26+ years). Abbreviations: UM: ultra-rapid metabolizer, RM: rapid metabolizer, NM: normal metabolizer, IM: intermediate metabolizer, PM: poor metabolizer. NM was the reference group. IRR were adjusted for: age, gender, region of index prescription, socio-economic status (SES), number of previous psychiatric diagnosis, CYP2C19/CYP2D6 inhibitor and inducer use within the last three months of index date, and calendar year of index prescription. For emergency department contact, we further adjusted for any hospital contacts within the previous year of index date. For the outcome of suicide attempt/self-harm, we also adjusted for previous suicide attempt/self-harm and for antiepileptic drug use within the last three months of index date.

The children and adolescents who were using (es)citalopram with a CYP2C19 PM status had an incident rate of switching of 41 per 100 PYs and a statistically significant increased risk of switching (IRR$_{PM}$ = 1.64 [95% CI: 1.10–2.43]) compared to those with CYP2C19 NM status. The children and adolescents who were using (es)citalopram with a CYP2C19 PM status had an incident rate of 23 per 100 PYs of attempted suicide/self-harm and had a statistically significant increased risk of suicide attempt/self-harm (IRR$_{PM}$ = 2.67 [95% CI; 1.57–4.52]), compared to those with CYP2C19 NM status (Figure 1a).

Among the young adults who were using sertraline with CYP2C19 PM status, 51 per 100 PYs switched to another drug, with a statistically significant increased risk of switching (IRR$_{PM}$ = 2.06 [95% CI; 1.03–4.11]) (Figure 1b) compared with CYP2C19 NMs. The young adults who were using fluoxetine with a CYP2D6 PM status had an IR of 55 psychiatric emergency department contacts per 100 PYs, with a more than three-fold increased risk of psychiatric emergency department contacts compared with CYP2D6 NMs (IRR$_{PM}$ = 3.28 [95% CI; 1.11–9.63]) (Figure 1b).

Among the adults, no statistically significant findings were detected, but associations indicating a U-shaped relationship across the phenotypes with higher risks in users of (es)citalopram with CYP2C19 PM and UM status were found (Figure 1c).

2.3. Potential Clinical Validity and Population Impact of PGx Testing

Overall, the clinical utility and population impact of PGx testing for all of the statistically significant associations of switching, suicide attempt, and self-harm among children and adolescents, and young adults were 1–2.5% for PAF, the NNG was between 460 and 503, according to their metabolizer phenotypes, and the NNT was between 10 and 11 in order to prevent one outcome, (Table 3).

Table 3. Measures of population impact of pharmacogenetic testing.

	Age Group	Children and Adolescents	Children and Adolescents	Young Adults	Young Adults
	Drug	(Es)citalopram	(Es)citalopram	Sertraline	Fluoxetine
	Phenotype	CYP2C19 PM	CYP2C19 PM	CYP2C19 PM	CYP2D6 PM
	Risk geno-/phenotype freq.	2.18%	2.18%	2.00%	4.30%
	Outcome	Switching	Suicide Attempt/Self-Harm	Switching	ER Contact
	IRR *	1.64	2.67	2.06	3.28
	RR	1.46	2.15	1.57	**
	RD	0.09	0.1	0.11	**
Population impact of PGx	PAF	1.00%	2.4%	1.12%	**
	NNT	11	11	10	**
	NNG	503	464	460	**

Abbreviations: PM: poor metabolizer, IRR: incidence rate ratio, RR: relative risk, RD: risk difference, PAF: population attributable fraction, NNT: number needed to treat, NNG: number needed to genotype. * Adjusted for: age, gender, region of index prescription, socio-economic status (SES), number of previous psychiatric diagnosis, CYP2C19/CYP2D6 inhibitor and inducer use within the last three months of index date, and calendar year of index prescription. For emergency room contact, we further adjusted for any hospital contacts within the previous year of index date. For the outcome of suicide attempt/self-harm, we also adjusted for previous suicide attempt/self-harm and for antiepileptic drug use within the last three months of index date. ** Numbers cannot be calculated because there were <5 cases for at least one of the needed numbers. See Supplementary Table S8 for the underlying numbers for the calculation.

3. Discussion

We have studied the association between CYP2C19 and CYP2D6 gene variants and the treatment outcomes in children and adolescents, young adults, and adults with depression who were using (es)citalopram, sertraline, or fluoxetine. The associations were most pronounced in the children and adolescents with statistically significant results in PM of CYP2C19 who were using (es)citalopram, with regard to switching and suicide attempts/self-harm. We found U-shaped associations from UM to PM of CYP2C19 in both the children and adolescents, and the adults who were using (es)citalopram, related to suicide attempt/self-harm. The association measures that were translated into measures of clinical utility were nominally modest, which may be partly because CYP2C19 and CYP2D6 PM are rare phenotypes in a multifactorial setting of drug response.

Compared with the previous findings of CYP2C19 genetic variability and switching, a study among adults [4] found a more than 3-fold increased frequency of switching within one year in CYP2C19 PM and RM/UM status who were using escitalopram compared with the none finding among PM in adults who were using (es)citalopram and the borderline non-significant association in the RM and UM adults in our study. In addition, we found a 64% significantly increased risk in the children and adolescents with CYP2C19 PM status who were using (es)citalopram. According to the authors, the increased risk of switching in CYP2C19 PMs and UM was explained by the increased (PM) and decreased (UM) drug-plasma concentrations [4], potentially leading to adverse events and an insufficient treatment response. Though pointing towards similar conclusions, our study differed from Jukic et al. in identifying the proxies for switching. The study by Jukic et al. was limited to data that was based on the therapeutic drug measurements, while our study was limited to prescription data. However, we were able to adjust for potential confounders and pheno-conversion, which may partly explain the differences in the sizes of the detected associations.

Regarding sertraline, we found that the young adults with PM status who were using sertraline were also more likely to switch. A systematic review and meta-analysis [5] showed that CYP2C19 PMs had higher sertraline plasma concentrations, while Poweleit et al. [18] showed that CYP2C19 status from PM to UM was inversely associated with sertraline doses at the beginning of treatment but not with doses in association with response. Overall, Jessel et al. [19] found that 10% of individuals tended to switch if they were using antidepressants that were not in line with their CYP2C19 and/or CYP2D6 status, compared with 6% of patients who were using antidepressants that were aligned with their metabolizer phenotype.

Regarding discontinuation, Aldrich et al. [20] found a significant association between the discontinuation of (es)citalopram in youth with anxiety and/or depression and CYP2C19 PM and IM status, which is partly in line with our study, where the children and adolescents who were using (es)citalopram with a CYP2C19 IM phenotype had a slightly increased, but statistically insignificant, risk for discontinuation. By contrast, meta-analyses of clinical trials have reported that those with CYP2C19 PM status who were using escitalopram had an improved treatment response, higher rates of side effects, but had less drop out from the clinical trials [6,21].

Suicidal behavior is a feared and severe outcome in young patients using SSRIs [22]. We have detected a more than a 2-fold increased risk of suicide attempt/self-harm in the children and adolescents who were using (es)citalopram with poor metabolizing capacity. In the young adults and the adults of our study, CYP2C19 PMs who were using (es)citalopram also showed a nominal increased risk of suicide attempt/self-harm, as well as CYP2C19 UMs, but this was not statistically significant. It should be noted that our definition included self-harm of both known and unknown suicidal intent [23]. By contrast, an international study of 243 patients found no differences between the phenotypes and suicidal behavior, as measured by clinical rating scales [24], while a post-mortem study showed an enrichment of CYP2C19 PMs and UMs among adult suicide victims who had tested positively for citalopram, compared with the population controls [25]. It should be noted that the use of (es)citalopram dropped to nearly 0 by 2021 [26] in children and adolescents since the warnings of the increased risk of suicidal behavior were issued in 2010 [22]. In 2021, fluoxetine and sertraline were the most frequently used antidepressants among children in Denmark [26]. The numbers were too small to assess the suicidality in the users of fluoxetine, while a nominally increased risk was seen among the children and adolescents with PM status who were using sertraline.

Regarding fluoxetine, according to previous reports, CYP2D6 metabolizer status showed no influence on 8- or 12-week fluoxetine treatment response, which was assessed with multiple disease severity scales in children and adolescents [27]. Here, we have found nominally decreased risks for all of the outcomes in the children and adolescents with CYP2D6 PM status, which may indicate a superior response to fluoxetine in CYP2D6 PMs, possibly due to higher drug-plasma concentrations in these patients [4], without the off-set of higher risks of adverse events leading to discontinuation or switching. In contrast to the children and adolescents, the young adults and the adults who were using fluoxetine with PM status in our study had an increased risk of switching and emergency room contacts, which is in line with a smaller study reporting that 33% of people with a CYP2D6 PM status discontinued the fluoxetine treatments compared with 14% of adults with a CYP2D6 NM status [28].

The metabolism of fluoxetine is complicated by the self-inhibition/pheno-conversion of CYP2D6 by fluoxetine enantiomers during chronic treatment, which increases the importance of alternative metabolic pathways, including CYP2C19 [13]. Thus, the CYP2C19 metabolism, and other alternative pathways, may compensate the limited CYP2D6 metabolism [29]. Due to the described complexity of the metabolic pathway, and the power issues regarding treatment outcomes, it would have been beyond the scope of the current study to evaluate the combinatorial effect of both the CYP2D6 and CYP2C19 variants, which should be addressed in future studies.

3.1. Potential Clinical Validity and Population Impact of PGx Testing

Despite the significant associations, translated to the clinical utility measures, these appear to be quite modest. This is partly because CYP2C19 and CYP2D6 PM are rare phenotypes in a multifactorial setting of drug response. Yet, regarding the suicide attempts/self-harm in association with (es)citalopram, the NNG was 464 and the NNT was 10, indicating the utility of pre-emptive PGx testing in those patients for whom fluoxetine is not an option. Overall, the limitation of the application of a simplified and mono-factorial approach of estimating the clinical utility highlights that the assessment/testing of PGx variability should be regarded as a clinical factor contributing to the full clinical assessment.

3.2. Strengths and Limitations

The population-based approach using the national health registries of a tax-financed health care system providing a free and equal health care service for everyone in Denmark, the relatively large sample size, the consistent and unambiguous data linkage of multiple registers, and the limited risk of selection bias are strengths of this study. The genotyping data with uniform quality control for the complete sample provides a solid foundation for unbiased phenotyping. Due to the data linkage, we were able to account for other independent factors and confounders that are related to drug response, including age, sex, co-medication, some somatic diseases, and pheno-conversion. We have accounted for the age differences in depression treatment and have included only the first-time use of the antidepressants of interest, which was possible due to the longitudinal design and prescription data availability going back to 1995.

Our study also has some limitations. First, we only had information on prescriptions that were redeemed at community pharmacies in order to identify antidepressant drug users, thus, any individuals who were solely treated with antidepressants at psychiatric hospitals were not included. Moreover, we do not know if the patients actually adhered to the treatment regimen as prescribed or if they discontinued the treatment during the prescription supply. Second, we focused on people with a life-time hospital diagnosis of depression from a psychiatric hospital based on the iPSYCH study design, therefore, people using antidepressants who were solely seen by their general practitioners or by private psychiatrists were not included. However, because antidepressants can also be used for other indications than depression, e.g., anxiety or other mental or neurological disorders, the focus on people with a depression diagnosis from a psychiatric hospital makes it more likely that antidepressants were actually used for the indication of depression of similar severity. Due to the case design of the iPSYCH sample, the index drug could have been prescribed before, during, or after the registered hospital-based depression diagnosis, with 50% of the study population having had a hospital contact due to depression at the time of their first antidepressant prescription redemption. Third, the data on dosage and drug-plasma-concentrations was not available in order to evaluate the clinical significance of the genetic variations in the drug-metabolizing enzymes on the drug metabolism and the drug-plasma-concentrations as intermediates for the investigated outcomes [4]. Fourth, only four out of the eight PGx relevant SNPs for the CYP2D6 gene were available in the genotyped iPSYCH sample, with the missing variants only accounting for a summed MAFs of 0.04 [23]. Fifth, due to the missing information on the functional duplications (CYP2D6*1xN and CYP2D6*2xN), the CYP2D6 UM phenotypes could not be determined, but the prevalence of these duplications is only 0.8% in the Danish population [30]. Sixth, we did not account for combinatorial pharmacogenetics between the CYP2D6 and CYP2C19 genetic variants [31]. Lastly, we analyzed escitalopram and citalopram in one group, although pharmacokinetic and pharmacodynamics differences exist [32].

4. Methods

4.1. Study Design and Setting

In this population- and register-based cohort study in Denmark, we investigated the one-year risks of developing clinical outcomes according to CYP2C19 or CYP2D6 genotypes/phenotypes in individuals with depression who had redeemed prescriptions for (es)citalopram, sertraline, or fluoxetine for the first time between 1 January 1996 and 31 December 2016.

4.2. Data Sources

We used data of the Integrative Psychiatric Research (iPSYCH) consortium, which has established a large Danish population-based case-cohort sample (iPSYCH2012) [33]. Details of iPSYCH2012 have been previously described [18]. In brief, the iPSYCH sample was selected from all individuals born as singletons between 1 May 1981 and 31 December 2005 who were alive and living in Denmark at their first birthday. iPSYCH2012 included (1) a randomly selected population-based cohort of 30,000 individuals, representative of the entire Danish population born between 1981 and 2005, and (2) all individuals (cases, n = 57,377) who had one or more hospital-based diagnoses of five selected severe mental disorders by 31 December 2012, including schizophrenia, affective disorders, bipolar disorder, attention-deficit/hyperactivity disorder (ADHD), and autism spectrum disorder [18].

iPSYCH2012 is linked via the anonymized personal identification number assigned to the residents of Denmark at birth or immigration to longitudinal data of the following: (i) The Danish Civil Registration System [34]; (ii) The Danish Psychiatric Central Research Register (PCRR) [35]; (iii) The Danish National Prescription Registry [36] holding information on prescriptions redeemed at community pharmacies since 1995; (iv) the Danish National Patient Register [37]; (v) the Danish Register of Causes of Death [38]; (vi) the socio-demographic and labor market-related data hosted at Statistics Denmark (DST) [39]; and (vii) the Danish Neonatal Screening Biobank [40], which stores dried blood spots from practically all neonates in Denmark.

4.3. Genotyping and Phenotyping

Genetic information of the individuals in iPSYCH2012 was collected from the dried blood spots retrieved from the Danish Neonatal Screening Biobank [40]. A total of 80,422 samples were genotyped using the Infinium PsychChip v1.0 array (Illumina, San Diego, CA, USA). The array-based genotyped SNPs were imputed using 1000 Genomes

Project phase 3, with GRCh37 as a reference. [41]. After sample and genotype QC using the Ricopilli bioinformatics pipeline [42], 6,361,597 high-quality best guess-genotypes were available. See Schorck et al. 2019 for a detailed description of the imputation and QC procedures [43].

4.4. Study Population and Study Period

From iPSYCH2012, we identified all individuals with a hospital-based depression diagnosis of F32–33 according to the International Classification of Diseases, 10th edition (ICD-10) as psychiatric inpatient, outpatient, or emergency department admissions at any time between 1 January 1996 and 31 December 2012 [44]. Of those. we included all individuals redeeming a first-time (i.e., incident new-use since 1995) prescription for (es)citalopram, sertraline, or fluoxetine between 1 January 1996 and 31 December 2016 (study period, Figure 2) [45]. Thus, we did not include individuals diagnosed with a mental disorder before the start of the study period (1 January 1996) or a prescription redemption for an SSRI of interest in 1995. We defined the date of the first prescription redemption of the respective drug as the index date.

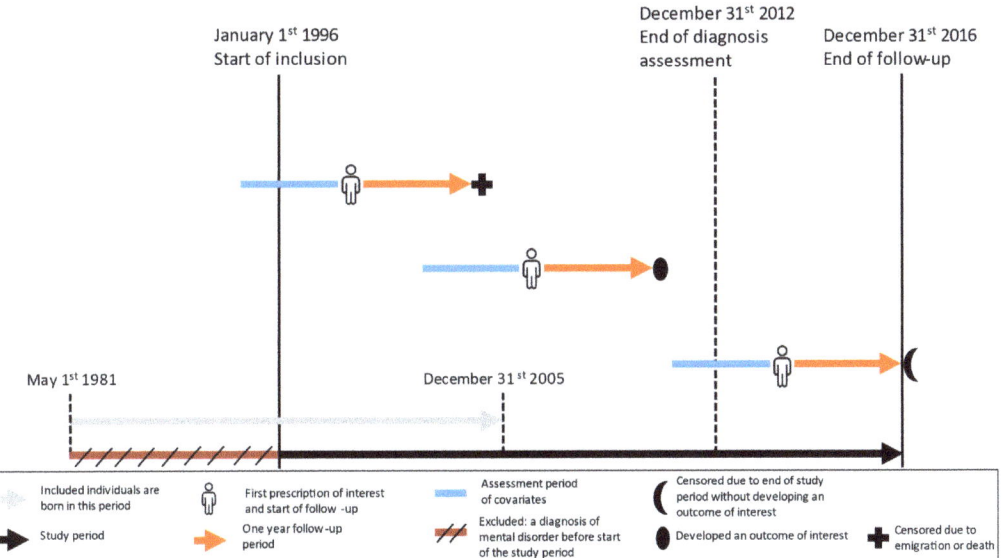

Figure 2. The selection of the study population, study design, and follow-up.

4.5. CYP2C19 and CYP2D6 Genotyping and Phenotyping

The exposure was defined as expression of any mutant CYP2C19 (UM, RM, IM, or PM) or CYP2D6 genotype/phenotype (IM or PM) based on the array-based SNP information [46,47]. Non-exposed individuals who did not carry a mutant CYP2C19 or CYP2D6 genetic variant and were classified as NM. The PGx phenotype translation procedure has been described in detail [46]. In short, the translation based on the 2019 Ubiquitous-PGx (U-PGx) panel [23] included 9 variants for CYP2C19 and 8 variants for CYP2D6, including CYP2D6 duplication and deletion. The SNPs were linked to star (*) allele nomenclature, which standardizes genetic polymorphism annotations for cytochrome P450 genes to simplify the translations of a patient's genotype into a predicted clinical phenotype [48–50]. For CYPC19, the star-alleles *2, *8, and *17 variants and the CYPCD6 the star-alleles *4, *10, *17, and *41 were available. Based on the individuals' genotypes, the diplotypes were translated into the PGx phenotypes (Tables S1 and S2).

4.6. Outcomes

Outcomes were assessed within one year of the index date (Figure 1) as follows: (1) Switching from the index prescription to any other antidepressant (ATC: N06A); (2) Discontinuation, defined as less than three prescriptions of the index antidepressant; (3) Emergency department contact at a psychiatric hospital; (4) Suicide attempt/self-harm, which was identified according to the algorithm as described by Gasse et al. [51].

4.7. Covariates

Detailed definitions of all the covariates and confounders are shown in Table S3. Covariates included the following: age, gender, region of index prescription, socio-economic status (SES, assessed for the adults of the study population and for the parents of the children of the study population), number of previous psychiatric diagnoses, prescription drug use acting as CYP2C19/CYP2D6 inhibitor/inducer within the last three months of the index date, calendar year of index prescription, any hospital contacts within the previous year of index date, previous suicide attempt/self-harm, and antiepileptic drug use within the last three months prior to the index date.

4.8. Statistical Analyses

The analysis was performed separately for the three age groups (children and adolescents, young adults, adults) because of the differences in disease states, enzyme activity, experience of adverse events, and choice of antidepressant treatment in children and adults. Children and adolescents with depression must be referred to a pediatric psychiatrist before treatment initiation, irrespective of the severity of depression, according to Danish guidelines [13]. Young adults with depression should be referred to a psychiatrist within one week after the start of antidepressant treatment. Adults are often treated solely by general practitioners and are only recommended to be referred to a psychiatric department if treatment with two different antidepressants has failed or suicidality is suspected, in diagnostic doubts, and/or the presence of psychotic symptoms or somatic disorders that complicate treatment with antidepressants [52].

We described the characteristics of the study population at the index date as proportions (%). We followed all individuals from the index date for one year. Individuals were censored at end of follow-up, outcome events, emigration, or death, whichever came first. We calculated incidence rates (IR) using SAS %Lexis macro [53]. The IRs were modeled in a Poisson regression analysis (using follow-up as offset) to investigate the association between CYP2C19/CYP2D6 phenotype status and clinical outcomes, which was presented as incidence rate ratios (IRR) with 95% confidence intervals (CI). We considered a 95% CI that did not overlap 1.00 to be statistically significant.

All analyses were adjusted for the following potential covariates and confounders: age, gender, region of index prescription, socio-economic status (SES, assessed for the adults of the study population and for the parents of the children of the study population (Table S3), number of previous psychiatric diagnoses, CYP2C19/CYP2D6 inhibitor/inducer use within the last three months of the index date, and calendar year of index prescription. For emergency department contact, we further adjusted for any hospital contacts within the previous year of the index date. For the outcome of suicide attempt/self-harm, we additionally adjusted for previous suicide attempt/self-harm and for antiepileptic drug use within the last three months of index date.

We have reported the potential clinical utility of PGx testing for CYP2C19 and CYP2D6 genetic variability by calculating the population attributable fraction (PAF), number needed to treat (NNT), and number needed to genotype (NNG) for all significant associations, based on Tonk et al. [16].

All data processing and analyses were carried out using SAS statistical software version 9.4 (SAS Institute Inc., Cary, NC, USA).

4.9. Data Protection

Data permissions have been granted to iPSYCH2012 by The Danish Scientific Ethics Committee (EC: 1-10-72-287-12), the Danish Health Data Authority, the Danish data protection agency, and the Danish Neonatal Screening Biobank Steering Committee. Danish Data Protection Agency: Journal number 2015-57-0002 /Journal number: 62908 (Umbrella permission Aarhus University) and National Board of Health: FSEID 00000098. Researchers can access anonymous individual-level data only through secure servers where the download of individual-level information is prohibited, which protects the privacy of the individuals included in the study. Due to data protection, we do not report numbers below five, but state '<5', or combine categories to achieve larger counts than five.

5. Conclusions

Our study adds new knowledge of the associations between CYP2C19 and CYP2D6 phenotypes and antidepressant switching, discontinuation, emergency department contacts, and suicide attempt/self-harm in children, adolescents, and adults with depression with incident new-use of (es)citalopram, sertraline, or fluoxetine, which indicates the clinical utility of PGx in patients with depression. Even though the associations were strong and pronounced from a population perspective, the nominal clinical utility remains low, due to the multifactorial contribution of many factors to the outcomes. Children and adolescents seem to be a relevant target group benefitting from PGx testing where clinical data is still rare and urgently needed, because a large part of the existing evidence is deduced from adult data.

Supplementary Materials: The following supporting information can be downloaded at: https://www.mdpi.com/article/10.3390/ph15070870/s1.

Author Contributions: Conceptualization, D.J.M. and C.G.; Data curation, E.A. and C.A.T.C.L.; Formal analysis, K.I.-A. and J.P.T.; Funding acquisition, C.G., C.A.T.C.L. and L.S.T.; Investigation, L.S.T.; Methodology, L.S.T., K.I.-A., C.A.T.C.L. and C.G.; Project administration, C.G.; Supervision, D.J.M. and C.G.; Writing—original draft, L.S.T.; Writing—review & editing, K.I.-A., J.P.T., E.A., D.J.M. and C.G. All authors have read and agreed to the published version of the manuscript.

Funding: The study was funded by unrestricted grants received by C. Gasse of the Alfred Benzon foundation, Denmark, and the Novo Nordisk foundation, Denmark (NNF17OC0029488), by C.A.T.C. Lunenburg of the Lundbeck foundation, Denmark (R322-2019-2404), and by L.S. Thiele of the Lundbeck foundation, Denmark (F-61171-19-27). The funders had no role in the study design, data collection and analysis, decision to publish, or preparation of the manuscript. The genotyping of the iPSYCH2012 samples was supported by grant numbers R102-A9118 and R155-2014-1724 from the Lundbeck Foundation, the Stanley Foundation, the Simons Foundation (SFARI 311789), and the National Institutes of Mental Health (NIMH 5U01MH094432-02). The Danish National Biobank resource is supported by the Novo Nordisk Foundation.

Institutional Review Board Statement: Data permissions have been granted to iPSYCH2012 by The Danish Scientific Ethics Committee (EC: 1-10-72-287-12), the Danish Health Data Authority, the Danish data protection agency, and the Danish Neonatal Screening Biobank Steering Committee. Danish Data Protection Agency: Journal number 2015-57-0002 /Journal number: 62908 (Umbrella permission Aarhus University) and National Board of Health: FSEID 00000098.

Informed Consent Statement: Patient consent was waived due to researchers can access anonymous individual-level data only through secure servers where the download of individual-level information is prohibited, which protects the privacy of the individuals included in the study. Due to data protection, we do not report numbers below five, but state '<5', or combine categories to achieve larger counts than five.

Data Availability Statement: Data is contained within the article and Supplementary Material.

Acknowledgments: The authors would like to thank the primary investigators of the iPSYCH consortium and members of the iPSYCH consortium for data acquisition and access.

Conflicts of Interest: The authors declare no competing interests.

References

1. Malhi, G.S.; Mann, J.J. Depression. *Lancet* **2018**, *392*, 2299–2312. [CrossRef]
2. McAllister-Williams, R.H.; Arango, C.; Blier, P.; Demyttenaere, K.; Falkai, P.; Gorwood, P.; Hopwood, M.; Javed, A.; Kasper, S.; Malhi, G.S.; et al. The identification, assessment and management of difficult-to-treat depression: An international consensus statement. *J. Affect Disord.* **2020**, *267*, 264–282. [CrossRef] [PubMed]
3. Bousman, C.A.; Bengesser, S.A.; Aitchison, K.J.; Amare, A.T.; Aschauer, H.; Baune, B.T.; Behroozi Asl, B.; Bishop, J.R.; Burmeister, M.; Chaumette, B.; et al. Review and consensus on pharmacogenomic testing in psychiatry. *Pharmacopsychiatry* **2021**, *54*, 5–17. [CrossRef] [PubMed]
4. Jukić, M.M.; Haslemo, T.; Molden, E.; Ingelman-Sundberg, M. Impact of CYP2C19 genotype on escitalopram exposure and therapeutic failure: A retrospective study based on 2087 Patients. *Am. J. Psychiatry* **2018**, *175*, 463–470. [CrossRef] [PubMed]
5. Milosavljevic, F.; Bukvic, N.; Pavlovic, Z.; Miljevic, C.; Pešic, V.; Molden, E.; Ingelman-Sundberg, M.; Leucht, S.; Jukic, M.M. Association of CYP2C19 and CYP2D6 poor and intermediate metabolizer status with antidepressant and antipsychotic exposure: A systematic review and meta-analysis. *JAMA Psychiatry* **2021**, *78*, 270–280. [CrossRef]
6. Fabbri, C.; Tansey, K.E.; Perlis, R.H.; Hauser, J.; Henigsberg, N.; Maier, W.; Mors, O.; Placentino, A.; Rietschel, M.; Souery, D.; et al. Effect of cytochrome CYP2C19 metabolizing activity on antidepressant response and side effects: Meta-analysis of data from genome-wide association studies. *Eur. Neuropsychopharmacol.* **2018**, *28*, 945–954. [CrossRef]
7. Lunenburg, C.A.; Gasse, C. Pharmacogenetics in psychiatric care, a call for uptake of available applications. *Psychiatry Res.* **2020**, *292*, 113336. [CrossRef]
8. Schmidt, M.; Hallas, J.; Laursen, M.; Friis, S. Data Resource Profile: Danish online drug use statistics (MEDSTAT). *Int. J. Epidemiol.* **2016**, *45*, 1401–1402g. [CrossRef]
9. Mars, B.; Heron, J.; Kessler, D.; Davies, N.M.; Martin, R.M.; Thomas, K.H.; Gunnell, D. Influences on antidepressant prescribing trends in the UK: 1995–2011. *Soc. Psychiatry Psychiatr. Epidemiol.* **2017**, *52*, 193–200. [CrossRef]
10. Milani, S.A.; Raji, M.A.; Chen, L.; Kuo, Y.-F. Trends in the Use of Benzodiazepines, Z-Hypnotics, and Serotonergic Drugs Among US Women and Men Before and During the COVID-19 Pandemic. *JAMA Netw. Open* **2021**, *4*, e2131012. [CrossRef]
11. Whirl-Carrillo, M.; Huddart, R.; Gong, L.; Sangkuhl, K.; Thorn, C.F.; Whaley, R.; Klein, T.E. An Evidence-Based Framework for Evaluating Pharmacogenomics Knowledge for Personalized Medicine. *Clin. Pharmacol. Ther.* **2021**, *110*, 563–572. [CrossRef]
12. Dutch Pharmacogenetics Working Group. Dutch Pharmacogenetics Working Group Guidelines 2018. Available online: https://api.pharmgkb.org/v1/download/file/attachment/DPWG_November_2018.pdf (accessed on 10 July 2022).
13. Retsinformation. Vejledning om Medikamentel Behandling af Børn og Unge Med Psykiske Lidelse. 2019. Available online: https://www.retsinformation.dk/eli/retsinfo/2019/9733 (accessed on 10 July 2022).
14. Ramsey, L.B.; Bishop, J.R.; Strawn, J.R. Pharmacogenetics of treating pediatric anxiety and depression. *Pharmacogenomics* **2019**, *20*, 867–870. [CrossRef] [PubMed]
15. Jürgens, G.; Jacobsen, C.B.; Rasmussen, H.B.; Werge, T.; Nordentoft, M.; Andersen, S.E. Utility and adoption of CYP2D6 and CYP2C19 genotyping and its translation into psychiatric clinical practice. *Acta Psychiatr. Scand.* **2012**, *125*, 228–237. [CrossRef] [PubMed]
16. Tonk, E.C.M.; Gurwitz, D.; Der Zee, A.-H.M.-V.; Janssens, A.C.J.W. Assessment of pharmacogenetic tests: Presenting measures of clinical validity and potential population impact in association studies. *Pharmacogenomics* **2017**, *17*, 386–392. [CrossRef] [PubMed]
17. Jansen, M.E.; Rigter, T.; Rodenburg, W.; Fleur, T.M.C.; Houwink, E.J.F.; Weda, M.; Cornel, M.C. Review of the reported measures of clinical validity and clinical utility as arguments for the implementation of pharmacogenetic testing: A case study of statin-induced muscle toxicity. *Front. Pharmacol.* **2017**, *8*, 555. [CrossRef]
18. Poweleit, E.A.; Aldrich, S.L.; Martin, L.J.; Hahn, D.; Strawn, J.R.; Ramsey, L.B. Pharmacogenetics of sertraline tolerability and response in pediatric anxiety and depressive disorders. *J. Child Adolesc. Psychopharmacol.* **2019**, *29*, 348–361. [CrossRef]
19. Jessel, C.D.; Mostafa, S.; Potiriadis, M.; Everall, I.P.; Gunn, J.M.; Bousman, C.A. Use of antidepressants with pharmacogenetic prescribing guidelines in a 10-year depression cohort of adult primary care patients. *Pharm. Genom.* **2020**, *30*, 145–152. [CrossRef]
20. Aldrich, S.L.; Poweleit, E.A.; Prows, C.A.; Martin, L.J.; Strawn, J.R.; Ramsey, L.B. Influence of CYP2C19 Metabolizer status on escitalopram/citalopram tolerability and response in youth with anxiety and depressive disorders. *Front. Pharmacol.* **2019**, *10*, 99. [CrossRef]
21. Campos, A.I.; Byrne, E.M.; Mitchell, B.L.; Wray, N.R.; Lind, P.A.; Licinio, J.; Medland, S.E.; Martin, N.G.; Hickie, I.B.; Rentería, M.E. Impact of CYP2C19 metaboliser status on SSRI response: A retrospective study of 9500 participants of the Australian Genetics of Depression Study. *Pharm. J.* **2022**, *22*, 130–135. [CrossRef]
22. Chen, Q.-H.; Li, Y.-L.; Hu, Y.-R.; Liang, W.-Y.; Zhang, B. Observing time effect of SSRIs on suicide risk and suicide-related behaviour: A network meta-analysis protocol. *BMJ Open* **2021**, *11*, e054479. [CrossRef]
23. Van der Wouden, C.H.; Cambon-Thomsen, A.; Cecchin, E.; Cheung, K.C.; Dávila-Fajardo, C.L.; Deneer, V.H.; Dolžan, M.; Ingelman-Sundberg, M.; Jönsson, S.; Karlsson, M.O.; et al. Implementing pharmacogenomics in Europe: Design and implementation strategy of the ubiquitous pharmacogenomics consortium. *Clin. Pharmacol. Ther.* **2017**, *101*, 341–358. [CrossRef] [PubMed]
24. Höfer, P.; Schosser, A.; Calati, R.; Serretti, A.; Massat, I.; Kocabas, N.A.; Konstantinidis, A.; Linotte, S.; Mendlewicz, J.; Souery, D.; et al. The impact of Cytochrome P450 CYP1A2, CYP2C9, CYP2C19 and CYP2D6 genes on suicide attempt and suicide risk—A European multicentre study on treatment-resistant major depressive disorder. *Eur. Arch. Psychiatry Clin. Neurosci.* **2013**, *263*, 385–391. [CrossRef] [PubMed]

25. Rahikainen, A.L.; Vauhkonen, P.; Pett, H.; Palo, J.U.; Haukka, J.; Ojanperä, I.; Niemi, M.; Sajantila, A. Completed suicides of citalopram users-the role of CYP genotypes and adverse drug interactions. *Int. J. Legal Med.* **2019**, *133*, 353–363. [CrossRef] [PubMed]
26. Available online: https://medstat.dk/ (accessed on 8 June 2022).
27. Gassó, P.; Rodríguez, N.; Mas, S.; Pagerols, M.; Blázquez, A.; Plana, M.T.; Torra, M.; Lázaro, L.; Lafuente, A. Effect of CYP2D6, CYP2C9 and ABCB1 genotypes on fluoxetine plasma concentrations and clinical improvement in children and adolescent patients. *Pharm. J.* **2014**, *14*, 457–462. [CrossRef] [PubMed]
28. Roberts, R.L.; Mulder, R.T.; Joyce, P.R.; Luty, S.E.; Kennedy, M.A. No evidence of increased adverse drug reactions in cytochrome P450CYP2D6 poor metabolizers treated with fluoxetine or nortriptyline. *Hum. Psychopharmacol. Clin. Exp.* **2004**, *19*, 17–23. [CrossRef]
29. Hicks, J.B.; Sangkuhl, K.; Muller, D.J.; Ji, Y.; Leckband, S.G.; Leeder, J.S.; Graham, R.L.; Chiulli, D.L.; LLerena, A.; Skaar, T.C.; et al. Clinical Pharmacogenetics Implementation Consortium (CPIC) Guideline for CYP2D6 and CYP2C19 Genotypes and Dosing of Selective Serotonin Reuptake Inhibitors. 2015. Available online: https://files.cpicpgx.org/data/guideline/publication/SSRI/2015/25974703.pdf (accessed on 10 July 2022).
30. Petrović, J.; Pešić, V.; Lauschke, V.M. Frequencies of clinically important CYP2C19 and CYP2D6 alleles are graded across Europe. *Eur. J. Hum. Genet.* **2020**, *28*, 88–94. [CrossRef] [PubMed]
31. Shelton, R.C.; Parikh, S.V.; Law, R.A.; Rothschild, A.J.; Thase, M.E.; Dunlop, B.W.; DeBattista, C.; Conway, C.R.; Forester, B.P.; Macaluso, M.; et al. Combinatorial pharmacogenomic algorithm is predictive of citalopram and escitalopram metabolism in patients with major depressive disorder. *Psychiatry Res.* **2020**, *290*, 113017. [CrossRef]
32. Montgomery, S.; Hansen, T.; Kasper, S. Efficacy of escitalopram compared to citalopram: A meta-analysis. *Int. J. Neuropsychopharmacol.* **2011**, *14*, 261–268. [CrossRef]
33. Pedersen, C.B.; Bybjerg-Grauholm, J.; Pedersen, M.G.; Grove, J.; Agerbo, E.; Bækvad-Hansen, M.; Poulsen, J.B.; Hansen, C.S.; McGrath, J.J.; Als, T.D.; et al. The iPSYCH2012 case–cohort sample: New directions for unravelling genetic and environmental architectures of severe mental disorders. *Mol. Psychiatr.* **2018**, *23*, 6–14. [CrossRef]
34. Pedersen, C.B.; Gøtzsche, H.; Møller, J.O.; Mortensen, P.B. The Danish Civil Registration System. A cohort of eight million persons. *Dan. Med. Bull.* **2006**, *53*, 441–449. [CrossRef]
35. Mors, O.; Perto, G.P.; Mortensen, P.B. The Danish Psychiatric Central Research Register. *Scand. J. Public Health* **2011**, *39*, 54–57.
36. Kildemoes, H.W.; Sørensen, H.T.; Hallas, J. The Danish national prescription registry. *Scand. J. Public Health* **2011**, *39* (Suppl. 7), 38–41. [CrossRef] [PubMed]
37. Lynge, E.; Sandegaard, J.L.; Rebolj, M. The Danish national patient register. *Scand. J. Public Health* **2011**, *39* (Suppl. 7), 30–33. [CrossRef] [PubMed]
38. Helweg-Larsen, K. The Danish Register of Causes of Death. *Scand. J. Public Health* **2011**, *39* (Suppl. 7), 26–29.
39. Statistics Denmark. Data for Research. Available online: https://www.dst.dk/en/TilSalg/Forskningsservice) (accessed on 10 July 2022).
40. Nørgaard-Pedersen, B.; Hougaard, D.M. Storage policies and use of the Danish Newborn Screening Biobank. *J. Inherit Metab. Dis.* **2007**, *30*, 530–536. [CrossRef]
41. 1000 Genome Project. Available online: https://www.internationalgenome.org/category/phase-3/ (accessed on 10 July 2022).
42. Broad Institute. Ricopili. Available online: https://data.broadinstitute.org/mpg/ricopili/ (accessed on 10 July 2022).
43. Schork, A.J.; Won, H.; Appadurai, V.; Nudel, R.; Gandal, M.; Delaneau, O.; Revsbech Christiansen, M.; Hougaard, D.M.; Bækved-Hansen, M.; Bybjerg-Grauholm, J.; et al. A genome-wide association study of shared risk across psychiatric disorders implicates gene regulation during fetal neurodevelopment. *Nat. Neurosci.* **2019**, *22*, 353–361. [CrossRef]
44. World Health Organization. *ICD-10: International Statistical Classification of Diseases and Related Health Problems: Tenth Revision*, 2nd ed.; World Health Organization: Geneva, Switzerldand, 2004.
45. Suissa, S.; Moodie, E.E.M.; Dell'Aniello, S. Prevalent new-user cohort designs for comparative drug effect studies by time-conditional propensity scores. *Pharmacoepidemiol. Drug Saf.* **2017**, *26*, 459–468. [CrossRef]
46. Lunenburg, C.A.T.C.; Thirstrup, J.P.; Bybjerg-Grauholm, J.; Bækvad-Hansen, M.; Hougaard, D.M.; Nordentoft, M.; Werge, T.; Børglum, A.D.; Mors, O.; Mortensen, P.B.; et al. Pharmacogenetic genotype and phenotype frequencies in a large Danish population-based case-cohort sample. *Transl. Psychiatry* **2021**, *11*, 294. [CrossRef]
47. Caudle, K.E.; Dunnenberger, H.M.; Freimuth, R.R.; Peterson, J.F.; Burlison, J.D.; Whirl-Carrillo, M.; Scott, S.A.; Rehm, H.L.; Williams, M.S.; Klein, T.E.; et al. Standardizing terms for clinical pharmacogenetic test results: Consensus terms from the Clinical Pharmacogenetics Implementation Consortium (CPIC). *Genet. Med.* **2017**, *19*, 215–223. [CrossRef]
48. Robarge, J.D.; Li, L.; Desta, Z.; Nguyen, A.; A Flockhart, D. The star-allele nomenclature: Retooling for translational genomics. *Clin. Pharmacol. Ther.* **2007**, *82*, 244–248. [CrossRef]
49. Botton, M.R.; Whirl-Carrillo, M.; Del Tredici, A.L.; Sangkuhl, K.; Cavallari, L.H.; Agúndez, J.A.G.; Duconge, J.; Lee, M.T.M.; Woodahl, E.L.; Claudio-Campos, K.; et al. PharmVar GeneFocus: CYP2C19. *Clin. Pharmacol. Ther.* **2021**, *109*, 352–366. [CrossRef] [PubMed]
50. Nofziger, C.; Turner, A.J.; Sangkuhl, K.; Whirl-Carrillo, M.; Agúndez, J.A.G.; Black, J.L.; Dunnenberger, H.M.; Ruano, G.; Kennedy, M.A.; Phillips, M.S.; et al. PharmVar GeneFocus: CYP2D6. *Clin. Pharmacol. Ther.* **2020**, *107*, 154–170. [CrossRef] [PubMed]

51. Gasse, C.; Danielsen, A.A.; Pedersen, M.G.; Pedersen, C.B.; Mors, O.; Christensen, J. Positive predictive value of a register-based algorithm using the Danish National Registries to identify suicidal events. *Pharmacoepidemiol. Drug Saf.* **2018**, *27*, 1131–1138. [CrossRef] [PubMed]
52. Sundhedsstyrelsen. Den Nationale Rekommandationsliste (NRL): Unipolar Depression. 2019. Available online: https://sst.dk/da/viden/laegemidler/anbefalinger/den-nationale-rekommandationsliste-_nrl_/unipolar-depression (accessed on 14 June 2022).
53. Carstensen, B.; Dickman, P. Lexis Macro for Splitting Follow-Up 2003. Available online: http://bendixcarstensen/Lexis/ (accessed on 10 July 2022).

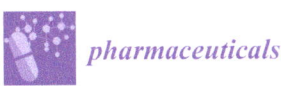 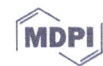

Article

Comparison of Multidrug Use in the General Population and among Persons with Diabetes in Denmark for Drugs Having Pharmacogenomics (PGx) Based Dosing Guidelines

Niels Westergaard [1,*], Lise Tarnow [2] and Charlotte Vermehren [3,4]

[1] Centre for Engineering and Science, Department of Biomedical Laboratory Science, University College Absalon, Parkvej 190, 4700 Naestved, Denmark
[2] Steno Diabetes Center, Birkevaenget 3, 3rd, 4300 Holbaek, Denmark; litar@regionsjaelland.dk
[3] Department of Clinical Pharmacology, University Hospital of Copenhagen, Bispebjergbakke 23, 2400 Copenhagen, Denmark; charlotte.vermehren@regionh.dk
[4] Department of Drug Design and Pharmacology, Faculty of Health and Medical Sciences, University of Copenhagen, Universitetsparken 2, 2100 Copenhagen, Denmark
* Correspondence: niew@pha.dk

Abstract: Background: This study measures the use of drugs within the therapeutic areas of antithrombotic agents (B01), the cardiovascular system (C), analgesics (N02), psycholeptics (N05), and psychoanaleptics (N06) among the general population (GP) in comparison to persons with diabetes in Denmark. The study focuses on drugs having pharmacogenomics (PGx) based dosing guidelines for CYP2D6, CYP2C19, and SLCO1B1 to explore the potential of applying PGx-based decision-making into clinical practice taking drug–drug interactions (DDI) and drug–gene interactions (DGI) into account. Methods: This study is cross-sectional, using The Danish Register of Medicinal Product Statistics as the source to retrieve drug consumption data. Results: The prevalence of use in particular for antithrombotic agents (B01) and cardiovascular drugs (C) increases significantly by 4 to 6 times for diabetic users compared to the GP, whereas the increase for analgesics (N02), psycholeptics, and psychoanaleptics (N06) was somewhat less (2–3 times). The five most used PGx drugs, both in the GP and among persons with diabetes, were pantoprazole, simvastatin, atorvastatin, metoprolol, and tramadol. The prevalence of use for persons with diabetes compared to the GP (prevalence ratio) increased by an average factor of 2.9 for all PGx drugs measured. In addition, the prevalence of use of combinations of PGx drugs was 4.6 times higher for persons with diabetes compared to GP. In conclusion, the findings of this study clearly show that a large fraction of persons with diabetes are exposed to drugs or drug combinations for which there exist PGx-based dosing guidelines related to CYP2D6, CYP2C19, and SLCO1B1. This further supports the notion of accessing and accounting for not only DDI but also DGI and phenoconversion in clinical decision-making, with a particular focus on persons with diabetes.

Keywords: pharmacogenomics; polypharmacy; persons with diabetes; drug–drug interactions; drug–gene interactions; cytochrome P450; SLCO1B1; drug interaction checkers

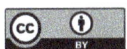

1. Introduction

Personalized medicine denotes a paradigm shift within medicine that addresses the patient's individual situation and, most notably, the genetic predispositions of patients in terms of metabolic differences in, e.g., the cytochrome P450 (CYP450) drug-metabolizing enzymes [1,2], leading to variability in drug response [1–3]. Diabetes is a complex, chronic illness requiring continuous medical care with multifactorial risk-reduction strategies beyond glycemic control [4]. The prevalence of diabetes continues to increase in virtually all regions of the world, with more than 415 million people worldwide now living with diabetes [5,6]. In Denmark, it is estimated to be 280.000 people [7]. Elderly people, in particular, are more prone to develop diabetes concomitantly leading to associated multiple chronic conditions such as hypertension, dyslipidaemia, coronary heart disease, depression and chronic kidney disease [6,8,9]. In order to prevent, treat and relieve these conditions the introduction of polypharmacy, including prescription cascades and inappropriate medication [8–10], is inevitable and so is the occurrence of adverse drug reactions (ADR) and drug–drug interactions (DDI) [8,9,11,12].

Not surprisingly, polypharmacy has been shown to be a significant precipitating factor in frequent hospital admissions [13] and increased risk of mortality [14]. Initiatives both internationally and in Denmark have been taken to incite the best clinical management of patients with multimorbidity and polypharmacy [15–17]. These initiatives are, however, often complicated by requiring multiple specialists to be involved in care planning and execution [18]. Therefore, any action that can improve the medical treatment of polypharmacy patients should be carefully considered as a valuable tool to obtain appropriate drug treatment.

CYP450 drug metabolising enzymes are responsible for catalysing the oxidative biotransformation of a large fraction of drugs in daily clinical use to either inactive metabolites or active substances from pro-drugs [19]. In particular, CYP2D6 and CYP2C19 have attracted considerable attention as the major targets for pharmacogenomics (PGx)-based testing because they are highly polymorphic and have been shown to affect both drug response and ADR [2,3,20]. The pharmacogenetic impact on the interaction between drug and CYP450 isozymes, referred to as drug–gene interaction (DGI), has been incorporated into clinical actionable dosing guidelines (AG) and non-actionable dosing guidelines (N-AG) for specific DGIs (see PharmGKB) [21]. Accordingly, a person can be scored as "poor metaboliser" (PM), "intermediate metaboliser" (IM), "extensive metaboliser" (EM; normal activity) and "rapid or ultra-rapid metaboliser" (RM and UM with UM having faster metabolic activity than RM [22–24]. In addition, single nucleotide polymorphisms (SNP) in the solute carrier organic anion transporter 1B1 (*SLCO1B1*) correlate with an increase in the plasma exposure to statins which can lead to muscle toxicity, a common statin-related ADR occurring in 1–5% of exposed users [25] in a dose-dependent fashion. Since statins are some of the most commonly prescribed drugs [25], many people are potentially affected by muscle-related ADR. PGx-based AGs are available for the phenotypes having an intermediate or low function of SLCO1B1 [25]. Daily exposure of patients to drugs having AG is not at all negligible as shown previously [26–30] and additionally makes a significant contribution to the occurrence of side effects [28,29]. In particular, the elderly part of the population is exposed to drugs or drug combinations for which there exist AGs related to PGx of CYP2D6 and CYP2C19 and SLCO1B1 [29,30]. Recently, we have demonstrated that the use of clopidogrel and proton pump inhibitors (PPIs), both having PGx-based AG and FDA annotations, either given alone or in combination is quite widespread, in particular among persons with diabetes and the elderly in Denmark [31]. The aim of this study is to further measure and scrutinize the use of drugs within the therapeutic areas of antithrombotic agents (B01), the cardiovascular system (C), analgesics (N02), psycholeptics (N05) and psycoanaleptics (N06) among the general population in comparison to persons with diabetes in Denmark and with a particular focus on of drugs having PGx-based dosing guidelines to further explore the potential of applying PGx-based decision-making into clinical practice.

2. Results

According to the ATC nomenclature, A10 denotes "drugs used in diabetes" which can be subdivided into A10A "insulins and analogues" and A10B "blood glucose lowering drugs excl. insulins". In this study, persons with diabetes are identified by looking at individuals who redeemed drug prescriptions of A10 during 2018 at a Danish pharmacy. Altogether, 258,494 persons were identified out of a total Danish population of 5,781,190 inhabitants. This corresponds to 4.5% of the Danish population. Table 1 shows the age distribution, as well as the total consumption of A10, A10A, A10B and A10A/B (persons who have redeemed both A10A and A10B), expressed as the number of users and prevalence of use (diabetic users/1000 inhabitants). The number of users is additive horizontally, so the total number of users of A10 is the sum of users of A10A, A10B, and A10A/B. The table illustrates how the number of users and the prevalence of use increase with age—in particular, for users of A10B. This group, as well as A10A/B, have a significant onset in drug use in the age group of 45–64 years. Relative to A10, 16.2% of the users with diabetes redeemed drug prescriptions of A10A, 67.5% of A10B and 16.3% the combination of A10A/B.

Table 1. Consumption of drugs used in diabetes.

Age Group	A10	A10A	A10B	A10A/B
0–17	3107 (2.7)	2987 (2.6)	105 (0.1)	15 (<0.1)
18–24	3695 (6.9)	2646 (5.0)	952 (1.8)	97 (0.2)
25–44	23,685 (16.4)	8311 (5.8)	13,153 (9.1)	2221 (1.5)
45–64	94,880 (62.2)	13,194 (8.7)	65,928 (43.2)	15,758 (10.3)
65–79	103,926 (120.9)	10,327 (12.0)	74,102 (86.2)	19,497 (22.7)
80+	29,201 (113.8)	4447 (17.3)	20,262 (78.9)	4492 (17.5)
All	258,494 (44.7)	41,912 (7.3)	174,502 (30.2)	42,080 (7.3)

Note: Data are presented as the total number of users who redeemed prescriptions of the ATC codes A10 (level 2) denoted as "drugs used in diabetes", A10A (insulins and analogues), A10B (blood glucose-lowering drugs excl. insulins) or the combination thereof 10A/B during 2018. The numbers in brackets show prevalence of use (number of users/1000 inhabitants).

Tables 2 and 3 show the use and prevalence of use of different pharmacological drug classes measured at different levels of ATC codes covering antithrombotic agent's (B01), the cardiovascular system (C), analgesics (N02), psycholeptics (N05) and psychoanaleptics (N06) both in the general population and among persons with diabetes. It is especially within these ATC groups that PGx-based AGs and N-AGs occur for CYP2D6, CYP2C19 and SLCO1B1. Examples of specific drugs (ATC level 5) having AGs representing each drug class are also given. The prevalence of use shown in Tables 2 and 3 is expressed relative to the total number of users of A10, A10A, A10B and A10A/B, respectively, as displayed at the bottom of Table 1. The prevalence of use in particular for antithrombotic agents (B01) and cardiovascular drugs (C) increases significantly by 4 to 6 times for users of A10 compared to the general population (Table 2), whereas the increase for analgesics (N02), psycholeptics and psychoanaleptics (N06) was somewhat less: 2–3 times, but still significant (Table 3). Comparison of users of A10A with users of A10B showed that the prevalence of use of the combinations of the different drug classes was mostly higher for users of A10B as shown in Tables 2 and 3, except for clopidogrel (same) and lower for antihypertensives, opioids, oxycodone, gabapentin, and amitriptyline. A similar comparison of users of A10B with users of A10A/B showed that the prevalence of use was higher and more pronounced for all drug combinations for users of A10A/B both when compared to users of A10A and A10B.

Table 2. Number of users and prevalence of platelet aggregation inhibitors and cardiovascular drugs.

	Denmark	A10	A10A	A10B	A10A/B
B01 (antithrombotic agents)	556,095 (96.2)	109,300 (422.8)	13,832 * (330.0)	71,648 ^ (410.6)	23,820 (566.0)
B01AC (platelet aggregation inhibitors)	395,373 (68.4)	84,862 (328.3)	10,994 * (261.1)	54,813 ^ (314.1)	19,105 (454.0)
B01AC04 Clopidogrel	127,480 (22.05)	21,746 (84.1)	3363 (80.2)	13,912 ^ (79.7)	4471 (106.3)
C (cardiovascular system)	1,413,160 (244.4)	221,472 (856.8)	26,665 * (636.1)	154,999 ^ (888.3)	39,808 (946.0)
C01 (cardiac therapy)	109,730 (19.0)	22,091 (85.5)	2760 * (65.9)	14,220 ^ (81.5)	5111 (121.5)
C02 (antihypertensives)	17,305 (3.0)	5151 (20.0)	1031 * (24.6)	2785 ^ (16.0)	1385 (31.7)
C03 (diuretics)	424,584 (73.4)	80,925 (313.1)	11,316 * (270.0)	52,129 ^ (298.7)	17,480 (415.4)
C07 (beta blocking agents)	385.920 (66.8)	71.406 (276.3)	7981 * (190.4)	48,563 ^ (278.3)	14,862 (353.2)
C07AB02 (Metoprolol)	279,767 (48.4)	52,559 (203.3)	5783 * (138.0)	35,906 ^ (205.8)	10,870 (258.3)
C08 (calcium channel blockers)	427,655 (74.0)	78,955 (305.4)	9551 * (227.8)	53,536 ^ (306.8)	15,868 (377.1)
C09 (agents acting on the renin-angiotensin system)	747,141 (129.2)	157,696 (610.1)	17,751 * (423.5)	108,958 ^ (624.4)	30,987 (736.4)
C10 (lipid modifying agents)	663,711 (114.8)	174,753 (676.0)	18,752 * (447.4)	122,359 ^ (701.2)	33,642 (799.5)
C10AA (statins)	649,020 (112.3)	171,188 (662.3)	18,039 * (430.4)	120,341 ^ (689.7)	32,808 (779.7)
C10AA01 (Simvastatin)	309,936 (53.6)	86,531 (334.8)	9106 * (217.3)	60,696 ^ (347.8)	16,729 (397.6)
C10AA05 (Atorvastatin)	304,764 (52.7)	76,599 (296.39)	7791 * (185.9)	54,606 ^ (312.9)	14,202 (337.5)

Note: Data are presented as the total number of users who redeemed drug prescriptions of the ATC codes A10, A10A, A10B and A10A/B in combination with antithrombotic agents (B01) and cardiovascular drugs (C). Numbers in brackets are prevalence (number of users/1000). * $p < 0.05$; A10A different from A10B; ^ $p < 0.05$ A10B different from A10A/B when compared horizontally (chi-square test).

Table 3. Number of users and prevalence of analgesics, psycholeptics, and psychoanaleptics.

	Denmark	A10	A10A	A10B	A10A/B
N02 (analgesics)	1,236,170 (213.8)	124,260 (480.7)	16,453 * (392,6)	83,676 ^ (479.5)	24,131 (573.5)
N02A (opiods)	390,614 (67.6)	47,006 (181.9)	7666 * (182.9)	29,130 ^ (166.9)	10,210 (242.6)
N02AA05 (Oxycodone)	79,328 (13.7)	9536 (36.9)	1856 * (44.3)	5469 ^ (31.3)	2211 (52.5)
N02AX02 (Tramadol)	211,591 (36.6)	26,302 (101.8)	3809 * (90.9)	16,697 ^ (95.7)	5796 (137.7)
R05DA05 (Codeine)	84,210 (14.6)	8987 (34.8)	1156 * (27.6)	6091 ^ (34.9)	1740 (41.4)
N02B (other analgesics and antipyretics)	1,089,807 (188.5)	113,995 (441.0)	14,711 * (351.0)	76,963 ^ (441.0)	22,321 (530.4)

Table 3. Cont.

	Denmark	A10	A10A	A10B	A10A/B
N03AX12 (Gabapentin)	78.048 (13.5)	11.559 (44.9)	1.958 * (46.7)	6.640 ^ (38.1)	3.001 (71.3)
N05 (psycoleptics)	407,387 (70.5)	37,461 (144.9)	5550 * (132.4)	25,042 ^ (143.5)	6869 (163.2)
N05A (antipsychotics)	131,836 (22.8)	13,355 (51.7)	1877 * (44.8)	8903 ^ (51.0)	2575 (61.2)
N05B (anxiolytics)	124,731 (21.6)	11,906 (46.1)	1802 * (42.9)	8079 (46.3)	2025 (48.2)
N05C (hypnotics and sedatives)	232,933 (40.3)	21,058 (81.5)	3407 * (81.3)	13,618 ^ (78,0)	4033 ^ (95.8)
N06 (psychoanaleptics)	471,341 (81.5)	44,440 (171.9)	6699 * (159.8)	28,961 ^ (166.0)	8780 (208.7)
N06A (antidepressants)	416,064 (72.0)	41,942 (162.3)	6188 * (147.6)	27,388 ^ (157.0)	8366 (198.8)
N06AA09 (Amitriptyline)	34,598 (6.0)	4334 (16.8)	693 * (16.5)	2555 ^ (14.6)	1086 (25.8)
N06AX21 (Duloxetin)	34,277 (5.9)	3852 (14.9)	533 * (12.7)	2514 ^ (14.4)	805 (19.1)

Note: Data are presented as the total number of users who redeemed drug prescriptions of the ATC codes A10, A10A, A10B and A10A/B in combination with analgesics (N02); gabapentin, psycoleptics (N05) and psychoanaleptics (N06). Numbers in brackets are prevalence (number of users/1000). * $p < 0.05$; A10A different from A10B; ^ $p < 0.05$ A10B different from A10A/B when compared horizontally (chi-square test).

Table 4 shows the use and prevalence of use of the most frequently prescribed PGx drugs having AGs or N-AGs for CYP2D6, CYP2C19 and SLCO1B1 in the general population and among persons with diabetes (A10) sorted by ATC codes. The five most used drugs both in the general population and among persons with diabetes were pantoprazole, simvastatin, atorvastatin, metoprolol, and tramadol, however, the order was different between the two groups. The prevalence of use for persons with diabetes compared to the general population (prevalence ratio) increased by an average factor of 2.9 for all drugs ranging from 1.7 for sertraline to as high as 6.2 for simvastatin except for methylphenidate and atomoxetine. Note that the number of users for the different drugs shown in the table is not additive (vertically) since dispensing to the same users can occur for the different drugs.

Table 4. Consumption of PGx drugs in the general population (GP) and among persons with diabetes (A10).

Drug Name	PGx-G	ATC	Users (GP)	Prevalence (GP)	Users (A10)	Prevalence (A10)	Prevalence Ratio
Pantoprazol	AG	A02BC02	329,222	56.95	39,287	151.98	2.7
Lansoprazol	AG	A02BC03	135,980	23.52	17,246	66.72	2.8
Omeprazol	AG	A02BC01	119,274	20.63	14,286	55.27	2.7
Esomeprazol	N-AG	A02BC05	32,295	5.59	3054	11.81	2.1
Ondansetron	AG	A04AA01	13,979	2.42	1341	5.19	2.2
Clopidogrel	AG	B01AC04	127,480	22.05	21,746	84.13	3.8
Amiodaron	N-AG	C01BD01	8582	1.48	1420	5.49	3.7
Metoprolol	AG	C07AB02	279,767	48.39	52,559	203.33	4.2
Carvedilol	N-AG	C07AG02	33,506	5.80	8004	30.96	5.3
Bisoprolol	N-AG	C07AB07	24,953	4.32	4860	18.80	4.4
Atenolol	N-AG	C07AB03	15,517	2.68	2859	11.06	4.1
Simvastatin	AG	C10AA01	309,936	53.61	86,531	334.75	6.2
Atorvastatin	AG	C10AA05	304,764	52.72	76,599	296.33	5.6

Table 4. *Cont.*

Drug Name	PGx-G	ATC	Users (GP)	Prevalence (GP)	Users (A10)	Prevalence (A10)	Prevalence Ratio
Tramadol	AG	N02AX02	211,591	36.60	26,302	101.75	2.8
Codein	AG	R05DA04	84,210	14.57	8987	34.77	2.4
Oxycodon	N-AG	N02AA05	79,328	13.72	9536	36.89	2.7
Quetiapine	N-AG	N05AH04	65,208	11.28	5540	21.43	1.9
Olanzapine	N-AG	N05AH03	17,584	3.04	1819	7.04	2.3
Risperidon	N-AG	N05AX08	16,066	2.78	1881	7.28	2.6
Aripiprazol	AG	N05AX12	12,381	2.14	1347	5.21	2.4
Sertraline	AG	N06AB06	110,671	19.14	8521	32.96	1.7
Citalopram	AG	N06AB04	90,460	15.65	9824	38.00	2.4
Mirtazapin	N-AG	N06AX11	83,603	14.46	9035	34.95	2.4
Venlafaxin	AG	N06AX16	48,398	8.37	5307	20.53	2.5
Methylphenida	N-AG	N06BA04	38,620	6.68	984	3.81	0.6
Amitriptyline	AG	N06AA09	34,598	5.98	4334	16.77	2.8
Duloxetine	N-AG	N06AX21	34,277	5.93	3852	14.90	2.5
Escitalopram	AG	N06AB10	23,607	4.08	2153	8.33	2.0
Nortriptyline	AG	N06AA10	14,339	2.48	1718	6.65	2.7
Paroxetine	AG	N06AB05	12,410	2.15	1332	5.15	2.4
Fluoxetine	N-AG	N06AB03	10,535	1.82	831	3.21	1.8
Atomoxetine	AG	N06BA09	9778	1.69	212	0.82	0.5

Note: Only drugs redeemed by more than 8000 users in the general population are shown and compared to persons with diabetes. Drugs are sorted by ATC categories. AG; actionable dosing guideline, N-AG; non-actionable dosing guideline, GP; general population.

Figure 1 shows the use of sertraline, having PGx-based AG for CYP2C19, and tramadol, having AG for CYP2D6, respectively, redeemed either alone or in combination, expressed as the total number of users and prevalence (numbers in brackets) in the general population and among persons with diabetes (A10). As can be seen, the prevalence of use of the combination of sertraline and tramadol was three times higher for persons with diabetes compared to the general population. When the prevalence of use of the combination of sertraline and tramadol was expressed relative to sertraline, 8.8% of the users of sertraline also obtain tramadol, whereas, when expressed relative to tramadol, it was less (4.6%). The same numbers for persons with diabetes were 15.4% and 5.0%, respectively. By calculating the relative risk (RR), it can be seen that persons with diabetes using sertraline have a 1.74 times higher risk of obtaining it in combination with tramadol compared to the general population whereas the same number for diabetic tramadol users is lower but still significant.

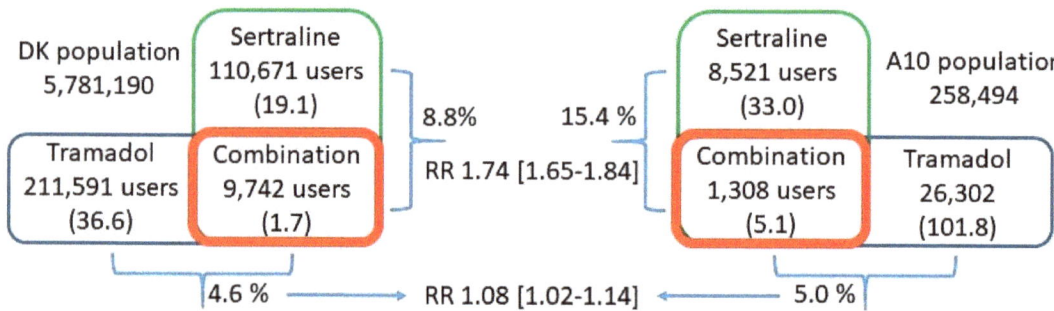

Figure 1. Prevalences of use and relative risks. Note: This figure illustrates the use of sertraline and tramadol either alone or in combination in the general population and among persons with diabetes. Numbers in brackets are prevalence (number of users/1000). Numbers in square brackets are relative risks (RR).

Table 5 is based on principles outlined in Figure 1, showing the prevalence of use of drug combinations of the most frequently redeemed drugs in each ATC category except for ondansetron and amiodarone (see Table 4) among the general population and among persons with diabetes. From the table, it can be calculated, based on the principles outlined above, that the prevalence of use of all combinations shown are on average 4.6 times higher for persons with diabetes compared to the general population, whereas the same number, when drugs are given alone (left column), is on average 3.3 higher. The lowest value was 1.6 for the combination of sertraline and quetiapine and the highest was 7.1 for the combination of simvastatin and quetiapine. Importantly, the RR of obtaining a combination of drugs was significantly higher for the majority of the combinations shown in the table for persons with diabetes compared to the general population. For, e.g., diabetic users of sertraline, the RR of obtaining it in combination with clopidogrel, metoprolol, or simvastatin was 2.35, 2.56, and 3.65, whereas for users of clopidogrel, metoprolol or simvastatin the RRs of obtaining these drugs in combination with sertraline were 1.06, 1.05, and 1.01. In addition, by using the drug interaction tracker by Medscape® [32], several of the combinations shown (in bold) are scored as "monitor close".

Table 5. Prevalences of use and relative risks (RR).

Drug Name	Alone	Clopidogrel	Metoprolol	Pantoprazole	Quetiapine	Sertraline	Tramadol	Simvastatin
Clopidogrel	84.1/22.1 (3.8)		25.7/4.7 (5.4)	20.4/4.4 (4.6)	2.1/0.5 (4.1)	4.0/1.0 (4.0)	12.1/2.6 (4.7)	31.5/7.1 (4.4)
RR			1.42 [1.39–1.45]	1.21 [1.18–1.24]	1.09 [0.99–1.19]	1.06 [1.00–1.13]	1.22 [1.18–1.26]	1.17 [1.14–1.19]
Metoprolol	203.3/48.4 (4.2)	25.7/4.7 (5.4)		41.7/8.4 (4.9)	3.6/0.8 (4.7)	6.8/1.5 (4.4)	26.7/5.2 (5.2)	76.2/11.6 (6.6)
RR		1.29 [1.26–1.32]		1.18 [1.16–1.20]	1.11 [1.04–1.20]	1.05 [1.00–1.10]	1.23 [1.20–1.26]	1.56 [1.54–1.59]
Pantoprazole	152.0/56.9 (2.7)	20.4/4.4 (4.6)	41.7/8.4 (4.9)		5.3/1.7 (3.2)	7.4/2.5 (3.0)	27.6/8.0 (3.4)	49.8/7.6 (6.6)
RR		1.73 [1.68–1.78]	1.85 [1.82–1.89]		1.18 [1.12–1.25]	1.11 [1.06–1.17]	1.29 [1.26–1.32]	2.47 [2.43–2.51]
Quetiapine	21.4/11.3 (1.9)	2.1/0.5 (4.1)	3.6/0.8 (4.7)	5.3/1.7 (3.2)		3.2/1.9 (1.6)	3.8/1.3 (3.0)	7.2/1.0 (7.1)
RR		2.18 [2.00–2.38]	2.47 [2.31–2.63]	1.66 [1.58–1.74]		0.86 [0.80–0.91]	1.57 [1.48–1.67]	3.72 [3.56–3.88]
Sertraline	33.0/19.1 (1.7)	4.0/1.0 (4.0)	6.8/1.5 (4.4)	7.4/2.5 (3.0)	3.2/1.9 (1.6)		5.1/1.7 (3.0)	10.9/1.7 (6.3)
RR		2.35 [2.21–2.51]	2.56 [2.45–2.68]	1.72 [1.66–1.80]	0.94 [0.88–1.01]		1.74 [1.65–1.84]	3.65 [3.52–3.78]
Tramadol	101.8/36.6 (2.8)	12.1/2.6 (4.7)	26.7/5.2/(5.2)	27.6/8.0 (3.4)	3.8/1.3 (3.0)	5.1/1.7 (3.0)		35.5/5.0 (7.0)
RR		1.67 [1.61–1.74]	1.86 [1.82–1.91]	1.24 [1.21–1.27]	1.07 [1.00–1.14]	1.08 [1.02–1.14]		2.53 [2.49–2.58]
Simvastatin	334.8/53.6 (6.2)	31.5/7.1 (4.4)	76.2/11.6 (6.6)	49.8/7.6 (6.6)	7.2/1.0 (7.1)	10.9/1.7 (6.3)	35.5/5.0 (7.0)	
RR		0.71 [0.70–0.73]	1.05 [1.04 1.07]	1.06 [1.04–1.08]	1.13 [1.07–1.19]	1.01 [0.97–1.05]	1.13 [1.10–1.15]	

Note: Data are presented as prevalence (users/1000) in persons with diabetes/in the general population (light blue rows) who redeemed combinations of drugs shown in the upper and left panel. The numbers in brackets are prevalence ratios, i.e., prevalence for the diabetes population divided by prevalence of the general population. The white rows show the relative risk (RR) for persons with diabetes who redeemed the drugs shown in the left panel to be exposed to the combinations of drugs (shown in upper panel). The numbers in the column "alone" are taken from Table 4 for comparison of prevalence's and prevalence ratio when the drugs are taken alone or in combination. Drug–drug interactions were scored by Medscape® [32] and bold indicates "monitor closely".

3. Discussion

In previous studies, it has been shown that the Danish Register of Medicinal Product Statistics constitutes a valuable tool to obtain detailed information, not only about the use of prescription drugs but also about the use of combinations, including drugs having PGx based AGs and N-AGs [28,31]. This offers a unique opportunity to measure drug use in specific disease areas such as diabetes. Based on nationwide registers, the number of persons with diabetes in Denmark in 2017 was estimated to be about 280.000, corresponding to 5% of the population, where type 1 diabetes (T1D) constituted about 28.000 (0.5%) and type 2 diabetes (T2D) about 252.000 (4.5%) [7]. In this study, we identified the total number of individual users of A10 drugs during 2018, which is assumed due to the length of the measured period, to represent a surrogate number for the total diabetes population in Denmark who are in medical antidiabetic treatment. With this assumption, and based on the pharmacological approaches and guidelines for the glycemic treatment of diabetes [33,34], users of solely A10A are T1D and users of solely A10B and both A10A/B are T2D. This assumption seems to be in good alignment with the numbers found by Carstensen et al. [7] both in terms of users, prevalence of use and age-specific prevalence [7]. However, our data on A10 users are slightly lower, somewhat higher for T1D and lower for T2D, which is mainly explained by the different approaches and epidemiological considerations used in this study and by Carstensen et al. [7]. Based on the above, we find it suitable throughout the discussion of the findings of this study to subdivide persons with diabetes into T1D (A10A users), T2D taking no insulin (A10B users) and T2D taking insulin (A10A/B.).

Persons with diabetes have increased platelet reactivity [35,36] and are more prone to cardiovascular disease (CVD) [37–39], although there are differences in the underlying pathophysiology between T1D and T2D [38]. This is reflected by the finding of 4–6 times higher prevalence of use of drugs within the drug classes of antithrombotic agents (B01) and the cardiovascular system (C) in persons with diabetes as shown in Table 2 compared to the general population. This clearly underscores the importance of these types of drugs in the prevention and treatment of cardiovascular diseases in persons with diabetes [35–40]. Interestingly, when looking at the prevalence's of use between T1D, T2D taking no insulin and T2D taking insulin it seems to be evident that across most of the ATC categories/drug classes shown, the prevalence of use of antithrombotic agents and CVD drugs was in the order of T2D taking insulin > T2D taking no insulin > T1D. In addition, depression, anxiety and neuropathy are common complications of both T1D and T2D. They affect a large fraction of persons with diabetes and are often associated with poor outcomes [40–43]. As seen for CVD the underlying pathophysiology for these comorbidities is not well understood, however, the pharmacotherapy for these complications have common features such as the use antidepressants (N06A), i.e., tricyclic antidepressants and serotonin-noradrenaline reuptake inhibitors in addition to gabapentin (and pregabalin)—anticonvulsants normally used to treat epilepsy, and opioids [41,43]. Note that in this study, we cannot discriminate between antidepressants used for neuropathy and depression. Although efficacious in the treatment of neuropathic pain, opioids are not considered to be the first choice because of concerns about abuse and addiction. As was the case with the CVD drugs, persons with diabetes have a 2–3 (for gabapentin 4 times) higher prevalence of use of analgesics including opioids, psycholeptics and psychoanaleptics compared to the general population and essentially follow the same order of prevalence of use as seen for CVD; T2D taking insulin > T2D taking no insulin > T1D. Depression and anxiety seem to be unrecognized and untreated in about two-thirds of persons with diabetes [40,41]. This may reflect the perception among clinicians that psychological matters are less important than physiological matters in persons with diabetes [44], which can explain the higher prevalence of use seen in the CVD area compared to the use of analgesics, psycholeptics and psychoanaleptics. Note that the number of users is not additive (vertical reading) for the different drugs shown in the tables since dispensing to the same users can occur for the different drugs.

However, the clinical relevance and justification of preventing and treating cardiovascular diseases, depression, anxiety and neuropathy by the use of multiple drug regimens also introduce the risk of inappropriate medication that may place persons with diabetes at an increased risk of ADR and poor outcomes [5,11]. Diabetes is inevitably associated with polypharmacy, in particular, among the elderly, and thereby increased risk of frequent hospital admissions [13] and increased risk of mortality [14]. Implementing PGx testing into daily clinical practice can provide a valuable tool to offer "appropriate polypharmacy" as previously suggested among others [3,20,45] and which is in alignment with the recent consensus report on precision medicine in diabetes [46]. In spite of supporting evidence and advances in PGx implementation in clinical practice, evidence on the cost-effectiveness of applying PGx-guided antiplatelet in cardiovascular diseases [47] and in polypharmacy have emerged [48] significant barriers still exist. Mainly concerning physicians' and pharmacists' awareness and education, but also evidence level, significance and cost-effectiveness are questioned [49].

The use of drugs in Denmark having PGx-based AGs and N-AGs are quite widespread, especially among the elderly, who often are exposed to several drug combinations having AGs, including combinations having warnings, according to drug–drug interaction checkers such as "monitor closely" or "serious use alternate" [28,29]. Stratifying the use of PGx drugs to persons with diabetes (A10 level) further substantiates the common and by on average 2.9 times more prevalent use of PGx drugs in persons with diabetes compared to the general population. In this study, we do not have data on the prevalence of use of PGx drugs as a function of age intervals. However, since we provide data on the age distribution of users of A10, A10A, A10B and A10A/B (Table 1) we assume that it is the elderly who are the most exposed to PGx drugs, further substantiating age as a key driver of polypharmacy [20,50]. Only in two instances, in the case of methylphenidate and atomoxetine, the prevalence of use was lower for persons with diabetes compared to the general population.

We further scrutinized the consumption of the most used PGx drugs in each drug class (see Figure 1 and Table 5) when drugs were redeemed either alone or in combination from a Danish pharmacy. The prevalence's of the use of PGx drugs in persons with diabetes were on average 3.3 times higher for diabetic users when given alone. Interestingly, when the PGx drugs were given in combinations, the prevalence ratios increased to an average of 4.6 further suggesting that persons with diabetes are much more exposed to PGx drugs than the general population and in particular, for PGx drug combinations, including drug combinations, for which there exist DDI warnings. Similar findings were also seen for the use of clopidogrel and proton pump inhibitors in persons with diabetes [31]. The frequency of DGI as recently reported for CYP2D6, CYP2C19 and SLCO1B1 [45] further implies that a significant proportion of persons with diabetes will have phenotypes for which actions in principle should be taken regarding dose adjustment or avoidance of the given drugs. Taking phenoconversion into consideration as well, i.e., the combination of DDI and DGI could potentially lead to additional changes in pharmacological responses as has been suggested elsewhere [3]. The differences in RR seen for diabetic users of, e.g., to obtain sertraline in combination with clopidogrel is twice as high as compared to users of obtaining clopidogrel in combination with sertraline, a pattern seen for several of the combinations shown in Table 5 and Figure 1. This suggests that users of certain drugs have a higher probability of obtaining it in combinations with certain other drugs and not necessarily vice versa. The fact that persons with diabetes are more exposed to PGx drugs, both when given alone and in combination, further substantiates that both DGI and DDI, so-called drug–drug-gene interactions (DDGI), are important measures to consider as previously suggested [28,29,31]. This calls for the need for the alignment of drug interaction trackers with regards to the incorporation of DGI and DDGI and thereby considering potential phenoconversion.

A limitation of this register study is a lack of information about dose, compliance, clinical effects as well as the duration of treatments and detailed demographics all of which should be taken into consideration in future research. For data on drug combinations, it cannot be assumed that all users are taking the drugs concomitantly, however, we have supporting data showing that around 50% of drug combinations were redeemed on the same day (unpublished results and [28,31]).

4. Materials and Methods

4.1. Register Data

This study is a cross-sectional study using The Danish Register of Medicinal Product Statistics [51], which comprises records of all prescriptions redeemed since 1st of January 1996, as the source. Drug consumption data was retrieved with the support of Statistics Denmark [52] for 2018. It is mandatory to report the sale of medicines, and therefore, the data cover all sales in Denmark. The personal identification number [53] (the CPR number) is a unique identifier to all Danish inhabitants which makes it possible to measure a person's drug consumption. Consumption is expressed as the number of users who redeemed prescriptions of drugs investigated by applying their ATC codes [54]. The drug use among persons with diabetes was identified by measuring inhabitants who redeemed prescriptions of the ATC code A10 (level 2) which solely includes "drugs used in diabetes" including users of A10A (level 3; insulins and analogues) and A10B (level 3; blood glucose-lowering drugs excl. insulins). In addition, the number of users of A10A, A10B and users of both A10A and A10B, referred to as A10A/B, were also measured. By combining the use of A10, A10A, A10B and A10A/B to ATC codes for the drug/drug classes investigated within the therapeutic areas of antithrombotic agents (B01), the cardiovascular system (C), analgesics (N02), psycholeptics (N05) and psychoanaleptics (N06) the number of persons using A10, A10A, A10B and A10A/B alone or in combination with the above-mentioned drug classes were identified and compared to the use in the general population. To convert the number of users to prevalence (users/1000 inhabitants), the total Danish population in 2018 was 5.781.190 and the age group distribution was as follow: 0–17 years 1,165,000; 18–24 years 532,622; 25–44 years 1,441,697; 45–64 years 1,525,308; 65–79 years 859,369 and 80+ years 256,694. The total number of persons who redeemed prescriptions of ATC-code A10 (persons with diabetes) was 258,494 (see Table 1).

Drug–drug interactions were scored in severity by using Medscape® drug interaction checker [32]. Warnings are displayed as "monitor closely" or "serious use alternate".

The dosing information, length of treatment and indication for prescribing were not recorded, and ethics approval was not applicable according to Danish law since the use of anonymized healthcare data for pharmacoepidemiological research does not require subject consent or approval from Ethics Committee.

4.2. Statistics

The relative risk (RR) was calculated by using the MedCalc Software Ltd. relative risk calculator. https://www.medcalc.org/calc/relative_risk.php (Version 20.0.5; accessed on 2 June 2021). The Chi-squared test was performed by using the CHI2.TEST function in Microsoft Excel version 2016.

4.3. Clinical Dosing Guidelines

The Clinical Pharmacogenetics Implementation Consortium (CPIC) and the Dutch Pharmacogenetics Working Group (DPWG) clinical dosing guidelines for specific gene-drug pairs were used as the source. The guidelines are available through the publicly available PharmGKB homepage (https://www.pharmgkb.org/ accessed on 15 August 2021). Drugs with guidelines were divided into drugs having an actionable guideline (AG) defined as at least one clinical recommendation (i.e., dose adjustment, dose monitoring or avoidance of the given drug) different from "extensive metaboliser" EM (normal situation) of any of the phenotypes PM, IM or RM. Drugs having a non-actionable guideline (N-AG) were defined as drugs with no clinical recommendation different from EM of any of the phenotypes based on current clinical knowledge.

5. Conclusions

The findings of this exploratory cross-sectional register study clearly show that a large fraction of the Danish population and in particular persons with diabetes, especially the elderly, are exposed to drugs or drug combinations for which there exists dosing guidelines as well as FDA annotation related to PGx of CYP2D6, CYP2C19 and SLCO1B1. In addition, it should be emphasized that T2D taking insulin seems to have a higher rate of use of drugs including PGx drugs compared to T2D taking no insulin and T1D. This further supports the notion of the emerging results of accessing and accounting for not only DDI but also DGI, DDGI and phenoconversion as supportive tools in clinical decision-making and appropriate polypharmacy. The focus should be on the elderly, nursing home residents and persons with diabetes due to their high exposure to PGx drugs. In spite of supporting evidence and advances in PGx implementation in clinical practice, including evidence on cost-effectiveness, significant barriers in the Danish healthcare system in implementing the use of PGx, mainly concerning awareness and education, but also at the evidence level which suggests initiatives should be taken focusing on these key barriers.

Author Contributions: Conceptualization, N.W., L.T. and C.V.; methodology, N.W., L.T. and C.V.; Software, N.W.; validation, N.W., L.T. and C.V.; formal analysis, N.W.; investigation, N.W., L.T. and C.V.; resources, N.W., L.T. and C.V.; data curation, N.W., L.T. and C.V.; writing—original draft preparation, N.W.; writing—review and editing, N.W., L.T. and C.V.; visualization, N.W.; supervision, N.W., L.T. and C.V.; project administration, N.W.; funding acquisition, none. All authors have read and agreed to the published version of the manuscript.

Funding: This research received no external funding.

Institutional Review Board Statement: Not applicable.

Informed Consent Statement: Not applicable and see Materials and Methods.

Data Availability Statement: The data presented in this study are available within the article.

Acknowledgments: The authors thank Merete Rasmussen and Caroline Louise Westergaard for valuable input throughout the preparation of this manuscript.

Conflicts of Interest: The authors declare no conflict of interest.

References

1. Cacabelos, R.; Cacabelos, N.; Carril, J.C. The role of pharmacogenomics in adverse drug reactions. *Expert Rev. Clin. Pharmacol.* **2019**, *12*, 407–442. [CrossRef]
2. Dong, A.N.; Tan, B.H.; Pan, Y.; Ong, C.E. Cytochrome P450 genotype-guided drug therapies: An update on current states. *Clin. Exp. Pharmacol. Physiol.* **2018**, *45*, 991–1001. [CrossRef] [PubMed]
3. Bahar, M.A.; Setiawan, D.; Hak, E.; Wilffert, B. Pharmacogenetics of drug–drug interaction and drug–drug–gene interaction: A systematic review on CYP2C9, CYP2C19 and CYP2D6. *Pharmacogenomics* **2017**, *18*, 701–739. [CrossRef] [PubMed]
4. Introduction: Standards of medical care in diabetes-2021. *Diabetes Care* **2021**, *44*, S1–S2. [CrossRef]
5. Harding, J.L.; Pavkov, M.E.; Magliano, D.J.; Shaw, J.E.; Gregg, E.W. Global trends in diabetes complications: A review of current evidence. *Diabeto* **2019**, *62*, 3–19. [CrossRef]
6. Ogurtsova, K.; Da, J.D.; Fernandes, R.; Huang, Y.; Linnenkamp, U.; Guariguata, L.; Cho, N.H.; Cavan, D.; Shaw, J.E.; Makaroff, L.E. IDF Diabetes Atlas: Global estimates for the prevalence of diabetes for 2015 and 2040. *Diabetes Res. Clin. Pract.* **2017**, *128*, 40–50. [CrossRef]
7. Carstensen, B.; Rønn, P.F.; Jørgensen, M.E. Prevalence, incidence and mortality of type 1 and type 2 diabetes in Denmark 1996-2016. *BMJ Open Diabetes Res. Care* **2020**, *8*, e001071. [CrossRef] [PubMed]
8. Dobrică, E.C.; Găman, M.A.; Cozma, M.A.; Bratu, O.G.; Stoian, A.P.; Diaconu, C.C. Polypharmacy in type 2 diabetes mellitus: Insights from an internal medicine department. *Medicina* **2019**, *55*, 436. [CrossRef] [PubMed]
9. Alwhaibi, M.; Balkhi, B.; Alhawassi, T.M.; Alkofide, H.; Alduhaim, N.; Alabdulali, R.; Drweesh, H.; Sambamoorthi, U. Polypharmacy among patients with diabetes: A cross-sectional retrospective study in a tertiary hospital in Saudi Arabia. *BMJ Open* **2018**, *8*, 20852. [CrossRef]
10. Brath, H.; Mehta, N.; Savage, R.D.; Gill, S.S.; Wu, W.; Bronskill, S.E.; Zhu, L.; Gurwitz, J.H.; Rochon, P.A. What Is Known About Preventing, Detecting, and Reversing Prescribing Cascades: A Scoping Review. *J. Am. Geriatr. Soc.* **2018**, *66*, 2079–2085. [CrossRef]

11. AL-Musawe, L.; Martins, A.P.; Raposo, J.F.; Torre, C. The association between polypharmacy and adverse health consequences in elderly type 2 diabetes mellitus patients; a systematic review and meta-analysis. *Diabetes Res. Clin. Pract.* **2019**, *155*, 107804. [CrossRef] [PubMed]
12. Noale, M.; Veronese, N.; Cavallo Perin, P.; Pilotto, A.; Tiengo, A.; Crepaldi, G.; Maggi, S. Polypharmacy in elderly patients with type 2 diabetes receiving oral antidiabetic treatment. *Acta Diabetol.* **2016**, *53*, 323–330. [CrossRef]
13. Sehgal, V.; Sehgal, R.; Bajaj, A.; Bajwa, S.J.; Khaira, U.; Kresse, V. Polypharmacy and potentially inappropriate medication use as the precipitating factor in readmissions to the hospital. *J. Fam. Med. Prim. Care* **2013**, *2*, 194. [CrossRef] [PubMed]
14. Leelakanok, N.; Holcombe, A.L.; Lund, B.C.; Gu, X.; Schweizer, M.L. Association between polypharmacy and death: A systematic review and meta-analysis. *J. Am. Pharm. Assoc.* **2017**, *57*, 729–738.e10. [CrossRef]
15. Muth, C.; Blom, J.W.; Smith, S.M.; Johnell, K.; Gonzalez-Gonzalez, A.I.; Nguyen, T.S.; Brueckle, M.-S.; Cesari, M.; Tinetti, M.E.; Valderas, J.M. Evidence supporting the best clinical management of patients with multimorbidity and polypharmacy: A systematic guideline review and expert consensus. *J. Intern. Med.* **2019**, *285*, 272–288. [CrossRef] [PubMed]
16. Høj, K.; Mygind, A.; Livbjerg, S.; Bro, F. Deprescribing of inappropriate medication in primary care. *Ugeskr. Laeger* **2019**, *181*, V01190027.
17. *Deprescribing.org—Optimizing Medication Use.* Available online: https://deprescribing.org/ (accessed on 3 April 2020).
18. Sinnott, C.; McHugh, S.; Browne, J.; Bradley, C. GPs' perspectives on the management of patients with multimorbidity: Systematic review and synthesis of qualitative research. *BMJ Open* **2013**, *3*, e003610. [CrossRef]
19. Zanger, U.M.; Schwab, M. Cytochrome P450 enzymes in drug metabolism: Regulation of gene expression, enzyme activities, and impact of genetic variation. *Pharmacol. Ther.* **2013**, *138*, 103–141. [CrossRef]
20. Sharp, C.N.; Linder, M.W.; Valdes, R. Polypharmacy: A healthcare conundrum with a pharmacogenetic solution. *Crit. Rev. Clin. Lab. Sci.* **2020**, *57*, 161–180. [CrossRef]
21. Barbarino, J.M.; Whirl-Carrillo, M.; Altman, R.B.; Klein, T.E. PharmGKB: A worldwide resource for pharmacogenomic information. *Wiley Interdiscip. Rev. Syst. Biol. Med.* **2018**, *10*, e1417. [CrossRef] [PubMed]
22. Gaedigk, A.; Dinh, J.C.; Jeong, H.; Prasad, B.; Leeder, J.S. Ten Years' Experience with the CYP2D6 Activity Score: A Perspective On Future Investigations to Improve Clinical Predictions for Precision Therapeutics. *J. Pers. Med.* **2018**, *8*, 15. [CrossRef]
23. Caudle, K.E.; Dunnenberger, H.M.; Freimuth, R.R.; Peterson, J.F.; Burlison, J.D.; Whirl-Carrillo, M.; Scott, S.A.; Rehm, H.L.; Williams, M.S.; Klein, T.E.; et al. Standardizing terms for clinical pharmacogenetic test results: Consensus terms from the Clinical Pharmacogenetics Implementation Consortium (CPIC). *Genet. Med.* **2017**, *19*, 215–223. [CrossRef]
24. Hicks, J.K.; Bishop, J.R.; Sangkuhl, K.; Müller, D.J.; Ji, Y.; Leckband, S.G.; Leeder, J.S.; Graham, R.L.; Chiulli, D.L.; LLerena, A.; et al. Clinical Pharmacogenetics Implementation Consortium (CPIC) Guideline for CYP2D6 and CYP2C19 Genotypes and Dosing of Selective Serotonin Reuptake Inhibitors. *Clin. Pharmacol. Ther.* **2015**, *98*, 127–134. [CrossRef] [PubMed]
25. Ramsey, L.B.; Johnson, S.G.; Caudle, K.E.; Haidar, C.E.; Voora, D.; Wilke, R.A.; Maxwell, W.D.; McLeod, H.L.; Krauss, R.M.; Roden, D.M.; et al. The Clinical Pharmacogenetics Implementation Consortium Guideline for SLCO1B1 and Simvastatin-Induced Myopathy: 2014 Update. *Clin. Pharmacol. Ther.* **2014**, *96*, 423–428. [CrossRef]
26. Bank, P.C.D.; Swen, J.J.; Guchelaar, H.J. Estimated nationwide impact of implementing a preemptive pharmacogenetic panel approach to guide drug prescribing in primary care in The Netherlands. *BMC Med.* **2019**, *17*, 110. [CrossRef]
27. Alshabeeb, M.A.; Deneer, V.H.M.; Khan, A.; Asselbergs, F.W. Use of Pharmacogenetic Drugs by the Dutch Population. *Front. Genet.* **2019**, *10*, 567. [CrossRef] [PubMed]
28. Westergaard, N.; Nielsen, R.S.; Jørgensen, S.; Vermehren, C. Drug use in Denmark for drugs having pharmacogenomics (PGx) based dosing guidelines from CPIC or DPWG for CYP2D6 and CYP2C19 drug–gene pairs: Perspectives for introducing PGx test to polypharmacy patients. *J. Pers. Med.* **2020**, *10*, 3. [CrossRef] [PubMed]
29. Vermehren, C.; Søgaard Nielsen, R.; Jørgensen, S.; Drastrup, A.M.; Westergaard, N. Drug Use among Nursing Home Residents in Denmark for Drugs Having Pharmacogenomics Based (PGx) Dosing Guidelines: Potential for Preemptive PGx Testing. *J. Pers. Med.* **2020**, *10*, 78. [CrossRef]
30. Lunenburg, C.A.T.C.; Hauser, A.S.; Ishtiak-Ahmed, K.; Gasse, C. Primary Care Prescription Drug Use and Related Actionable Drug-Gene Interactions in the Danish Population. *Clin. Transl. Sci.* **2020**, *13*, 798–806. [CrossRef]
31. Westergaard, N.; Tarnow, L.; Vermehren, C. Use of Clopidogrel and Proton Pump Inhibitors Alone or in Combinations in Persons with Diabetes in Denmark; Potential for CYP2C19 Genotype-Guided Drug Therapy. *Metabolites* **2021**, *11*, 96. [CrossRef]
32. *Medscape Drug Interactions Checker—Medscape Drug Reference Database.* Available online: https://reference.medscape.com/drug-interactionchecker (accessed on 7 July 2021).
33. Association, A.D. Pharmacologic approaches to glycemic treatment: Standards of medical care in diabetesd2021. *Diabetes Care* **2021**, *44*, S111–S124. [CrossRef]
34. Buse, J.B.; Wexler, D.J.; Tsapas, A.; Rossing, P.; Mingrone, G.; Mathieu, C.; D'Alessio, D.A.; Davies, M.J. 2019 update to: Management of hyperglycaemia in type 2 diabetes, 2018. A consensus report by the American Diabetes Association (ADA) and the European Association for the Study of Diabetes (EASD). *Diabetologia* **2020**, *63*, 221–228. [CrossRef]
35. Schilling, U.; Dingemanse, J.; Ufer, M. Pharmacokinetics and Pharmacodynamics of Approved and Investigational P2Y12 Receptor Antagonists. *Clin. Pharmacokinet.* **2020**, *59*, 545–566. [CrossRef] [PubMed]
36. Rivas Rios, J.R.; Franchi, F.; Rollini, F.; Angiolillo, D.J. Diabetes and antiplatelet therapy: From bench to bedside. *Cardiovasc. Diagn. Ther.* **2018**, *8*, 594–609. [CrossRef]

37. Angermayr, L.; Melchart, D.; Linde, K. Multifactorial lifestyle interventions in the primary and secondary prevention of cardiovascular disease and type 2 diabetes mellitus—A systematic review of randomized controlled trials. *Ann. Behav. Med.* **2010**, *40*, 49–64. [CrossRef] [PubMed]
38. Schofield, J.; Ho, J.; Soran, H. Cardiovascular Risk in Type 1 Diabetes Mellitus. *Diabetes Ther.* **2019**, *10*, 773–789. [CrossRef]
39. American Diabetes Association Cardiovascular disease and risk management: Standards of medical care in diabetesd 2021. *Diabetes Care* **2021**, *44*, S125–S150. [CrossRef]
40. Holt, R.I.G.; De Groot, M.; Golden, S.H. Diabetes and depression. *Curr. Diab. Rep.* **2014**, *14*, 491. [CrossRef] [PubMed]
41. Collins, M.M.; Corcoran, P.; Perry, I.J. Anxiety and depression symptoms in patients with diabetes: Original Article: Psychology. *Diabet. Med.* **2009**, *26*, 153–161. [CrossRef] [PubMed]
42. Schreiber, A.K. Diabetic neuropathic pain: Physiopathology and treatment. *World J. Diabetes* **2015**, *6*, 432. [CrossRef] [PubMed]
43. Attal, N. Pharmacological treatments of neuropathic pain: The latest recommendations. *Rev. Neurol.* **2019**, *175*, 46–50. [CrossRef]
44. Katon, W.J. The Comorbidity of Diabetes Mellitus and Depression. *Am. J. Med.* **2008**, *121*, 8–15. [CrossRef]
45. Samwald, M.; Xu, H.; Blagec, K.; Empey, P.E.; Malone, D.C.; Ahmed, S.M.; Ryan, P.; Hofer, S.; Boyce, R.D. Incidence of Exposure of Patients in the United States to Multiple Drugs for Which Pharmacogenomic Guidelines Are Available. *PLoS ONE* **2016**, *11*, e0164972. [CrossRef]
46. Chung, W.K.; Erion, K.; Florez, J.C.; Hattersley, A.T.; Hivert, M.F.; Lee, C.G.; McCarthy, M.I.; Nolan, J.J.; Norris, J.M.; Pearson, E.R.; et al. Precision medicine in diabetes: A Consensus Report from the American Diabetes Association (ADA) and the European Association for the Study of Diabetes (EASD). *Diabetologia* **2020**, *63*, 1671–1693. [CrossRef]
47. Zhu, Y.; Swanson, K.M.; Rojas, R.L.; Wang, Z.; St. Sauver, J.L.; Visscher, S.L.; Prokop, L.J.; Bielinski, S.J.; Wang, L.; Weinshilboum, R.; et al. Systematic review of the evidence on the cost-effectiveness of pharmacogenomics-guided treatment for cardiovascular diseases. *Genet. Med.* **2020**, *22*, 475–486. [CrossRef] [PubMed]
48. Brixner, D.; Biltaji, E.; Bress, A.; Unni, S.; Ye, X.; Mamiya, T.; Ashcraft, K.; Biskupiak, J. The effect of pharmacogenetic profiling with a clinical decision support tool on healthcare resource utilization and estimated costs in the elderly exposed to polypharmacy. *J. Med. Econ.* **2016**, *19*, 213–228. [CrossRef]
49. Klein, M.E.; Parvez, M.M.; Shin, J.G. Clinical Implementation of Pharmacogenomics for Personalized Precision Medicine: Barriers and Solutions. *J. Pharm. Sci.* **2017**, *106*, 2368–2379. [CrossRef] [PubMed]
50. Longo, M.; Bellastella, G.; Maiorino, M.I.; Meier, J.J.; Esposito, K.; Giugliano, D. Diabetes and aging: From treatment goals to pharmacologic therapy. *Front. Endocrinol.* **2019**, *10*, 45. [CrossRef] [PubMed]
51. Schmidt, M.; Hallas, J.; Laursen, M.; Friis, S. Data Resource Profile: Danish online drug use statistics (MEDSTAT). *Int. J. Epidemiol.* **2016**, *45*, 1401–1402g. [CrossRef] [PubMed]
52. *Statistics Denmark Statistics Denmark.* Available online: https://www.dst.dk/en# (accessed on 7 July 2021).
53. Schmidt, M.; Pedersen, L.; Sørensen, H.T. The Danish Civil Registration System as a tool in epidemiology. *Eur. J. Epidemiol.* **2014**, *29*, 541–549. [CrossRef]
54. *World Health Organization Collaborating Centre for Drug Statistics Methodology. WHOCC—ATC/DDD Index.* Available online: https://www.whocc.no/atc_ddd_index/ (accessed on 7 July 2021).

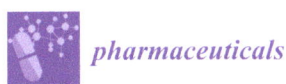

Systematic Review

Adverse Drug Reactions of Olanzapine, Clozapine and Loxapine in Children and Youth: A Systematic Pharmacogenetic Review

Diane Merino [1,2,3], Arnaud Fernandez [1,2,†], Alexandre O. Gérard [3,†], Nouha Ben Othman [3], Fanny Rocher [3], Florence Askenazy [1,2], Céline Verstuyft [4,5], Milou-Daniel Drici [3] and Susanne Thümmler [1,2,*]

1. Department of Child and Adolescent Psychiatry, Children's Hospitals of Nice CHU-Lenval, 06200 Nice, France; merino.d@chu-nice.fr (D.M.); fernandez.a@pediatrie-chulenval-nice.fr (A.F.); askenazy.f@pediatrie-chulenval-nice.fr (F.A.)
2. CoBTek Laboratory, Université Côte d'Azur, 06100 Nice, France
3. Department of Pharmacology and Pharmacovigilance Center, University Hospital of Nice, 06000 Nice, France; gerard.a@chu-nice.fr (A.O.G.); ben-othman.n@chu-nice.fr (N.B.O.); rocher.f@chu-nice.fr (F.R.); pharmacovigilance@chu-nice.fr (M.-D.D.)
4. Service de Génétique Moléculaire, Pharmacogénétique et Hormonologie, Hôpital Bicêtre, Groupe Hospitalier Paris Saclay, AP–HP, 94270 Le Kremlin-Bicêtre, France; celine.verstuyft@aphp.fr
5. CESP/UMR-S1178, Inserm, Université Paris-Sud, 92290 Paris, France
* Correspondence: thummler.s@pediatrie-chulenval-nice.fr
† These authors contributed equally to this work.

Abstract: Children and youth treated with antipsychotic drugs (APs) are particularly vulnerable to adverse drug reactions (ADRs) and prone to poor treatment response. In particular, interindividual variations in drug exposure can result from differential metabolism of APs by cytochromes, subject to genetic polymorphism. *CYP1A2* is pivotal in the metabolism of the APs olanzapine, clozapine, and loxapine, whose safety profile warrants caution. We aimed to shed some light on the pharmacogenetic profiles possibly associated with these drugs' ADRs and loss of efficacy in children and youth. We conducted a systematic review relying on four databases, following the Preferred Reporting Items for Systematic Reviews and Meta-Analyses (PRISMA) 2020 recommendations and checklist, with a quality assessment. Our research yielded 32 publications. The most frequent ADRs were weight gain and metabolic syndrome (18; 56.3%), followed by lack of therapeutic effect (8; 25%) and neurological ADRs (7; 21.8%). The overall mean quality score was 11.3/24 (±2.7). In 11 studies (34.3%), genotyping focused on the study of cytochromes. Findings regarding possible associations were sometimes conflicting. Nonetheless, cases of major clinical improvement were fostered by genotyping. Yet, *CYP1A2* remains poorly investigated. Further studies are required to improve the assessment of the risk–benefit balance of prescription for children and youth treated with olanzapine, clozapine, and/or loxapine.

Keywords: cytochromes; *CYP1A2*; adverse drug reaction; antipsychotics; olanzapine; clozapine; loxapine; pharmacogenetics; children; youth

1. Introduction

In child psychiatry, antipsychotic drugs (APs) are used to treat psychotic or mood disorders, as well as behavioral symptoms, despite limited evidence. Although APs are usually efficacious, the risk of adverse drug reactions (ADRs) associated with this class should be considered when initiating APs in this vulnerable population [1,2]. Treatment resistance is also a major concern [3]. Many intrinsic and extrinsic factors may influence the pharmacokinetics and pharmacodynamics of APs, such as sex, ancestry, puberty, dietary and smoking habits [4–7], potentially leading to ADRs or lack of therapeutic effects.

Furthermore, the *cytochrome P450 (CYP)* proteins, a superfamily of liver enzymes, are instrumental to drug metabolism. At least 57 human *CYPs* have been described [8], even if most reactions are undertaken by *CYP2C9, CYP2C19, CYP2D6*, and *CYP3A4* [9]. Major interindividual differences in their expression arise from genetic polymorphisms, leading to various metabolizing phenotypes [10] that determine the *CYPs'* level of activity. Furthermore, alterations in their activity by extrinsic inducers or inhibitors, can imbalance a previously well-tolerated treatment; conversely, it can potentiate a given medication [11]. As *CYP* metabolize most APs [12], some studies addressed the potential consequences of *CYP2D6* polymorphisms in children and youth treated with antipsychotics [13]. While *CYP1A2* represents approximately 15% of hepatic *CYP* content [14], it is nonetheless pivotal in the metabolism of the two atypical APs, olanzapine [15] and clozapine [16], as well as loxapine [17] (whose properties are closely related to those of atypical APs [18,19]).

Olanzapine, clozapine, and loxapine share a common tricyclic structure and belong to the thienobenzodiazepine, dibenzodiazepine, and dibenzoxazepine families, respectively [20]. Olanzapine [21] and clozapine [22] are currently used as second- to third-line therapy, while loxapine may allow symptomatic relief of acute agitation [23,24]. In child psychiatry, the Food and Drug Administration (FDA) has granted marketing authorization for olanzapine in acute mixed or manic episodes of bipolar I disorder and treatment of schizophrenia for adolescents aged from 13 to 17 years old [25]. Similarly, the FDA authorized use of olanzapine in cases of depressed bipolar I disorder, in combination with fluoxetine, in children and adolescents aged between 10 and 17 years old [25]. By contrast, the European Medicines Agency (EMA) did not recommend olanzapine for use in children and adolescents below 18 years of age, mainly because of a lack of data on safety and efficacy. Furthermore, the EMA highlighted a greater magnitude of weight gain, lipid, and prolactin alterations in short-term studies of adolescent patients, in comparison with studies of adult patients [26]. Regarding clozapine, its therapeutic indications are mainly represented by treatment-resistant schizophrenia and recurrent suicidal behaviors in schizophrenic disorders [27], without prejudice to the age, reflecting the lack of guidelines for use of clozapine in pediatric population [28]. The EMA stated that safety and efficacy of clozapine in children under the age of 16 have not been established yet, and therefore that it should not be used in this group until further data become available [29]. Likewise, regarding loxapine, both FDA and EMA mentioned that safety and effectiveness in pediatric patients have not been established [30,31]. However, in France, the National Drug Agency (Agence Nationale de Sécurité du Médicament et des produits de santé (ANSM)) granted authorization for loxapine in the treatment of acute and chronic psychotic disorders as from the age of 15 years [32].

Atypical APs tend to induce less extrapyramidal effects (compared to typical antipsychotics) [33] and may therefore be the preferred option when treating children and youth, despite these grey areas. However, their profile comes at the price of other prominent ADRs, such as metabolic changes (weight gain, hyperglycemia, and dyslipidemia) [34]. As they begin in childhood, they are likely to persist over lifetime. Off-label use being frequent in this population [35], children are also exposed to a plethora of ADRs, such as neuroleptic malignant syndrome, seizures, agranulocytosis, or hyperprolactinemia. The safety profile of olanzapine [36] and clozapine [1] shows major issues of concern, and the tolerability of loxapine scarcely has been investigated [37], especially in children and youth.

Increased knowledge of the intrinsic determinants of each patient's exposure to APs could pave the way to tailored therapy. Pharmacogenetics has been defined as the study of how genetic differences influence the variability in patient's responses to drugs [38]. On a large scale, genome-wide association studies (GWAS) allow to genotype all known single-nucleotide polymorphisms (SNPs) in the human genome. When a smaller set of SNPs are likely to affect treatment response, candidate gene studies can be conducted to detect a potential association [39]. Further, whole-genome sequencing approaches (WGS) may allow to identify rare gene variants, and therefore raises interesting prospects in psychiatric disorders [40,41]. The *in vivo* assessment of a cytochrome's phenotype relies on the administration of a selective enzyme substrate. These approaches brought us closer to personalized medicine, whereby the understanding of each patient's genetic profile may predict the occurrence of ADRs or lack of effect. This may be especially useful in specific populations [42], often excluded of clinical trials and of the classical field of evidence-based medicine.

Therefore, we aimed to review the pharmacogenetic variants underlying olanzapine, clozapine, and loxapine ADRs and/or efficacy in children and youth having undergone genotyping. Then, we assessed the most frequently investigated ADRs and genetic polymorphisms in this population. Finally, we assessed the specific effect of *CYP1A2* variants in the occurrence of ADRs and/or lack of therapeutic effect.

2. Materials and Methods

2.1. Research

The PROSPERO International prospective register of systematic reviews was checked for similar systematic reviews. Due to our issue of concern never having been addressed, we have submitted the research protocol to the INPLASY International platform of registered systematic review and meta-analysis protocols (INPLASY202250025).

We have, therefore, conducted this systematic review following the Preferred Reporting Items for Systematic Reviews and Meta-Analyses (PRISMA) 2020 recommendations and checklist [43]. We further followed special methodological considerations regarding pediatric systematic reviews [44]. The following query was used: ((((adolescent* OR youth OR child* OR pedia* OR paedia*) AND (clozapine OR olanzapine OR loxapine) AND (pharmacogen* OR allele OR genotype* OR cytochrome* OR CYP1* OR CYP2* OR CYP3* OR CYP4*) AND (adverse drug reaction* OR adverse event* OR adverse reaction* OR side effect* OR secondary effect* OR after effect* OR tolerability OR safety)))). Two authors (D.M. and A.O.G.) separately conducted the research in PubMed, EMBASE, PsycINFO, and PsycArticles. Our query retrieved publications registered in the four selected databases up to 21 March 2022.

Relying on four electronic bibliographic databases, our extraction retrieved for each publication the source database, publication year, language, full list of authors' names, article title, DOI (Digital Object Information), journal title, abstract, and Medical Subject Headings (MeSH) terms associated. Two authors independently performed the preliminary two steps of proper article screening, with the results shown in the PRISMA flowchart (Figure 1).

Before screening, duplicates were removed. First, the eligibility of the titles and abstracts of the articles identified by the initial query were checked. Next, full-text copies of the articles whose titles and abstracts met the inclusion criteria were retrieved. Then, to ensure compliance with the inclusion criteria, the yielded full-text articles were assessed for eligibility.

When the two reviewing authors could not obtain a consensus regarding an article, the disagreement was resolved through discussion. Lastly, data extraction was performed for all publications that met the inclusion criteria, including the study site(s), study type, characteristics of the subjects (age, sample size, sex distribution, ancestry, diagnosis), antipsychotic(s) of interest and its (their) dosing, other drugs administered, outcome(s) measured, gene variants assessed, their potential association(s) with the ADR(s), the pathophysiology involved, and the pharmacogenetic approach. For quality assessment needs, we also extracted data addressing the reasons for choosing the genes/SNPs to genotype (summaries of previous findings, reasons given for choosing the genes and SNPs genotyped, the adjustment methods for multiple testing, and the *p*-values provided for the associations), the sample size (details on calculation of sample size and on a priori power to detect effect sizes of varying degrees), the reliability of genotypes (description of the genotyping procedure, of the primers and of any quality control methods, previously reported genotype frequencies, blind of genotyping personnel to outcome status), missing genotype data (the extent and reasons for missing data, any checks for missingness at random performed, any imputation of missing genotype data, number of patients contributing to each analysis and consistence with sample size), population stratification (tests undertaken for cryptic population stratification and adjustment for in the analyses), Hardy–Weinberg Equilibrium testing (was it performed, and were deviating (or not) SNPs highlighted and excluded from further analysis where appropriate), and choice and definition of outcomes (clear definition of all outcomes investigated, justification, results shown).

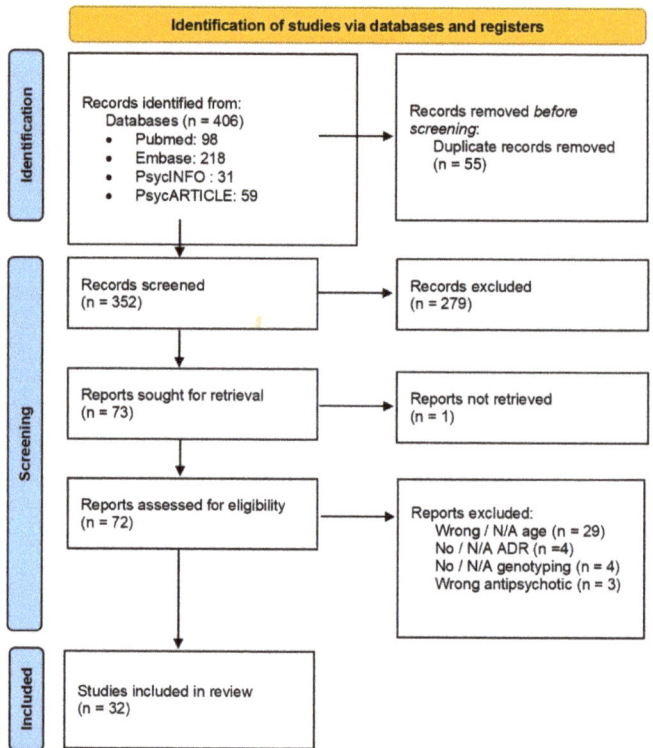

Figure 1. PRISMA 2020 flow diagram for identification of studies. N/A: Not applicable. From: Page MJ, McKenzie JE, Bossuyt PM, Boutron I, Hoffmann TC, Mulrow CD, et al. The PRISMA 2020 statement: an updated guideline for reporting systematic reviews. BMJ 2021; 372: n71. doi:10.1136/bmj.n71.

2.2. Selection Criteria

Data extraction relied on the following inclusion criteria:

1. Studies including at least one child and/or adolescent and/or youth, therefore aged under 25, following the United Nations definition [45].
2. Receiving at least one atypical antipsychotic that is metabolized by *CYP1A2* (clozapine, olanzapine, loxapine).
3. Having experienced an adverse drug reaction/a lack of therapeutic effect linked to at least one of these treatments.
4. Having undergone pharmacogenomic analysis/genotyping, the results of which are mentioned.
5. Record issued from an English-language and peer-reviewed journal, for which full-text was available

We therefore excluded books (and chapters), commentaries, but also any published material that did not meet the original research criteria (e.g., systematic reviews, meta-analyses) [46]. However, considering the foreseeable paucity of evidence informing the review, we decided to include conference abstracts and editorial pieces [47].

To serve the same purpose, we have chosen to include studies including 'mixed' (both adult and pediatric) populations [44], with due regard to the age criterion: 'Studies including at least one child and/or adolescent, therefore aged under 25'.

Then, identical or overlapping patient cohorts were detected by the analysis of study site(s) and characteristics of the subjects, among others. The objectives and genetic variants investigated tended to differ across the reports, based on overlapping or identical cohorts, so we have chosen to include publications presenting redundant cohorts [39].

When the ancestry of patients (whose consideration is pivotal in genetics concerns) was not provided in a study, we hypothesized that it could be consistent with the study site, and reported it as such.

Studies were classified according to their methodology: case reports or case series, cohort studies [48], and case–control (or cross-sectional) studies [49]. We distinguished 'pediatric' studies, exclusively relying on pediatric samples, and 'mixed-population' studies, to present their respective characteristics (Tables 1 and 2) and quality assessments (Tables S1 and S2). Then, the whole studies were grouped according to the main classes of ADRs investigated (Tables 3–5).

2.3. Quality Assessment

The quality of the included pharmacogenetic studies was independently assessed by D.M. and A.O.G, relying on a tool adapted from Maruf et al. [13] and the checklist developed by Jorgensen and Williamson [50]. As stated above, we considered each article (irrespective of the potential redundancy of its (their) cohort(s)) for quality assessment. Indeed, methods may vary from an article to another, relying on identical or overlapping patient cohorts. Any case of discrepancy between their assessments was resolved through discussion.

The used tool addressed different issues of methodological quality:

1. Choosing the genes/SNPs to genotype (4 binary questions).
2. Sample size (3 questions: 2 binary and 1 open).
3. Study design (1 open question).
4. Reliability of genotypes (5 binary questions).
5. Missing genotype data (6 binary questions).
6. Population stratification (2 binary questions).
7. Hardy–Weinberg Equilibrium (2 binary questions).
8. Choice and definition of outcomes (3 binary questions).

The purpose of open questions (sample size; study design) was to allow a quality visual check as a complement to the global score of each publication.

For each binary question, we answered:

- 'Yes' if the study provided an adequate response.
- 'No' if the response was not mentioned in the manuscript nor a method publication referenced by the authors.
- 'N/A' (not applicable) if the response to the main (first) question of the issue of concern addressed is 'No'.

Consequently, each study received a quality score between 0 and 24, based on the summation of the 'Yes' answers. According to this approach, the higher the score, the higher the quality of a given study.

3. Results

3.1. Study Selection

Selection and progressive elimination of the identified articles are summarized in the Preferred Reporting Items for Systematic Reviews and Meta-Analyses (PRISMA) flowchart provided in Figure 1. Our database query retrieved 406 records. Before screening, we removed 55 duplicates (see Methods). Then, 352 records were screened on the basis of their title and abstract. Among them, 72 publications were assessed for eligibility via the analysis of their full-text version. Finally, 32 records met the inclusion criteria of this systematic review.

3.2. Characteristics of Studies

3.2.1. General Characteristics

The most represented study type was cohort studies (20 reports; 62.5%). Sample sizes ranged from single cases (case reports) to 1445 patients (case–control study). Among articles for which the ancestry was provided, 90.9% involved Caucasian/European/White populations. It was not reported in 10 records (31.3%). Diagnosis of the included patients was provided in 32 records (96.9%), mainly represented by psychotic disorders (29 reports; 93.5%). In 11 studies (34.3%), genetic assessment relied on studying cytochromes. Olanzapine was the most commonly used AP (24 reports; 75.0%). The most frequent ADR was weight gain and metabolic syndrome (MetS), investigated in more than half of the studies (18 reports; 56.3%). Lack of therapeutic effect accounted for 8 reports (25.0%) and neurological ADRs for 7 reports (21.8%). Comparing study sites and characteristics of the populations, we noticed several overlaps between the included articles. Indeed, Nussbaum et al. in both studies ([51,52]), as well as Le Hellard et al. [53] and Jassim et al. [54] relied on identical cohorts, respectively. To a lesser extent, Le Hellard et al. included the Theisen et al. [55] cohort; the Gagliano et al. [56] cohort overlapped with the Tiwari et al. [57] cohort; and the Quteineh et al. [58] and Saigi et al. [59] cohorts were both overlapping the Choong et al. [60] cohort.

The mean quality assessment score (see Methods) of the 32 included studies was 11.3/24 ($\pm$2.7). The scores ranged from 6 (a case series) to 18 (a cohort study). In all studies, a literature review was undertaken, whose findings were summarized, as well as the reasons for choosing the genes and SNPs genotyped. The method of adjustment for multiple testing was described in 13 records (40.6%). Precise p-values were provided for all associations in 25 records (78.1%). Regarding sample size, details on its calculation were given in one (3.1%) study (a cohort study). Details were given regarding the a priori power to detect effect sizes of varying degrees in 5 publications (15.6%). Almost all records described the genotyping procedure (31; 96.9%). Primers and quality control methods were described in 8 (25.0%) and 6 (18.8%) studies, respectively. Previously reported genotype frequencies were quoted in 9 publications (28.1%). Genotyping personnel was blinded to outcome status in one study (a cohort study) (3.1%). The extent of missing data was summarized in 9 studies (28.1%), among which 6 gave the reasons for missing data (66.7%). No study reported checks for missingness at random, nor imputed missing genotype data. All studies quoted the number of patients contributing to each analysis (32; 100%), which agreed to samples sizes in 24 studies (75.0%). No study presented tests for cryptic population stratification. Hardy–Weinberg Equilibrium (HWE) was tested in 18 reports (56.3%). Among them, the presence (or the absence) of deviating SNPs was highlighted and excluded from further analysis in 17 studies (94.4%). Finally, all studies provided definitions, justifications for their choices, and results for all outcomes investigated (32; 100%).

3.2.2. Pediatric Studies

Cohort studies accounted for 41.6% of pediatric studies ($n = 5$), followed by case reports and case series (4 studies; 33.3%). Sample sizes ranged from single cases (2 case reports) to 279 patients (a cohort study). The population was aged 3 to 20 years old. Ancestry was not reported in most publications (7 studies; 58.3%). All studies in which ethnicity was reported included Caucasian/European/White populations and African/Black populations (5; 100%). Patients' diagnosis was mentioned in 11 studies (91.6%); psychotic disorders in 8 of them (72.7%) and mood disorders in 5 of them (45.5%). Cytochromes were genotyped in a great majority of reports (9; 75.0%). Olanzapine was mentioned in nearly all the publications (11; 91.6%). Among the studied ADRs, 5 studies were related to inadequate efficacy (41.7%), 4 (33.3%) to weight gain or MetS, and 3 (25.0%) to neurological symptoms. Detailed characteristics of the included pediatric studies are provided in Table 1.

For pediatric studies, the average quality assessment score was 9.1/24 (±1.7), ranging from 6 (a case series) to 13 (a cohort study). The adjustment for multiple testing was described in one-fourth of the studies (3; 25.0%), and precise p-values were provided for all associations in one-half of the studies (6; 50.0%). No pediatric study provided details on the calculation of the sample size nor on the a priori power to detect effect sizes of varying degrees. The genotyping procedure was described in nearly all the publications (11; 92.0%). However, no study described the primers nor the quality control methods used. Previously reported genotype frequencies were quoted in 4 studies (33.3%). No study reported blinding of the genotyping personnel to outcome status. One study (1; 8.3%) summarized the extent of missing data (a cohort study), but justifications were not provided. The number of patients contributing to analyses agreed to the sample size in 10 studies (83.3%). HWE was tested in one study (a cohort study), where the absence of deviation was highlighted (1; 8.3%). The comprehensive quality assessment for pediatric studies is displayed in Table S1.

Table 1. Characteristics of the studies (pediatric population).

Study	Design	N	Age (Years)	Male (%)	Ancestry	Diagnosis	Antipsychotic	Gene Variant	ADR	Quality
Baumann et al. (2006)	Case Report	1	14	0	Swiss?	OCD	Olanzapine	CYP2D6 XN; *4; CYP3A5 *3; CYP2B6 *6; CYP2C9 *1; CYP2C19 *1	Generalized tonic-clonic seizure	8
Prows et al. (2009)	Cohort study	279 (18 OLZ)	3 to 18; mean (12.7 ± 3.2)	50.9%	White 72.4%; Black 22.6%; Other 5.0%	Mood disorders; Disruptive behavior; Anxiety, ICD; Psychotic disorders; PDD; ED; Adjustment disorders; Other	Olanzapine	CYP2D6 *1, *3, *4, *5, Dup; CYP2C19 *1, *2	Sleep disturbances; gastro-intestinal symptoms; headache, difficulty concentrating; mood change; dizziness; extrapyramidal symptoms; aggressive behavior; rash; shortness of breath; lack of therapeutic effect	9
Devlin et al. (2012)	Case-control study	105 (4 OLZ)	mean (12.58 ± 3.14)	66.7%	European 74%; Asian 8.7%; Aboriginal 2.9%; South Asian 2.9%; African/Caribbean 10.7%; Hispanic 4.8%	Non provided	Olanzapine	MTHFR (rs1801133) C677T C;T	Metabolic syndrome	9
Nussbaum et al. (2014)	Cohort study	81	9 to 20; median (15.74)	46%	Romanian?	Schizophrenia; BD	Olanzapine	CYP2D6 *4	Weight gain	9
Nussbaum et al. (2014)	Cohort study	81	9 to 20; median (15.74)	46%	Romanian?	Schizophrenia; BD	Olanzapine	CYP2D6 *4	Lack of therapeutic effect	8
Butwicka et al. (2014)	Case Report	1	16	100%	Polish?	Schizophreniform disorder	Olanzapine	CYP2D6 *4	Neuroleptic Malignant Syndrome	8
Cote et al. (2015)	Case-control study	134 (5 OLZ)	mean (12.5 ± 3.1)	68.7%	European 73.9%; African 7.5%; Asian 9.0%; Hispanic 5.2%; South Asian 2.2%; First Nations 2.2%	Anxiety, Depression, ADHD, Mood disorder, Psychotic disorder, Adjustment disorder, PDD, Other	Olanzapine	COMT Val158Met (rs4680) Met; Val	Cardiometabolic risk factors	10
Ocete-Hita et al. (2017)	Case-control study	92: 30 cases (1 OLZ); 62 controls	0 to 15; mean (8.3 ± 3)	36.7%	White 90%; Black 3.3%; Other 6.6%	ADHD	Olanzapine	Class I HLA-A, B, C* loci, class II HLA-DRB1, DQB1, DQA1, DP loci, KIR: 14 KIR genes and 2 pseudo-KIR genes; TNFα (rs1800629); TGFβ1 (-10T/A; 25C/G); IL-10 ((rs1800896); -819T/C; -(rs1800872)); IL-6 (rs1800795); IFNγ (rs2430561)	DILI: Idiosyncratic Drug-Induced Liver Injury	10
Thümmler et al. (2018)	Case series	9 (3 OLZ, CLZ, LOX)	11 to 16; mean (14.1 ± 1.8) (13 to 16 OLZ, CLZ, LOX)	55.5% (33% OLZ, CLZ, LOX)	French?	COS, ASD, ODD (OLZ, CLZ, LOX); COS, PTSD, behavioral disorder, ASD, ODD, ID	Olanzapine; Clozapine; Loxapine	CYP2D6 *3, *4, *5, *6, *41, Dup	EPS, weight gain, hepatic cytolysis, akathisia, dystonia, galactorrhea, binge eating, weight gain, constipation, lack of therapeutic effect	9

153

Table 1. Cont.

Study	Design	N	Age (Years)	Male (%)	Ancestry	Diagnosis	Antipsychotic	Gene Variant	ADR	Quality
Grădinaru et al. (2019)	Cohort study	81	9 to 20; median (15.74)	54%	Romanian?	Schizophrenia; BD	Olanzapine	CYP2D6 *3, *4, *5, *41	Hyperprolactinemia	10
Ivashchenko et al. (2020)	Cohort study	53 (6 CLZ) (5 OLZ)	mean (15.08 ± 1.70)	52.8%	Russian?	BPD; schizophrenia; schizoaffective disorder; schizotypal disorder; MDD; delusional disorders	Clozapine; Olanzapine	CYP2D6 *4, *9, *10; CYP3A4 *22, CYP3A5 *3; ABCB1 (rs1128503, rs2032582, rs1045642); DRD2 (rs1800497); DRD4 (rs1800955); HTR2A (rs6313)	Lack of therapeutic effect; decreased/increased salivation, increased/reduced duration of sleep, tremor, constipation, subjective akathisia; polyuria/polydipsia; increased dream activity	13
Berel et al. (2021)	Case series	4	9; 10; 11; 14;	75%	2 Caucasian, 1 Caucasian/Indian, 1 African	Tourette syndrome and ID; behavioral disorders and neurodevelopmental delay; EOS; ASD with catatonia	Clozapine	CYP1A2 *1F, *1; CYP2D6 *1, *4, *10, *41; CYP2C19 *1, *2; CYP3A5 *1, *3; CYP3A4 *1; CYP2C9 *1, *3	Lack of therapeutic effect (low concentrations)	6

OLZ: Olanzapine; CLZ: Clozapine; LOX: Loxapine; OCD: Obsessive Compulsive Disorder; ICD: Impulse Control Disorder; PDD: Pervasive Development Disorder; ED: Eating Disorder; ADHD: Attention Deficit Hyperactivity Disorder; COS: Childhood Onset Schizophrenia; ASD: Autism Spectrum disorder; ODD: Oppositional Defiant Disorder; ID: Intellectual Disability; PTSD: Post-Traumatic Stress Disorder; BDP: Brief Psychotic Disorder; MDD: Major Depressive Disorder; EOS: Early Onset Schizophrenia; EPS: Extrapyramidal Syndrome ?: when the ancestry of the patients was not provided in a study, we hypothesized that it could be consistent with the study site, and reported it as such.

3.2.3. Mixed Population Studies

Among mixed-population studies, cohort studies were prevailing (15; 75.0%). The sample sizes ranged from 21 to 1445 (both case–control studies). Age ranged from 10 to 75 years old. Ancestry was available in 17 reports (85.0%), among which Caucasian/European/White populations accounted for 88.2% (15 reports). All studies included patients suffering from schizophrenia-spectrum disorders (20 reports; 100%). Serotonin receptors or transporters, genes coding for proteins involved in energy and lipid homeostasis, and COMT Val158Met (rs4680) polymorphism were assessed in 3 studies each (15.0%). Regarding antipsychotics of interest, 15 studies involved clozapine (75.0%), and 13 studies involved olanzapine (65.0%). Weight gain and MetS were studied in 14 studies (70.0%), followed by lack of therapeutic effect (3; 15.0%) and extrapyramidal syndrome (EPS) (2; 10.0%). Detailed characteristics of the mixed population studies are provided in Table 2.

For mixed population studies, the mean quality assessment score was 12.6/24 ($\pm$ 2.4), lying between 8 (a case–control study) and 18 (a cohort study). The method used to adjust for multiple testing was described in one-half of the studies (10; 50.0%). Precise p-values were provided for all associations in almost all studies (19; 95.0%).The calculation of sample size was detailed in one study (1; 5.0%) and the a priori power to detect effect sizes of varying degrees was detailed in 5 studies (5; 20.0%). All studies described the genotyping procedure (20; 100%). Primers were described in 8 studies (40.0%), and quality control methods in 6 studies (30.0%). Previously reported genotype frequencies were quoted in one-fourth of the studies (5; 25.0%). Genotyping personnel was blinded to outcome status in one study (a cohort study) (5.0%). The extent of missing data was summarized in 8 reports (40.0%), among which 6 justified it (75.0%). The number of patients contributing to the analyses agreed to sample size in 14 studies (70.0%). HWE was tested in 17 reports (85.0%), among which almost all (16; 94.1%) underlined the presence (or absence) of deviating SNPs and excluded them from further analysis when appropriate. The comprehensive quality assessment for mixed population studies is displayed in Table S2.

Table 2. Characteristics of the studies (mixed population).

Study	Design	N	Age (Years)	Male (%)	Ancestry	Diagnosis	Antipsychotic	Gene Variant	ADR	Quality
Vandel et al. (1999)	Case-control study	65: 22 cases (1 OLZ); 43 controls	16 to 75; mean (41.9 ± 1.9)	35%	French?	MDD, dysthymia, OCD, schizophrenia	Olanzapine	CYP2D6 *1A, *2, *2B, *3, *4A, *4D *5, *6B, *9, *10B	EPS: akathisia, dystonia, parkinsonism, dyskinesia	8
Hong et al. (2002)	Cohort study	88	18 to 66; mean (37.1 ± 8.2)	66%	Han Chinese	schizophrenic disorders	Clozapine	H1 receptor (rs2067467) Glu, Asp	Weight gain	11
Mosyagin et al. (2004)	Case-control study	159: 81 cases (49 CLZ), (2 OLZ); 78 controls	Female: 22 to 85; mean (48); Male: 18 to 77; mean (47)	36%	German Whites	schizophrenia paranoid type	Clozapine, Olanzapine	MPO (rs2333227) G,A; CYBA (rs4673) C,T; (rs1049255) A,G	Agranulocytosis	13
Theisen et al. (2004)	Cohort study	97	14 to 45; mean (22.1 ± 7.7)	59%	German	schizophrenia spectrum disorders	Clozapine	5-HT2CR (rs3813929)-759C/T C,T	Weight gain	11
Kohlrausch et al. (2008)	Cohort study	121: (55 NR), (27 NOGS)	16 to 64: mean (34.02 ± 8.79) total; mean (34.13 ± 9.84) NR; mean (34.37 ± 9.41) NOGS	total 83.5%; NR 81.8%; NOGS 70.4%	European	schizophrenia	Clozapine	GNB3 (rs5443) 825C > T	Lack of therapeutic effect, NOGS: new onset generalized seizures	12
Godlewska et al. (2009)	Cohort study	107	mean (29.3 ± 10.0)	49%	Caucasian, Polish	schizophrenia (mostly paranoid)	Olanzapine	5-HT2CR (rs3813929) 759C/T C,T; 5-HT2CR (rs518147) 697G/C G,C	Weight gain	13
Le Hellard et al. (2009)	Cohort study	160	10 to 64; mean (21.9 ± 8.9)	61%	German	schizophrenia spectrum disorders	Clozapine	44 SNPs: 3 SNPs in INSIG1; 21 SNPs in INSIG2; 3 SNPs in SCAP; 4 SNPs in SREBF1; 13 SNPs in SREBF2	Weight gain	14
Tiwari et al. (2010)	Cohort study	183	18 to 60; mean (36.12 ± 10.17)	67.8%	European-American 63.9%; African-American 30.1%; Others 6.0%	schizophrenia or schizoaffective disorders	Clozapine, Olanzapine	20 SNPs in CNR1	Weight gain	17
Lencz et al. (2010)	Cohort study	58	16 to 38; mean (23.5 ± 4.9)	76.8%	African-American 40%; Caucasian (European) 28%; Hispanic 19%; Asian 5%; Other 8%	schizophrenia, schizoaffective or schizophreniform disorder	Olanzapine	DRD2 (rs1799732) 141C Ins; Del	Weight gain	12
Kohlrausch et al. (2010)	Cohort study	116 (52 NR)	16 to 64; mean (33.82 ± 8.51)/R: mean (33.89 ± 8.04)/NR: mean (33.73 ± 9.14)	85.3%/R 85.9%/NR 84.6%	European	schizophrenia	Clozapine	5-HTT HTTLPR (rs25531) LA, LG, S; VNTR Stin2 9, 10, 12 repeats	Lack of therapeutic effect	11
Jassim et al. (2011)	Cohort study	160	10 to 64; mean (21.9 ± 8.9)	61%	Central European	schizophrenia spectrum disorders	Clozapine	96 SNPs: 13 for ADIPOQ; 10 for FABP3; 7 for PRKAA1; 14 for PRKAA2; 3 for PRKAB1; 4 for PRKAG1; 40 for PRKAG2; 4 for PRKAG3; 1 for FTO	Weight gain	12
Choong et al. (2013)	Cohort study	444; S1: 152; S2: 174; S3: 118	S1: 19 to 64, median (42); S2: 12 to 69, median (35); S3: 19 to 69, median (42)	S1: 52%; S2: 49%; S3: 67%	Swiss?	Psychotic disorders, mood disorders, others	Clozapine, Olanzapine	3 CRTC1 SNPs: rs10402536 G > A; rs8104411 C > T; rs3746266 A > G	Weight gain	13
Gagliano et al. (2014)	Cohort study	99	18 to 65 median (34)	44%	Caucasian	schizophrenia or schizoaffective disorders	Clozapine, Olanzapine	16 PRKAR2B SNPs	Weight gain	18
Dong et al. (2015)	Cohort study	536: D: 328; R: 208	D: 18 to 45 mean (29.1 ± 7.6); R: 18 to 60 mean (21.3 ± 8.2)	D: 48.7%; R 57.2%	Chinese Han	schizophrenia	Olanzapine	4 A2BP1 SNPs: rs10500331, rs4786847, rs8048076, rs1478697, rs10500331	Weight gain	14
Pouget et al. (2015)	Case-control study	1445: 670 cases; 775 controls	18 to 60; (38.54 ± 10.4)	71%	European	schizophrenia of schizoaffective disorders	Clozapine, Olanzapine	TSPO 8 SNPs: rs739092, rs5759197, rs138911, rs113515, rs6971, rs6973, rs80411, rs138926	Weight gain; lack of therapeutic effect	16

Table 2. Cont.

Study	Design	N	Age (Years)	Male (%)	Ancestry	Diagnosis	Antipsychotic	Gene Variant	ADR	Quality
Quteineh et al. (2015)	Cohort study	834: 478 + 168 + 188	main: 12 to 97 median 50; S1 19.5 to 64, median (42.2); S2: 19 to 69, median (42.3)	main: 43.7%; S1 52.9%; S2 62.2%	White	Psychotic disorders, mood disorders, schizoaffective disorders, others	Clozapine, Olanzapine	HSD11B1 7 variants: rs12565406 G > T, rs10863782 G > A, rs846910 G > A, rs375319 G > A, rs12086634 T > G, rs4844488 A > G, rs84690 C > T	MetS	11
Saigi et al. (2016)	Cohort study	750: S1: 425; S2:148; S3: 177	combined 13 to 97 median 45; S1 13 to 97 median 51; S2 19 to 64 median 42; S3 18 to 69 median 42	combined 50%; s1 43% s2 55% s3 62%	White	psychotic disorders, schizoaffective disorders, BD, depression, other	Clozapine, Olanzapine	52 SNPs previously associated with BMI/21 associated with type 2 diabetes/9 associated with psychiatric disorders	Weight gain	14
Nelson et al. (2018)	Case-control study	71: cases 32 (1 OLZ); controls 39	15 to 55 Met FEP mean 25.15 ± 7.20, Val FEP mean 22.92 ± 7.08	FEP Met 75%; FEP Val 58%	Caucasian, African American, Other	schizophrenia spectrum, BD with psychosis, MDD with psychosis, psychotic disorder NOS	Olanzapine	COMT Val158Met (rs4680) Met; Val	alteration of cognitive flexibility	11
Menus et al. (2020)	Cohort study	96	18 to 74, median (39)	40%	Hungarian?	schizophrenia	Clozapine	CYP1A2 *1C, *1F, *1; CYP3A5 *1, *3; CYP3A4 *1, *1B, *22	MetS, altered concentration, hypersalivation, blurred vision, constipation, fatigue	11
Nicotera et al. (2021)	Case-control study	21: 4 cases; 17 controls	16 to 46	62%	Caucasian	ID, psychotic disorder, schizophrenia spectrum, gait disorder, specific learning disorder, schizotypal personality disorder	Clozapine, Olanzapine	COMT Val158Met (rs4680) Met; Val COMT L136L (rs4818) G,C	Dystonia	11

OLZ: Olanzapine; CLZ: Clozapine; NR: Non responders; FEP: First episode psychosis; OCD: Obsessive Compulsive Disorder; ID: Intellectual Disability; MDD: Major Depressive Disorder; BD: Bipolar Disorders; SNP: Single-Nucleotide Polymorphism; EPS: extrapyramidal syndrome; MetS: Metabolic Syndrome. Ancestry: '?' when the ancestry of the patients was not provided in a study, we then hypothesized that it could be consistent with the study site, and reported it as such.

3.3. Main Adverse Drug Reactions

3.3.1. Weight Gain and Metabolic Syndrome

While 14 studies (43.8%) investigated solely weight gain, 4 studies (12.5%) addressed the potential correlations of MetS with genetics, as shown in Table 3. Among studies specifically assessing antipsychotic-induced weight gain (AIWG), 2 were pediatric studies (14.3%) and 12 were mixed-population studies (85.7%). Both pediatric and mixed studies accounted for half (2; 50.0%) of the reports addressing MetS.

In 2014, Nussbaum et al. [51] found that *CYP2D6 wt/*4 (intermediate metabolizer–IM)* children had a significant increase in weight gain when compared to the patients without **4 allele*, after six months of administration of atypical APs ($p < 0.001$). Likewise, Thümmler et al. [3] reported the case of a *CYP2D6 *4/*41 (poor metabolizer–PM)* 14-year-old female who showed weight gain and binge-eating behaviors when treated with clozapine and loxapine. According to the findings of Menus et al. [61], a moderate/high risk of obesity in patients treated with clozapine was significantly more frequent in *low CYP3A4 expressers* (13.6% of *CYP3A4 low expressers*, 1.5% of *CYP3A4 normal/high expressers*, OR = 13.5 (95% CI 1.2–147.9), n = 87, $p = 0.045$). However, there was no association between *CYP1A2* or *CYP3A4* expression and blood glucose or lipid levels ($p > 0.1$). By contrast, in *low CYP3A4 expressers*, a significant correlation was found between the clozapine serum concentration and blood glucose level (r = 0.52, n = 20, $p = 0.02$).

Few studies investigated the potential link between lipid homeostasis and polymorphisms of genes involved in energy. Indeed, Le Hellard et al. [53] found a strong association ($p = 0.0003–0.00007$) between three genetic polymorphisms localized within or near the *INSIG2 gene (rs17587100, rs10490624,* and *rs17047764)* and AIWG in patients treated with clozapine. Choong et al. [60] found that carriers of the *CRTC1 (rs3746266) G allele* had a lower BMI than noncarriers *(AA genotype)* ($p = 0.001$, $p = 0.05$, and $p = 0.0003$, respectively, in the three samples). When excluding patients taking other weight gain-inducing drugs, *G allele* carriers ($n = 98$) had a 1.81 kg/m^2 lower BMI than noncarriers ($n = 226$; $p < 0.0001$). This association was more marked in women aged under 45 years, with a 3.87 kg/m^2 lower BMI in *G allele* carriers ($n = 25$) compared with noncarriers ($n = 48$; $p < 0.0001$). In patients treated with clozapine, Jassim et al. [54] found a marked association between AIWG and 6 genetic polymorphisms in *ADIPOQ*, among which only 2 showed both allelic and genotypic association. Body Mass Index (BMI) changes were, to a lesser extent, associated with one marker in *PRKAA1 (rs10074991)*, by an allelic ($p = 0.011$) and genotypic ($p = 0.004$) association, as well as three markers in *PRKAA2 (rs4912411*, $p = 0.044$; *rs7519509*, $p = 0.043$; *rs10489617*, $p = 0.036$). In *PRKAG2*, one marker (*rs17714947*, $p = 0.020$) displayed allelic association with AIWG, while another marker (*rs7800069*, $p = 0.0008$) showed genotypic association. By contrast, Gagliano et al. [56] analyzed 16 tag SNPs across the *PRKAR2B* gene in a sample of patients treated with clozapine or olanzapine. Patients displaying the minor allele of the polymorphism *PRKAR2B (rs9656135)* had a mean weight increase of 4.1%, whereas patients without this allele had an increase of 3.4%, but this association did not remain significant after correcting for multiple testing. Quteineh et al. [58] found that only male carriers of the *HSD11β1 (rs846906) T allele* had significantly higher waist circumference and triglycerides (TG), and lower high-density lipoprotein cholesterol (HDL) ($p_{corrected} = 0.028$). This allele was also associated with a higher risk of antipsychotic-induced MetS at 3 months of follow-up (OR = 3.31 (95% CI 1.53–7.17), $p_{corrected} = 0.014$). When studying patients treated with APs, the impact of 52 SNPs previously associated with BMI changes, Saigi et al. [59] found that *CADM2 (rs13078807)* showed a nominal association with BMI over time ($p = 0.01$), with a 1.04 increase in BMI per additional risk allele after 12 months of treatment. The genetic polymorphisms *HSD11β1 (rs3753519)* ($p = 0.00001$) and *CRTC2 (rs8450)* ($p = 0.04$) were also associated with a risk of an increase in BMI.

Regarding genotyping of *5-HT2C* (serotonin) *receptor*, Theisen et al. [55] found no association between the *5-HT2C receptor (rs3813929)-759C allele* and weight gain after 12 weeks of clozapine treatment in 97 patients with schizophrenia. Notwithstanding, among patients treated with olanzapine and genotyped for *5-HT2C receptor (rs518147)*, Godlewska et al. [62] found that significantly less patients with -697C (3/51, $p \leq 0.0006$) and no patient with -759T (0/28, $p \leq 0.002$) *alleles* experienced a BMI increase $\geq 10\%$. In an analysis of body weight change after 4 months of clozapine treatment, Hong et al. [63] showed no relationship with the histamine receptor H1 genotype (rs2067467). The analysis of *DRD2 -141C (rs1799732)* by Lencz et al. [64] in patients treated with APs showed that *deletion carriers* gained significantly more weight over time (time-by-genotype interaction, $p = 0.024$). Tiwari et al. [57] showed a nominal association of the CNR1 (rs806378) polymorphism with weight gain in patients treated with clozapine or olanzapine. *T allele* (minor allele) carriers gained more weight (5.96%) than the CC carriers (2.76%, $p \leq 0.008$), which can be translated into approximately 2.2 kg more weight gain in patients carrying the *T allele* (CC vs. CT + TT, 2.21 ± 4.51 vs. 4.33 ± 3.89 kg; $p \leq 0.022$). When searching for an association of *COMT Val158Met (rs4680)* variants with MetS, Cote et al. [65] found that atypical AP-treated children with the Met allele had higher systolic ($p = 0.014$) and diastolic ($p = 0.034$) blood pressure, and higher fasting glucose concentrations ($p = 0.030$) compared with children with the Val/Val genotype.

In atypical AP-treated children, Devlin et al. [66] found an association between the *MTHFR (rs1801133) 677T allele* with MetS ($p \leq 0.05$) (OR 5.75 [95% CI 1.18–28.12]). Dong et al. [67] found that the *A2BP1 (rs1478697)* polymorphism was significantly associated with AIWG caused by olanzapine ($p = 0.0012$, Bonferroni corrected $p = 0.0048$). This association was replicated in another sample, including 208 first-episode and drug-naïve patients presenting with schizophrenia after a 4-week treatment with olanzapine ($p = 0.0092$, Bonferroni corrected $p = 0.0368$). Pouget et al. [68] found no association between *TSPO (rs739092, rs5759197, rs138911, rs113515, rs6971, rs6973, rs80411 and rs138926)* polymorphisms and weight change.

Table 3. Synthesis of studies investigating metabolic adverse drug reactions.

Study	Diagnosis	Antipsychotic	Dosing	Outcome Measured	Gene Variant	Role of the Genes	Association	Pathophysiology
Devlin et al. (2012)	Not provided	Olanzapine	Not provided	MetS: weight; waist circumference; BMI; DBP and SBP; plasma glucose, insulin, TC, LDL; HDL; TG; ALAT; ASAT	MTHFR (rs1801133) C677T C;T	Conversion of folate to 5-methyltetrahydrofolate (active form)	SGA-treated children with T-allele: ↑ prevalence of MetS, ↑ diastolic blood pressure Z-scores, and fasting plasma glucose	Changes in DNA methylation + gene expression profile that favors development of MetS characteristics.
Nussbaum et al. (2014) A	Schizophrenia; BD	Olanzapine	Not provided	Weight gain; BMI; insulin variations	CYP2D6 *4	Drug and steroid metabolism	Patients with the genotype wt/*4, IM have significantly ↑ WG values than the patients without *4 allele.	Nonfunctional CYP2D6 alleles increase exposure to antipsychotics.
Cote et al. (2015)	Anxiety, Depression, ADHD, Mood disorder, Psychotic disorder, Adjustment disorder, PDD, Other	Olanzapine	Not provided	Cardiometabolic risk factors: Plasma glucose, insulin, TC, LDL, HDL, TG; weight, waist circumference, BMI, DBP and SBP	COMT Val158Met (rs4680) Met; Val	Degradation of catecholamines	No significant findings. Interaction observed for SBP z-score. Children with Met allele had ↑ fasting plasma glucose and ↓ HDL.	COMT Val158Met genotype may influence epigenetic regulation and ↓ activity of COMT = deleterious effect on cardiometabolic dysfunction and BP regulation.
Thümmler et al. (2018)	COS, ASD, ODD (OLZ, CLZ, LOX); COS, PTSD, behavior disorders, ASD, ODD, ID	Olanzapine; Clozapine; Loxapine	Not provided	Lack of therapeutic effect, various ADRs (weight gain, dystonia...)	CYP2D6 *3, *4, *5, *6, *41, Dup	Drug and steroid metabolism	Major adverse events in 4/9 patients	Accumulation of metabolites, CYP expression variation with age, drugs which are CYP inhibitors
Hong et al. (2002)	schizophrenic disorders	Clozapine	Not provided	Body weight change; BMI	H1 (rs2067467): Glu, Asp	H1 (histamine) receptor	No significant correlation between BWC and H1 genotypes.	In animal studies, blocking the H1 receptor = stimulation of feeding behaviors, and ↑ weight gain.
Theisen et al. (2004)	schizophrenia spectrum disorders	Clozapine	mean clozapine dose: 302 ± 128 mg/day (range 100–800 mg/day)	Weight gain; BMI change	5-HT2CR (rs3813929)-759C/T C,T	5-HT2CR: serotonin receptor	Higher proportion of patients with the CC genotypes with weight gain when compared with those with a T allele, this result was not significant.	Serotonin has been suggested to play an important role in the regulation of feeding behavior.
Godlewska et al. (2009)	schizophrenia (mostly paranoid)	Olanzapine	Olanzapine monotherapy: range 20–25mg/day	Weight gain; BMI change	5-HT2CR (rs3813929) 759C/T C,T; 5-HT2CR (rs518147) 697G/C G,C	5-HT2CR: serotonin receptor	A protective effect of -759T and -697C alleles was found: significantly less patients with -697C and no patient with -759T alleles experienced body mass index increase above 10%.	Serotonin could play an important role in the regulation of feeding behavior, especially particular through 5-HT2C receptors.
Le Hellard et al. (2009)	schizophrenia spectrum disorders	Clozapine	range 20–25 mg/day	Weight gain; BMI	44 SNPs: 3 SNPs in INSIG1; 21 SNPs in INSIG2; 3 SNPs in SCAP; 4 SNPs in SREBF1; 13 SNPs in SREBF2	INSIG1; INSIG2; SCAP; SREBF1 and SREBF2: regulation of biosynthesis and uptake of lipids	Strong association between 3 markers localized within or near the INSIG2 gene (rs17587100, rs10490624 and rs17047764) and AIWG.	SREBP mediated activation of lipid biosynthesis in cultured cells. INSIG2 has recently been implicated as a susceptibility gene in obesity
Tiwari et al. (2010)	schizophrenia or schizoaffective disorders	Clozapine, Olanzapine	mean clozapine dose: 285 ± 121 mg/day (range 50–800 mg/day)	Weight gain	20 SNPs in CNR1	CNR1: cannabinoid receptor	No association of any of the polymorphisms with weight change. In the European subgroup, the polymorphism rs806378 was the only significant SNP in genotypic comparison. Carriers of the 'T' allele gained more weight than the CC genotype carriers. In African-Americans a significant association was observed only for rs1049353 (increased risk for CT vs. CC).	The T allele created a binding site for arylhydrocarbon receptor translocator, a member of the basic helix–loop–helix/Per–Arnt–Sim protein family. Genetic polymorphisms in the CNR1 gene have been associated with basal metabolic index, obesity and various metabolic parameters.
Lencz et al. (2010)	schizophrenia, schizoaffective or schizophreniform disorder	Olanzapine	Patients randomly assigned to receive either clozapine (500 mg/day), olanzapine (20 mg/day)	Weight gain; BMI change	DRD2 (rs1799732) 141C Ins;Del	DRD2: dopamine receptor	Deletion carriers gained significantly more weight; they began to separate from Ins/Ins homozygotes after 6 weeks of treatment on either medication.	Liability to antipsychotic-induced weight gain may be related to variation in density of D2 receptors.

158

Table 3. *Cont.*

Study	Diagnosis	Antipsychotic	Dosing	Outcome Measured	Gene Variant	Role of the Genes	Association	Pathophysiology
Jassim et al. (2011)	schizophrenia spectrum disorders	Clozapine	Not provided	Weight gain; BMI change as BMI-1_2 (from the start of the AP until prior to the clozapine administration), Δ BMI-2_3 (during the clozapine administration) and Δ BMI-1_3 (the whole AP treatment) period	96 SNPs: 13 for ADIPOQ; 10 for FABP3; 7 for PRKAA1; 14 for PRKAA2; 3 for PRKAB1; 4 for PRKAG1; 40 for PRKAG2; 4 for PRKAG3; 1 for FTO	ADIPOQ; FABP3; PRKAA1; PRKAA2; PRKAB1; PRKAG1; PRKAG2; PRKAG3; FTO: regulation of lipid and energy homeostasis	Allelic and genotypic association between rs17300539 in the ADIPOQ gene and Δ BMI-1_2 and Δ BMI-1_3. 4 other ADIPOQ markers showed nominal allelic association to Δ BMI-1_2 (rs17373414) or Δ BMI-2_3 (rs864265, rs1501299 and rs6773957). rs6773957 also displayed genotypic association for Δ BMI-2_3, together with rs3821799. 1 marker in PRKAA1 (rs10074991) displayed allelic and genotypic association to Δ BMI-1_3. In PRKAA2, 3 markers demonstrated weak association either to Δ BMI-1_2 (rs4912411) or Δ BMI-1_3 (rs7519509 and rs10489617). In PRKAG2, one marker (rs17714947) demonstrated allelic, and another marker (rs7800069) genotypic association with Δ BMI-2_3.	Adiponectin has recently been suggested as a biomarker for AP-induced metabolic disturbances: negative correlation between circulating levels of adiponectin and BMI, TG and insulin levels in patients taking AP. Variants of AMPK-encoding genes influence the baseline BMI, with limited if any direct effects upon AIWG.
Choong et al. (2013)	Psychotic disorders, mood disorders, others	Clozapine, Olanzapine	Not provided	Weight gain; BMI change	3 CRTC1 SNPs: rs10402536 G > A; rs8104411 C > T; rs3746266 A >G	CREB co-activator (mood, memory, energy metabolism...)	Significant association between CRTC1 rs3746266 A > G and BMI, with G carriers having a lower BMI. After adjustment for the severity of the psychiatric disorder, the association between BMI and CRTC1 rs3746266 A > G is even stronger. Stronger association in women, especially < 45 years. The T allele of rs6510997C > T (a proxy of the rs3746266 G allele) was associated with lower BMI and fat mass.	Role for the CRTC1 gene in the regulation of human bodyweight and fat mass consistent with animal models. Psychiatric illness and/or weight gain-inducing psychotropic drugs might play a role in genetically mediated energy homeostasis
Gagliano et al. (2014)	schizophrenia or schizoaffective disorders	Clozapine, Olanzapine	Not provided	Weight gain	16 PRKAR2B SNPs	PRKAR2B: regulation of lipid homeostasis	One SNPs in PRKAR2B (rs9656135) was significantly associated with AIWG before correcting for multiple testing, but lost significance when adjusting for the 176 effective tests.	Evidence was provided by animal studies suggesting a role of the PRKAR2B gene in energy metabolism.
Dong et al. (2015)	schizophrenia	Olanzapine	Not provided	Weight gain; BMI	4 A2BP1 SNPs: rs10500331, rs4786847, rs8048076, rs1478697, rs10500331	A2BP1: regulates tissue-specific splicing, involved in neurological function	The SNP rs1478697 in the A2BP1 gene was associated with olanzapine-induced WG. The association of rs8048076 did not remain significant after correction for multiple comparisons.	A2BP1 gene was preferentially expressed in the human brain; it might affect adiposity via the hypothalamic MC4R pathway, explaining the role of A2BP1 in olanzapine induced AIWG.

Table 3. Cont.

Study	Diagnosis	Antipsychotic	Dosing	Outcome Measured	Gene Variant	Role of the Genes	Association	Pathophysiology
Pouget et al. (2015)	schizophrenia of schizoaffective disorders	Clozapine, Olanzapine	Olanzapine dose (mg/d) D: 10.2 ± 2.3 R: 11.8 ± 3.1	Weight gain; lack of therapeutic effect through treatment response (BPRS)	TSPO 8 SNPs: rs739092, rs5759197, rs138911, rs113515, rs6971, rs6973, rs80411, rs138926	TSPO: translocator protein, peripheral benzodiazepine receptor	No association between any of the TSPO SNPs and change in overall BPRS. Non significant trend for association between rs6971 and WG, with an increase in weight for each Thr allele an individual carried. In the subset of 78 subjects treated with clozapine or olanzapine, rs6971 was nominally associated with weight gain, but did not remain significant after multiple testing correction.	Unknown mechanism by which TSPO influences glucose lowering and activation of fasting metabolism, possibilities include the altering of steroid synthesis, cytokine production or ROS levels.
Quteineh et al. (2015)	Psychotic disorders, mood disorders, schizoaffective disorders, others	Clozapine, Olanzapine	Not provided	Weight gain, blood pressure and the other components of MetS	HSD11B1 7 variants: rs12565406 G > T, rs10863782 G > A, rs846910 G > A, rs375319 G > A, rs12086634 T > G, rs4844488 A > G, rs84690 C > T	HSD11B1: cortisone reductase, reduces cortisone to the active hormone cortisol	Carriers of the variant rs846910-A, rs375319-A, and rs4844488-G alleles showed lower BMI values and lower WC, compared with patients with the wild-type genotypes. Association was exclusively detected in women. For the rs846906C > T SNP, only men carrying the T-allele showed higher WC compared with noncarriers. Among women, carriers of the rs846910-A, rs375319-A, and rs4844488-G alleles had lower DBP compared with noncarriers. Among men, carriers of the T-allele had higher TG levels compared with noncarriers. Men carrying the T-allele of rs846906C > T showed lower HDL-C levels compared with noncarriers.	A direct relationship between aromatase activity and body weight was proposed + estrogen may increase cortisone to cortisol conversion mediated by 11 β-HSD1 and cortisol may increase aromatase activity = more estrogen in the tissues. Findings between rs846906C > T and lipid traits and BWC in men are not explained.
Saigi et al. (2016)	psychotic disorders, schizoaffective disorders, BD, depression, other	Clozapine, Olanzapine	Not provided	Weight gain, waist circumference, serum lipids, glucose	52 SNP's previously associated with BMI	Weight regulation; glycemia regulation; psychiatric disorders	w-GRS of 32 polymorphisms significantly associated with BMI in men 1 SNP in CADM2 gene showed a nominal association with BMI over time. At 12 months of treatment, the rs13078807 polymorphism showed an increase in BMI for each additional risk allele. HSD11β1 rs3753519 showed an association with lower BMI for rs3753519 in patients homozygous for the variant allele compared to wild types.	The HSD11β1 gene codes for a microsomal enzyme-catalyzing tissue regeneration of active cortisol from the inactive form cortisone. It is highly expressed in metabolic tissues such as the liver and adipose tissue. ↑ plasma cortisol levels have been associated with visceral obesity and metabolic syndrome. An overexpression of this gene has been associated with hyperphagia and obesity in mice. CADM2 plays an important role in systemic energy homeostasis.

Table 3. Cont.

Study	Diagnosis	Antipsychotic	Dosing	Outcome Measured	Gene Variant	Role of the Genes	Association	Pathophysiology
Menus et al. (2020)	schizophrenia	Clozapine	Clozapine daily dose (mg): 194.3 ± 130.5	Structured questionnaire + BMI, bodyweight (obesity), fasting glucose concentrations, TG, TC, HDL, LDL	CYP1A2 *1C, *1F, *1; CYP3A5 *1, *3; CYP3A4 *1, *1B, *22	Drug and steroid metabolism	No association between CYP1A2 or CYP3A4 expression and blood glucose, TG or cholesterol levels in patients. Moderate/high risk obesity was significantly more frequent in low CYP3A4 expressers. In low CYP3A4 expressers, a significant correlation was found between clozapine serum concentration (or daily dose) and blood glucose level	The relative activity of CYP1A2 and CYP3A4 is assumed to determine which enzyme has a greater role in clozapine metabolism. 5-HT2C antagonism has been reported to be a mechanism underlying atypical AIWG + norclozapine has a greater antagonist effect on 5-HT2C receptors than the parent compound = positive correlation between BMI and norclozapine/clozapine ratios.

OLZ: Olanzapine; CLZ: Clozapine; LOX: Loxapine; PDD: Pervasive Development Disorder; ADHD: Attention Deficit Hyperactivity Disorder; COS: Childhood Onset Schizophrenia. ASD: Autism Spectrum disorder; ODD: Oppositional Defiant Disorder; ID: Intellectual Disability; PTSD: Post-Traumatic Stress Disorder; BD: Bipolar Disorders; SNP: Single-Nucleotide Polymorphism; MetS: Metabolic syndrome; DBP: Diastolic Blood pressure; SBP: Systolic Blood Pressure; SGA: Second-Generation Antipsychotic; IM: Intermediate Metabolizer; BWC: Body Weight Change; AIWG: Antipsychotic-Induced Weight Gain.

3.3.2. Neurological Symptoms: Movement Abnormalities and Seizures

Our query retrieved two studies investigating seizures (28.6%) and five studies addressing movement abnormalities (71.4%), as shown in Table 4. One pediatric and one mixed population study assessed antipsychotic-induced seizures (50%). In addition, two pediatric (40%) and thee mixed studies (60%) investigated movement abnormalities.

Baumann et al. [69] reported an epileptiform seizure, which occurred in a 16-year-old female treated with sertraline and olanzapine. She was found to be CYP3A5 *3/*3 (though, with a preserved CYP3A activity), CYP2B6 *6/*6, and CYP2D6 *4/*4 (PM). Indeed, the resulting high sertraline plasma levels added to the olanzapine treatment could have contributed to the onset of the seizure. Prows et al. [70] found that patients' combined phenotype (generated via CYP2C19 and CYP2D6 phenotypes) was associated with the number of ADRs ($p = 0.03$). Combined PMs treated with psychotropics had the highest number of ADRs (among which EPS was classified as a severe ADR), and *combined ultrarapid metabolizers (UMs)* had the lowest number of ADRs. By contrast, Thümmler et al. [3] reported the case of a CYP2D6 (>2N) UM 16-year-old male that presented EPS when treated by olanzapine and clozapine. Their case series also mentioned the case of a 14-year-old female, CYP2D6 *4/*41 (PM), who presented numerous ADRs, including EPS, akathisia, and dystonia, when treated with clozapine and loxapine. In patients treated with psychotropic drugs, Vandel et al. [71] observed a higher percentage of carriers of a genotype with CYP2D6 unfunctional alleles in the group of patients suffering from extrapyramidal ADRs than in the symptom-free patient group ($p < 0.00001$).

Beyond cytochromes, Kohlrausch et al. (2008) [72] found that, in patients treated with clozapine, carriers of the *T825 allele* of the *GNB3 (rs5443)* polymorphism had a higher risk to present a convulsion episode ($p = 0.007$). Ivashchenko et al. [73] observed that patients with *HTR2A (rs6313) C allele* (42.1 vs. 0%, $p = 0.003$), but also patients with *DRD2 (rs1800497) T allele*, more often complained of tremor (50 vs. 21.6%, $p = 0.039$). However, these associations could not be confirmed because of coincidence with higher dosing of antipsychotics. In patients treated with APs, Nicotera et al. [74] found that the COMT Val158Met (rs4680) G/A (Val/Met) genotype was almost exclusively represented in patients presenting with persistent dystonia.

Table 4. Synthesis of studies investigating neurological adverse drug reactions.

Study	Diagnosis	Antipsychotic	Dosing	Outcome Measured	Gene Variant	Role of the Genes	Association	Pathophysiology
Baumann et al. (2006)	OCD	Olanzapine	Olanzapine at 2.5 mg/d (day 1) and titrated until 10 mg/d on day 42	Epileptiform seizure	CYP2D6 *4; CYP3A5 *3; CYP2B6 *6; CYP2C9 *1; CYP2C19 *1	Drug and steroid metabolism	CYP3A5: PM 100% (but normal CYP3A activity); CYP2B6: PM 100% and CYP2D6: PM 100% (may explain high sertraline plasma levels)	Seizure favored by high sertraline concentrations + olanzapine
Prows et al. (2009)	Mood disorders; Disruptive behavior; Anxiety, ICD; Psychotic disorders; PDD; ED; Adjustment disorders; Other	Olanzapine	Not provided	Behavioral Intervention Score (BIS); number of PRN doses; LOS; change in GAF from admission to discharge; number of ADRs (sleep disturbances, EPS...)	CYP2D6 *1, *3, *4, *5, Dup; CYP2C19 *1, *2	Drug and steroid metabolism	Significant relationship between combined predicted phenotype and the number of ADRs. Relationship between CYP2C19-predicted metabolizing phenotype and number and severity of ADRs.	Increased metabolizing capacity leads to a decrease in drug efficacy and number of ADRs. Regarding CYP2C19, its decreased metabolizing ability led to an increase in the number/severity of ADRs
Thümmler et al. (2018)	COS, ASD, ODD (OLZ, CLZ, LOX); COS, PTSD, behavioral disorders, ASD, ODD, ID	Olanzapine; Clozapine; Loxapine	Not provided	Lack of therapeutic effect, various ADRs (EPS, dystonia...)	CYP2D6 *3, *4, *5, *6, *41, Dup	Drug and steroid metabolism	Major adverse events were described in 4/9 patients representing 1/2 of PM and 2/3 of UM	Accumulation of metabolites + CYP expression patterns alter with age + some drugs are inhibitors of CYP = might be related to pharmacoresistance.
Ivashchenko et al. (2020)	BPD; schizophrenia; schizoaffective disorder; schizotypal disorder; MDD; delusional disorders	Clozapine; Olanzapine	mean (SGA) (50 [50; 180] mg/day)	Tolerability of psychopharmacology: UKU SERS (salivation, duration of sleep, tremor, akathisia...), SAS, BARS; effectiveness of antipsychotics: PANSS;	CYP2D6 *4, *9, *10; CYP3A4 *22, CYP3A5 *3; ABCB1 (rs1128503, rs2032582, rs1045642); DRD2 (rs1800497); DRD4 (rs1800955); HTR2A (rs6313)	CYP2D6, CYP3A4, CYP3A5: drug and steroid metabolism. ABCB1: ATP-dependent efflux pump; DRD2 and DRD4: dopamine receptors; HTR2A: serotonin receptor	Patients with HTR2A rs6313 more often complained of tremor. DRD2 rs1800497 was significantly associated with tremor.	Associations of DRD2 rs1800497 and HTR2A rs6313 with ADEs could not be confirmed because there was coincidence with higher daily doses of antipsychotics.
Vandel et al. (1999)	MDD, dysthymia, OCD, schizophrenia	Olanzapine	Olanzapine 10	EPS (SAS, Leo's criteria)	CYP2D6 *1A, *2, *2B, *3, *4A, *4D *5, *6B, *9, *10B	Drug and steroid metabolism	Higher % of genotypes with no (extensive) functional alleles in the group of patients suffering from extrapyramidal side effects.	Increased exposure
Kohlrausch et al. (2008)	schizophrenia	Clozapine	Mean daily dose of clozapine: 540.91 mg/day, but varied from 100 to 900 mg/day	Clozapine response (BPRS ↓ 30% = appropriate response); occurrence of clozapine-induced NOGS (clinical interviews)	GNB3 (rs5443) 825C > T	GNB3: G-protein (G-protein-coupled receptors GPCRs)	Carriers of the T825 allele showed an increased risk for a convulsive episode.	Since dopamine and serotonin receptor subtypes activate intracellular pathways through GPCRs, the effect of the variability in the GNB3 gene might affect CNS toxicity of clozapine.
Nicotera et al. (2021)	ID, psychotic disorder, schizophrenia spectrum, gait disorder, specific learning disorder, schizotypal personality disorder	Clozapine, Olanzapine	Not provided	Dystonia (review of medical records)	COMT Val158Met (rs4680) Met; Val COMT L136L (rs4818) G,C	Degradation of catecholamines	G/G and A/A genotype polymorphisms of COMT gene are associated with a protective effect for developing EPS. G/A genotype, almost exclusively present in sensible patients, could be a risk factor for developing dystonia after administration of APs.	The V158M polymorphism of the COMT = low enzymatic activity and ↑ dopamine levels in the CNS = this can cause or aggravate EPS in these patients (including parkinsonism, akathisia, dystonia, and dyskinesia).

OCD: Obsessive Compulsive Disorder; ICD: Impulse Control Disorder; PDD: Pervasive Developmental Disorder; ED: Eating Disorder; COS: Childhood onset schizophrenia; ASD: Autism spectrum disorder; ODD: Oppositional Defiant Disorder; PTSD: Post-Traumatic Stress Disorder; ID: Intellectual Disability; BPD: Brief Psychotic Disorder; MDD: Major Depressive Disorder; OLZ: Olanzapine; CLZ: Clozapine; LOX: Loxapine; PRN: Pro re nata, "as needed" basis; LOS: Length of Stay; GAF: Global Assessment of Functioning; UKU SERS: UKU Side Effect Self-Rating Scale; SAS: Simpson-Angus Scale; BARS: Barnes Akathisia Rating Scale; PANSS: Positive And Negative Syndrome Scale; BPRS: Brief Psychiatric Rating Scale; NOGS: New Onset Generalized Seizures; EPS: Extrapyramidal Syndrome; CNS: Central Nervous System.

3.3.3. Lack of Therapeutic Effect

Among studies addressing lack of therapeutic effect (Table 5), pediatric and mixed studies each accounted for a half (4; 50%).

Berel et al. [11] reported four cases of children (1: *CYP1A2 *1F/*1F* (UM), 2: *CYP2D6 *1/*41* (IM) *CYP3A5 *1/*1*, 3: *CYP2C9 *1/*3* (IM), 4: *CYP1A2 *1/*1F* (UM)) presenting with behavioral disorders of various causes. In all these cases, low clozapine plasma levels led to a lack of therapeutic effect, corrected with fluvoxamine (*CYP1A2* inhibitor) addition. Among children treated with psychotropic drugs, Prows et al. [70] found that the combined phenotype of *CYP2D6* and *CYP2C19* was associated with behavior intervention score (BIS), which is a measure of aggression severity (depending on the number of recorded timeouts/seclusions, therapeutic holds, and physical restraints). In this context, combined PMs had the lowest BIS (highest efficacy), and combined UMs had the highest BIS (lowest efficacy). There was no difference among groups in change in GAF (Global Assessment of Functioning) scores ($p = 0.90$). In children treated with atypical APs, Nussbaum et al. [52] found a significant correlation between the *CYP2D6 wt/*4* genotype and higher PANSS (Positive And Negative Syndrome Scale, used in schizophrenia) scores, indicating a poor clinical outcome and a bad response to the atypical antipsychotics ($p = 0.001$). In line with these findings, Thümmler et al. [3] noted that in their case series, five patients out of nine with pharmacoresistant mental health disease presented functional CYP2D6 abnormalities (three patients > 2N (UM), one patient *4/*41 (PM), and one patient *3/*4 (PM)). Conversely, Ivashschenko et al. [73] observed that *CYP2D6*, *CYP3A5*3*, and *ABCB1 (rs1128503, rs2032582, rs1045642)* genetic polymorphisms were not significantly associated with a change in the mean score of PANSS between 1 and 14 days of treatment. Yet, the carriers of *DRD2 C2137T (rs1800497)* had a higher degree of the PANSS "productive symptoms" subscale score change (M = −7.5 (−9; −4.5) vs. M = −4 (−7; −2), $p = 0.005$). In addition, for *HTR2A T102C (rs6313)* polymorphism, the improvement of C-allele carriers in PANSS subscale "negative symptoms" was significantly lower than in *TT homozygotes* (M = −1 (−3.25; 0.25) vs. M = −3 (−6; −1), $p = 0.037$, respectively).

Regarding other genes, Kohlrausch et al. (2008) [72] found an increased frequency of homozygosity for the *GNB3 (rs5443) T825* allele among non-responders to clozapine ($p = 0.021$). In 2010, Kohlrausch et al. [75] found significant differences between responders and non-responders to clozapine involving the *5-HTT HTTLPR (rs25531)* polymorphism. Non-responders displayed a higher frequency of *S'-allele* ($p = 0.01$) and were more likely to *be S'/S' homozygous* or *S'/L' heterozygous* than the responders ($p = 0.04$). In patients treated with APs, Pouget et al. [68] found no association between investigated SNPs for TSPO *(rs739092, rs5759197, rs138911, rs113515, rs6971, rs6973, rs80411,* and *rs138926)* and change in Brief Psychiatric Rating Scale (BPRS) (all $p_{uncor} > 0.05$).

Figure 2A,B summarizes the number of studies evaluating the drug–ADR association, for pediatric and mixed population studies, respectively.

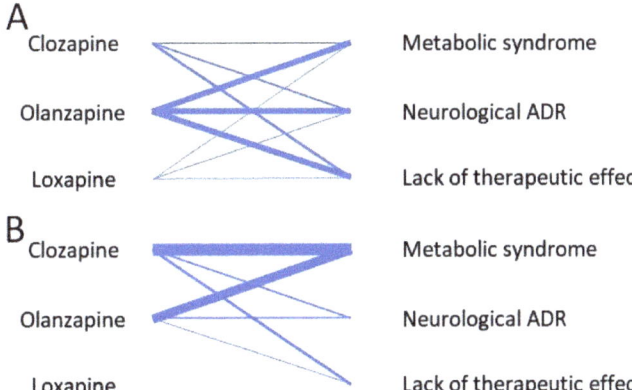

Figure 2. (**A**) Network diagram for pediatric pharmacogenetic studies regarding CYP1A2-metabolized AP and their adverse drug reactions. (**B**) Network diagram for mixed population pharmacogenetic studies regarding CYP1A2-metabolized AP and their adverse drug reactions. The thickness of the connecting lines corresponds to the number of studies evaluating the drug–ADR association.

Table 5. Synthesis of studies investigating lack of therapeutic effect.

Study	Diagnosis	Antipsychotic	Dosing	Outcome Measured	Gene Variant	Role of the Genes	Association	Pathophysiology
Prows et al. (2009)	Mood disorders; Disruptive behavior; Anxiety, ICD; Psychotic disorders; PDD; ED; Adjustment disorders; Other	Olanzapine	Not provided	Behavioral Intervention Score (BIS); number of PRN doses; LOS; change in GAF from admission to discharge; number of ADRs (including sleep disturbances, EPS...)	CYP2D6 *1, *3, *4, *5, Dup; CYP2C19 *1, *2	Drug and steroid metabolism	C-PM group had lower BIS (higher efficacy), C-UM group had highest BIS (lowest efficacy). Significant relationship between combined predicted phenotype and the number of ADRs. Relationship between CYP2C19-predicted metabolizing phenotype and number and severity of ADRs.	Increased metabolizing -> decrease in drug efficacy and number of ADRs. CYP2C19's decreased metabolizing ability -> ↑ in the number/severity of ADRs
Nussbaum et al. (2014) B	Schizophrenia; BD	Olanzapine	Not provided	Lack of therapeutic effect: change in PANSS	CYP2D6 *4	Drug and steroid metabolism	Significant correlations between wt/*4 genotype, ↑ PANSS scores, a poor clinical outcome and a bad drug response	Drug response to atypical APs correlated with the CYP2D6 genotype
Thümmler et al. (2018)	COS, ASD, ODD (OLZ, CLZ, LOX); COS, PTSD, behavioral disorders, ASD, ODD, ID	Olanzapine; Clozapine; Loxapine	Not provided	Lack of therapeutic effect, various ADRs (weight gain, dystonia...)	CYP2D6 *3, *4, *5, *6, *41, Dup	Drug and steroid metabolism	5/9 patients with pharmacoresistant mental health disease presented functional CYP2D6 abnormalities.	CYP expression patterns varies with age, in addition to direct metabolism by CYP2D6, some drugs are inhibitors of CYPs
Ivashchenko et al. (2020)	BPD; schizophrenia; schizoaffective disorder; schizotypal disorder; MDD; delusional disorders	Clozapine; Olanzapine	mean (SGA) (50 [50; 180] mg/day)	Tolerability of psychopharmacology: UKU SERS, SAS, BARS; effectiveness of antipsychotics: PANSS; salivation, duration of sleep, tremor, akathisia...	CYP2D6 *4, *9, *10; CYP3A4 *22; CYP3A5 *3; ABCB1 (rs1128503, rs2032582, rs1045642); DRD2 (rs1800497); DRD4 (rs1800955); HTR2A (rs6313)	CYP2D6, CYP3A4, CYP3A5: drug and steroid metabolism; ABCB1: ATP-dependent efflux pump; DRD2 and DRD4: dopamine receptors; HTR2A: serotonin receptor	Carriers of DRD2 C2137T (rs1800497) had higher degree of productive symptoms subscale score change. Significant associations between the HTR2A T102C polymorphism (rs6313) and the subscale negative symptoms: the improvement in C-allele carriers significantly lower than in TT homozygotes.	DRD2 rs1800497 T-allele is associated with ↓ activity of D2 receptors (↓ binding to the ligand). ↓ in HTR2A expression in CNS may alter antipsychotics' effect in terms of reducing negative symptoms.
Berel et al. (2021)	Tourette syndrome and ID; behavioral disorders and neurodevelopmental delay; EOS; ASD with catatonia	Clozapine	clozapine dosage (500 mg/day); clozapine dosage (300 mg/day); clozapine dosage between 400 and 500 mg/day; clozapine dosage (200 mg/day)	Clozapine plasma levels and clinical improvement (SAPS, ABC) with adjunction of fluvoxamine	CYP1A2 *1F, *1; CYP2D6 *1, *4, *10, *41; CYP2C19 *1, *2; CYP3A5 *1, *3; CYP3A4 *1; CYP2C9 *1, *3	Drug and steroid metabolism	CYP1A2 UM: low clozapine plasma levels, ↑ with fluvoxamine addition (clinical improvement) CYP2D6 IM; CYP3A5 UM: low clozapine plasma levels -> fluvoxamine addition clozapine levels ↑ (clinical improvement) CYP2C9 PM: low clozapine plasma levels, ↑ with fluvoxamine addition (clinical improvement) CYP1A2 UM CYP2D6 IM CYP2C19 IM: low clozapine plasma levels, ↑ with fluvoxamine addition (clinical improvement)	Genotypes explaining low clozapine plasma level + lack of improvement with previous treatments
Kohlrausch et al. (2008)	schizophrenia	Clozapine	Mean daily dose of clozapine: 540.91 mg/day, but varied from 100 to 900 mg/day	Clozapine response (BPRS, reduction 30% = appropriate response); occurrence of clozapine induced new onset generalized seizures (clinical interviews)	GNB3 (rs5443) 825C > T	GNB3: G-protein (G-protein-coupled receptors GPCRs)	Homozygosity for the T825 allele more frequent among NR Homozygosity for the C825 allele more frequent among responders.	Dopamine and serotonin receptor subtypes activate intracellular pathways through GPCRs, the variability in GNB3 gene might affect medication response.

Table 5. Cont.

Study	Diagnosis	Antipsychotic	Dosing	Outcome Measured	Gene Variant	Role of the Genes	Association	Pathophysiology
Kohlrausch et al. (2010)	schizophrenia	Clozapine	Patients received clozapine at doses ranging from 100 to 900 mg daily; mean daily dose of clozapine: 540.91 mg/day.	Lack of therapeutic effect: non responders/responders (30% reduction BPRS)	5-HTT HTTLPR (rs25531) LA, LG, S; VNTR Stin2 9, 10, 12 repeats	5-HTT: serotonin transporter	The S'-allele of HTTLPR/rs25531 was more frequent in NR. No significant association between the polymorphisms of VNTR Stin2 and clozapine response.	Carriers of the low expression allele S' would be under increased risk for poor response to clozapine, through the influence in availability of extracellular serotonin concentrations at all synapses. Since the action of clozapine is by antagonism of serotonin receptors, the serotonin transporter coded by the L'L' genotype (higher expression compared with the S' allele), mediates more active re-uptake of serotonin –> less serotonin would be available to compete with clozapine for the serotonin receptors, facilitating its action.
Pouget et al. (2015)	schizophrenia of schizoaffective disorders	Clozapine, Olanzapine	Not provided	Weight gain; lack of therapeutic effect through treatment response (BPRS)	TSPO 8 SNPs: rs739092, rs5759197, rs138911, rs113515, rs6971, rs6973, rs80411, rs138926	TSPO: translocator protein, peripheral benzodiazepine receptor	We found no association between any of the TSPO SNPs and change in overall BPRS. Nonsignificant trend for association between rs6971 and weight gain, with an increase in weight for each Thr allele an individual carried. In the subset of 78 subjects treated with clozapine or olanzapine, rs6971 was nominally associated with weight gain, but did not remain significant after multiple testing correction.	TSPO may act as a modifier gene, affecting clinical features of schizophrenia not investigated in the study. Although the mechanism by which TSPO influences glucose lowering and activation of fasting metabolism is unknown, possibilities include the altering of steroid synthesis, cytokine production or ROS levels.

ICD: Impulse Control Disorder; PDD: Pervasive Developmental Disorder; ED: Eating Disorder; COS: Childhood Onset Schizophrenia; ASD: Autism spectrum disorder; ODD: Oppositional Defiant Disorder; PTSD: Post-Traumatic Stress Disorder; ID: Intellectual Disability; BPD: Brief Psychotic Disorder; MDD: Major Depressive Disorder; OLZ: Olanzapine; CLZ: Clozapine; LOX: Loxapine; PRN: Pro re nata, "as needed" basis; LOS: Length of Stay; GAF: Global Assessment of Functioning; UKU SERS: UKU Side Effect Self-Rating Scale; SAS: Simpson-Angus Scale; BARS: Barnes Akathisia Rating Scale; PANSS: Positive and Negative Syndrome Scale; BPRS: Brief Psychiatric Rating Scale; ABC: Aberrant Behavior Checklist; SAPS: Scale for the Assessment of Positive Symptoms; EPS: Extrapyramidal Syndrome.

3.3.4. Others

Studies investigating other ADRs were represented by a majority of pediatric studies (5; 62.8%), the remaining 3 (37.5%) relying on mixed-population samples.

Butwicka et al. [76] reported the case of a patient who presented a neuroleptic malignant syndrome when treated with olanzapine. His CYP2D6 genotype was CYP2D6*4/*4 (PM), indicating a lack of activity. Likewise, Thümmler et al. mentioned the case of a CYP2D6 (>2N) (UM) adolescent presenting a clozapine-induced hepatic cytolysis. They also reported a case of a CYP2D6 *4/*41 (PM) adolescent with, among other ADRs, galactorrhea and constipation, treated with clozapine and loxapine. In patients treated with atypical APs, Grădinaru et al. [77] found that the mean level of prolactin was higher for IMs than for extensive (normal) metabolizers (EMs) at each time point except baseline. Menus et al. [61] noted a significant effect of CYP3A4 expression on constipation (47.1% in normal/high CYP3A4 expressers, 71.4% in low CYP3A4 expressers, OR = 3.6 (95% CI = 0.9–14.1), $p = 0.06$). Ivashschenko et al. [73] found a significantly more frequent increased dream activity in CYP2D6 IMs compared to EMs (54 vs. 22%, $p = 0.043$). Increased duration of sleep was more frequent among TT homozygotes of ABCB1 (rs2032582) polymorphism (50 vs. 15.8%, $p = 0.006$) and TT of ABCB1 (rs1045642) polymorphism (41.7 vs. 8.2%, $p = 0.007$). DRD2 (rs1800497) T allele was significantly associated with constipation (25 vs. 5.4%, $p = 0.039$).

Beyond cytochromes assessments, Mosyagin et al. [78] studied a population of schizophrenic patients having presented a drug-induced agranulocytosis. They found that for *MPO (rs2333227)* polymorphism, the *AA carriers* (low activity) were overrepresented among cases (OR = 4.16 (95% CI 0.86–20.3), $p = 0.056$). This finding was even more marked in clozapine-induced agranulocytosis ($p = 0.04$). Ocete-Hita et al. [79] investigated idiosyncratic Drug-Induced Liver Injury (DILI) in a pediatric sample, in which one case has been imputed to olanzapine. The human leucocyte antigens *HLA-DRB*12* (OR = 9.3 (95% CI 1–88.1), $p = 0.05$) and *HLA-DQA*0102* (OR = 2.51 (95% CI 0.9–6.5), $p = 0.058$) were more commonly found in children presenting DILI. Using the Penn Conditional Exclusion Test (PCET), Nelson et al. [80] investigated the relationship of performance errors (as a reflection of cognitive flexibility alteration) with *COMT Val158Met (rs4680)* genotype in patients treated with atypical APs. *Met carriers* displayed significant changes for error type ($F(1,62) = 14.874$, $p < 0.001$) and time ($F(1,62) = 14.068$, $p < 0.001$), characterized by a decrease in perseverative and regressive errors following AP treatment. Among the *Val homozygotes*, the perseverative error rate was not modified after treatment, while regressive errors rate increased ($F(1,36) = 6.26$, $p = 0.017$).

3.4. Main Implications of Cytochromes Genotyping

Among studies involving cytochrome genotyping, nine relied on exclusively pediatric samples (81.8%), while two (18.2%) were based on mixed populations. Most of the studies (10; 90.9%) investigating a potential cytochrome involvement were genotyping at least one *CYP2D6* genetic polymorphism. Then, *CYP3A5* genetic polymorphisms were assessed in four studies (36.3%), followed by *CYP2C19* and *CYP3A4* (3; 27.2%), *CYP2C9* and *CYP1A2* (2; 18.1%), and *CYP2B6* (1; 9.1%).

Vandel et al. [71] showed a higher percentage of genotypes, including at least one allele characterized by an extensive enzyme metabolic capacity for *CYP2D6* in the symptom-free group (86%) in comparison with 45.4% in the group suffering from EPS. The genotypes deprived from extensive functional alleles were more frequent (54.4%) in the group of patients suffering from EPS than in the other group (14%).

Butwicka et al. [76] reported the case of a 16-year-old male who experienced a neuroleptic malignant syndrome while being treated by olanzapine. This patient displayed a *CYP2D6 *4/*4* (PM) genotype, leading to a decreased *CYP2D6* activity. Nussbaum et al. [51] found that patients showing a *CYP2D6 wt/*4* genotype presented a higher BMI than patients showing a *wt/wt* genotype. A difference across these groups was also noted for insulin values. Nussbaum et al. [52] further noted that the PANSS score in the *CYP2D6 wt/*4* group was higher than in the *wt/wt* group. Indeed, the first patients would have exhibited no adequate drug response.

As stated above, Thümmler et al. [3] described five young patients with pharmacoresistant mental health disease who displayed *CYP2D6* abnormalities: three patients were >2N UM and two patients were PM with **4/*41* and **3/*4* polymorphisms. Major psychotropic ADRs were found in four patients (EPS, akathisia, dystonia, binge eating and weight gain, hepatic cytolysis, galactorrhea, and constipation inter alia).

Grădinaru et al. [77] found that, in *CYP2D6* poor and intermediate metabolizers, the use of atypical APs led to a significant increase in prolactin levels from baseline to 18 months. In IMs, the mean level of prolactin was higher than in EMs at each time point except baseline. After 6 months of AP treatment, IMs displayed a significant increase in prolactin level, over EMs.

Ivashschenko et al. [73] noted an increased dream activity in *CYP2D6* IMs compared to NMs (54 vs. 22%; $p = 0.043$). *CYP2D6* was not significantly associated with a change in the mean score of the PANSS between 1 and 14 days of treatment.

Prows et al. [70] found a relationship between *CYP2D6*-predicted metabolizing phenotype and BIS ($p = 0.01$). Indeed, they noted a statistically significant relationship between combined phenotype (*CYP2D6* and *CYP2C19*) and BIS ($p = 0.01$).

In the case series of Berel et al. [11], the second patient presented a *CYP2D6* IM phenotype and a *CYP3A5 *1/*1* polymorphism, and these profiles could have contributed to previous high aripiprazole and low haloperidol plasma levels.

In Ivashschenko et al.'s study [73], *CYP3A5*3* polymorphism was not significantly associated with changes in the mean score of the PANSS between 1 and 14 days of treatment.

In Prows et al.'s study [70], while a significant association between combined phenotype (*CYP2D6* and *CYP2C19*) and BIS was found, no relationship was detected between *CYP2C19*-predicted metabolizing phenotype and BIS ($p = 0.57$). Nonetheless, a relationship between *CYP2C19*-predicted metabolizing phenotype and the number of ADRs was observed ($p = 0.01$). *CYP2C19*-predicted metabolizing phenotype has also been linked to the type of ADRs (severe vs. mild vs. none, $p = 0.04$).

In the study of Menus et al. [61], exaggerated clozapine concentrations (>600 ng/mL) were more frequently noted in low *CYP3A4* expressers (22%) than in normal/high expressers (2.7%) (low vs. normal/high expressers: OR = 9.8 (95% CI 1.8–55.0), $p = 0.009$). They also noted an association between norclozapine formation and *CYP3A4* expression (0.56 ± 0.17 vs. 0.98 ± 0.62, $p < 0.0001$). However, no association was found between *CYP3A4* expression and blood glucose, TG, or cholesterol (total, HDL, and LDL) levels in patients ($p > 0.1$). Still, moderate/high risk obesity was significantly more frequent in low *CYP3A4* expressers than in normal expressers (13.6% of *CYP3A4* low expressers, 1.5% of *CYP3A4* normal/high expressers, OR = 13.5 (95% CI 1.2–147.9), $p = 0.045$). *CYP3A4* low expressers more frequently reported constipation, as stated before. In low *CYP3A4* expressers only, significant correlations were found between clozapine serum concentration and blood glucose level ($r = 0.52$, $p = 0.02$), and between glucose concentrations and the daily dose of clozapine ($r = 0.49$, $p = 0.03$). In normal/high *CYP3A4* expressers, fasting glucose ($r = 0.27$, $p = 0.03$) and TG levels ($r = 0.26$, $p = 0.048$) significantly correlated with norclozapine/clozapine ratios.

In the study of Berel et al. [11], the third patient was found to display a *CYP2C9*1/*3* heterozygous genotype. Leading to a *CYP2C9* IM phenotype, it could partly explain the low clozapine plasma levels.

Berel et al. [11] reported in their case series two 11-year-old patients with low clozapine plasma levels, which were found to be *CYP1A2* UM (*CYP1A2*1F/*1F* and *CYP1A2*1/*1F*, respectively). Therefore, this issue has been corrected by the adjunction of fluvoxamine, a potent *CYP1A2* inhibitor. Menus et al. [61] demonstrated a contribution of *CYP1A2* to norclozapine production (0.86 ± 0.55 vs. 1.17 ± 0.70, $p = 0.0007$). Yet, no association was found between *CYP1A2* expression and blood glucose, TG, or cholesterol (total, HDL, and LDL) levels in patients ($p > 0.1$). Similarly, *CYP1A2* expression has not been linked with obesity ($p > 0.1$). None of the ADRs reported by patients was influenced by their *CYP1A2* expression ($p > 0.1$).

In the case report of Baumann et al. [69], *CYP2B6 *6/*6 homozygosity* added to a PM *CYP2D6* phenotype and to an olanzapine co-prescription, may have favored the occurrence of the epileptiform seizure.

4. Discussion

Our review aimed to assess whether pharmacogenetic mechanisms underly the occurrence of olanzapine, clozapine, and loxapine ADRs in children and youth. Several included publications investigated the genes involved in neurotransmission (COMT [65,74,80], serotonin receptors/transporters [55,62,73], dopamine receptors [64,73]), and in energy and lipid homeostasis (AMP-K related genes [54,56], *HSD11β1* [58,59]), mostly regarding weight gain (or MetS). However, findings regarding possible associations were sometimes conflicting. While *COMT Val158Met (rs4680)* genetic polymorphism may have influenced epigenetic regulation and, therefore, decreased activity of COMT, contributing to a deleterious effect in adults [81], Cote et al. [65] found no significant association in children. Whereas Theisen et al. [55] retrieved no association between the *5-HT2C receptor gene (rs3813929)* polymorphism and clozapine-induced weight gain, Godlewska et al. [62] found a protective effect of -759T and -697C alleles. In antipsychotic-naive patients, Houston et al. [82] did not find similar associations. However, highlighting the possible association of *DRD2* polymorphisms with increased weight gain, their findings supported Lencz et al.'s [64] conclusions. Otherwise, while our query yielded one study addressing the role of *HLA* gene variations in DILI (Ocete-Hita et al.) [79], we did not retrieve similar approaches regarding clozapine-induced neutropenia and agranulocytosis that formerly have been investigated [83].

Cytochromes genotyping (and phenotyping) was the preferred approach when investigating ADRs, especially in pediatric studies. Studies relying on large sample size underlined increased weight gain [51], prolactin levels [77], risk of EPS [71], and impaired treatment response [52] in patients deprived from at least one functional allele for *CYP2D6*, resulting in increased drug exposure. While the findings regarding movement abnormalities and lack of therapeutic effect concur with existing evidence [84,85], AIWG [86] and hyperprolactinemia [87] were not consistently linked with *CYP2D6* impairments. However, olanzapine is mostly metabolized by *CYP1A2* (and to a lesser extent by *CYP2D6* and *CYP3A4*) [88,89], clozapine is mainly metabolized by *CYP3A4* and *CYP1A2* (with *CYP2D6* playing a minor role) [16,90], and loxapine is primarily metabolized by *CYP1A2* (then by *CYP3A4* and *CYP2D6*) [19]. Despite the fact that Menus et al. [61] found no association between *CYP1A2* expression and any ADR, some variants have been formerly linked to tardive dyskinesia [91,92] and to an increased risk of insulin and lipid elevation [93].

Indeed, some of these discrepancies may originate from several limitations of the evidence included in our review. First, we chose to focus on studies involving children and youth, often characterized by smaller samples and thus lack of power to show an existing difference, and lower-evidence study designs (case reports/series). Several large cohorts were (at least partially) overlapping, therefore lowering the total size of the investigated population. Second, we aimed to assess the pharmacogenetic causes of ADRs related to olanzapine, clozapine, and loxapine, whereas several of our largest sample size studies investigated atypical APs indiscriminately. Furthermore, Thümmler et al. [3] only reported a case of patients treated with loxapine, which may be due to French-specific prescription behaviors [23,24]. Third, apart from metabolic changes, ADRs were subject to heterogeneous outcome measurements (EPS, clinical improvement), which may have prevented us from direct comparisons between different studies. Fourth, most studies lacked consideration for potential interacting factors with AP-induced side effects, such as co-treatments, inflammation, weight change, dietary habits, smoking, and/or consumption of caffeine. These factors may be prevailing, especially in transitioning-age youths, and are important to consider. Fifth, our quality assessment of the studies (see Methods), relying on a tool adapted from the checklist by Jorgensen and Williamson [50], yielded an average score of 11.3/24. Overall, some issues of concern were the lack of information upon quality control methods, handling of missing data, and population stratification. In studies including children and youth only, lack of adjustments for multiple testing and of HWE testing were frequent additional flaws, therefore lowering the mean quality score of these studies (9.1/24). Furthermore, the quality assessment tool we relied on may be used as a checklist for further pharmacogenetic studies, to improve the comprehensiveness of the presented results.

In fact, in addition to proper pediatric studies, and considering the foreseeable scarce body of evidence among this population, we accepted to include studies involving at least one youth patient (see Methods) [44]. Thus, while broadening the study population, it may have lowered the impact of the children's metabolic characteristics. As stated above, the features of the included studies did not permit a strict comparison, preventing any meta-analysis. Nevertheless, our grouping strategy, relying on the main ADR classes (see Methods), enabled qualitative assessments. As a flaw inherent to systematic reviews, reporting bias limits the interpretation of our findings, even if several studies showed negative results. Furthermore, as the overall quality of evidence could not be estimated with reference methods such as GRADE [94], the methodological quality of our included pharmacogenetic studies was assessed via a tool adapted from the checklist of Jorgensen and Williamson [50] (see Methods). Then, a quality assessment was conducted among pediatric and mixed-population studies, allowing us to detect the main issues of concern in each study category. For each database query, the two screening steps and the quality scoring were subject to a dual assessment (D.M. and A.O.G.), which may have limited sources of bias.

While findings in children and youth pharmacogenetics are conflicting regarding olanzapine, clozapine, and loxapine, the benefits of genotyping in clinical use may be limited by lack of sufficient evidence, the barriers to routine use, and overall impact [95]. However, the dose–effect relationship is significantly influenced by cytochromes, holding sway over exposure to the medication [96]. Yet, in comparison with *CYP2D6*, *CYP1A2* remains less investigated, while olanzapine and clozapine's ADRs are serious. Furthermore, cases of major clinical improvement were fostered by *CYP1A2* genotyping [11], although its benefit is not collective yet. The use of advanced technologies, such as WGS, might provide an interesting complement, broadening the research spectrum in psychiatric disorders [40,41]. From this perspective, further studies addressing the cytochromes' and other genes' (involved in energy homeostasis, metabolism, neurotransmission *inter alia*) impact should consider potential polypharmacy and intercurrent modifications in the metabolism of children and youth. Further studies may provide insights into possible cross-talks between the pathways associated with ADRs and GABA-A signaling, identifying new drug targets and therefore paving the way for the development of new antipsychotic drugs with variable receptor affinities. These drugs could constitute alternatives to thienobenzodiazepines, dibenzodiazepines, and dibenzoxazepines, and improve the acceptability of treatments. Phenotypical variations due to ancestry and/or infrequent cytochrome variants should also be taken into account by studying larger pediatric samples that originate from different countries. Determined by genetics, but influenced by the environment, *CYP1A2* and its interactions should be further investigated, to improve assessment of the risk–benefit balance in children and youth treated with olanzapine, clozapine, and loxapine.

Supplementary Materials: The following supporting information can be downloaded at: https://www.mdpi.com/article/10.3390/ph15060749/s1, Table S1 Quality assessment of included pediatric studies; Table S2 Quality assessment of included mixed population studies.

Author Contributions: Conceptualization, D.M., A.F. and S.T.; methodology, D.M., A.O.G., C.V. and S.T.; validation, D.M., A.O.G., M.-D.D. and S.T.; formal analysis, investigation, resources, data curation, D.M., A.O.G. and N.B.O.; writing—original draft preparation, D.M., A.O.G. and S.T.; writing—review and editing, A.F., F.A., C.V., F.R., M.-D.D. and S.T.; visualization, D.M. and S.T.; supervision, M.-D.D. and S.T.; project administration, D.M. and S.T. All authors have read and agreed to the published version of the manuscript.

Funding: This research received no external funding.

Institutional Review Board Statement: Not applicable.

Informed Consent Statement: Not applicable.

Data Availability Statement: Data sharing not applicable.

Conflicts of Interest: The authors declare no conflict of interest.

References

1. Krause, M.; Zhu, Y.; Huhn, M.; Schneider-Thoma, J.; Bighelli, I.; Chaimani, A.; Leucht, S. Efficacy, acceptability, and tolerability of antipsychotics in children and adolescents with schizophrenia: A network meta-analysis. *Eur. Neuropsychopharmacol.* **2018**, *28*, 659–674. [CrossRef] [PubMed]
2. Minjon, L.; van den Ban, E.; de Jong, E.; Souverein, P.C.; Egberts, T.C.; Heerdink, E.R. Reported Adverse Drug Reactions in Children and Adolescents Treated with Antipsychotics. *J. Child Adolesc. Psychopharmacol.* **2019**, *29*, 124–132. [CrossRef] [PubMed]
3. Thümmler, S.; Dor, E.; David, R.; Leali, G.; Battista, M.; David, A.; Askenazy, F.; Verstuyft, C. Pharmacoresistant Severe Mental Health Disorders in Children and Adolescents: Functional Abnormalities of Cytochrome P450 2D6. *Front. Psychiatry* **2018**, *9*. [CrossRef] [PubMed]

4. Aichhorn, W.; Whitworth, A.B.; Weiss, E.M.; Marksteiner, J. Second-Generation Antipsychotics: Is There Evidence for Sex Differences in Pharmacokinetic and Adverse Effect Profiles? *Drug Saf.* **2006**, *29*, 587–598. [CrossRef]
5. Becker, A.L.; Epperson, C.N. Female Puberty: Clinical Implications for the Use of Prolactin-Modulating Psychotropics. *Child Adolesc. Psychiatr. Clin. N. Am.* **2006**, *15*, 207–220. [CrossRef]
6. Sagud, M.; Mihaljević-Peles, A.; Mück-Seler, D.; Pivac, N.; Vuksan-Cusa, B.; Brataljenović, T.; Jakovljević, M. Smoking and Schizophrenia. *Psychiatr. Danub.* **2009**, *21*, 371–375. [CrossRef]
7. Barrangou-Poueys-Darlas, M.; Guerlais, M.; Laforgue, E.-J.; Bellouard, R.; Istvan, M.; Chauvin, P.; Guillet, J.-Y.; Jolliet, P.; Gregoire, M.; Victorri-Vigneau, C. CYP1A2 and tobacco interaction: A major pharmacokinetic challenge during smoking cessation. *Drug Metab. Rev.* **2021**, *53*, 30–44. [CrossRef]
8. David, R.N.; Nebert, D.W. Comparison of Cytochrome P450 (CYP) Genes from the Mouse and Human Genomes, Including Nomenclature Recommendations for Genes, Pseudogenes and Alternative-Splice Variants. *Pharm. Genom.* **2004**, *14*, 1–18.
9. Waring, R.H. Cytochrome P450: Genotype to phenotype. *Xenobiotica* **2020**, *50*, 9–18. [CrossRef]
10. Gaedigk, A.; Sangkuhl, K.; Whirl-Carrillo, M.; Klein, T.; Leeder, J.S. Prediction of CYP2D6 phenotype from genotype across world populations. *Genet. Med.* **2017**, *19*, 69–76. [CrossRef]
11. Berel, C.; Mossé, U.; Wils, J.; Cousin, L.; Imbert, L.; Gerardin, P.; Chaumette, B.; Lamoureux, F.; Ferrafiat, V. Interest of Fluvoxamine as an Add-On to Clozapine in Children with Severe Psychiatric Disorder According to CYP Polymorphisms: Experience from a Case Series. *Front. Psychiatry* **2021**, *12*. [CrossRef] [PubMed]
12. Altar, C.A.; Hornberger, J.; Shewade, A.; Cruz, V.; Garrison, J.; Mrazek, D. Clinical validity of cytochrome P450 metabolism and serotonin gene variants in psychiatric pharmacotherapy. *Int. Rev. Psychiatry* **2013**, *25*, 509–533. [CrossRef] [PubMed]
13. Maruf, A.A.; Stein, K.; Arnold, P.D.; Aitchison, K.J.; Müller, D.J.; Bousman, C. CYP2D6 and Antipsychotic Treatment Outcomes in Children and Youth: A Systematic Review. *J. Child Adolesc. Psychopharmacol.* **2021**, *31*, 33–45. [CrossRef] [PubMed]
14. Desta, Z.; Flockhart, D.A. Pharmacogenetics of Drug Metabolism. In *Clinical and Translational Science*, 2nd ed.; Robertson, D., Williams, G.H., Eds.; Academic Press: Cambridge, MA, USA, 2017; pp. 327–345. ISBN 978-0-12-802101-9. Chapter 18.
15. Callaghan, J.T.; Bergstrom, R.F.; Ptak, L.R.; Beasley, C. Olanzapine. Pharmacokinetic and Pharmacodynamic Profile. *Clin. Pharmacokinet.* **1999**, *37*, 177–193. [CrossRef] [PubMed]
16. Dean, L.; Kane, M. Clozapine Therapy and CYP Genotype. In *Medical Genetics Summaries*; Pratt, V.M., Scott, S.A., Pirmohamed, M., Esquivel, B., Kane, M.S., Kattman, B.L., Malheiro, A.J., Eds.; National Center for Biotechnology Information (US): Bethesda, MD, USA, 2012.
17. Luo, J.P.; Vashishtha, S.C.; Hawes, E.M.; McKay, G.; Midha, K.K.; Fang, J. In vitro identification of the human cytochrome p450 enzymes involved in the oxidative metabolism of loxapine. *Biopharm. Drug Dispos.* **2011**, *32*, 398–407. [CrossRef]
18. Glazer, W.M. Does loxapine have "atypical" properties? Clinical evidence. *J. Clin. Psychiatry* **1999**, *60* (Suppl. 10), 42–46.
19. Popovic, D.; Nuss, P.; Vieta, E. Revisiting loxapine: A systematic review. *Ann. Gen. Psychiatry* **2015**, *14*, 15. [CrossRef]
20. Diazepines, Oxazepines and Thiazepines. Available online: https://www.pharmgkb.org/chemical/PA164712682 (accessed on 26 April 2022).
21. Volavka, J. Violence in schizophrenia and bipolar disorder. *Psychiatr. Danub.* **2013**, *25*, 24–33.
22. Wang, P.S.; Ganz, D.A.; Benner, J.S.; Glynn, R.J.; Avorn, J. Should clozapine continue to be restricted to third-line status for schizophrenia?: A decision-analytic model. *J. Ment. Health Policy Econ.* **2004**, *7*, 77–85.
23. Lesem, M.D.; Tran-Johnson, T.K.; Riesenberg, R.A.; Feifel, D.; Allen, M.H.; Fishman, R.; Spyker, D.A.; Kehne, J.H.; Cassella, J.V. Rapid acute treatment of agitation in individuals with schizophrenia: Multicentre, randomised, placebo-controlled study of inhaled loxapine. *Br. J. Psychiatry* **2011**, *198*, 51–58. [CrossRef]
24. Bourdinaud, V.; Pochard, F. Survey of management methods for patients in a state of agitation at admission and emergency departments in France. *Encephale* **2003**, *29*, 89–98. [PubMed]
25. FDA-Approved Drugs: Olanzapine. Available online: https://www.accessdata.fda.gov/scripts/cder/daf/index.cfm?event=overview.process&ApplNo=020592 (accessed on 11 April 2022).
26. EMA Zyprexa. Available online: https://www.ema.europa.eu/en/medicines/human/EPAR/zyprexa (accessed on 15 April 2022).
27. FDA-Approved Drugs: Clozapine. Available online: https://www.accessdata.fda.gov/scripts/cder/daf/index.cfm?event=overview.process&ApplNo=019758 (accessed on 11 April 2022).
28. Rachamallu, V.; Elberson, B.W.; Vutam, E.; Aligeti, M. Off-Label Use of Clozapine in Children and Adolescents—A Literature Review. *Am. J. Ther.* **2019**, *26*, e406–e416. [CrossRef]
29. EMA EMA: Leponex (Clozapine). Available online: https://www.ema.europa.eu/en/medicines/human/referrals/leponex (accessed on 11 April 2022).
30. FDA-Approved Drugs: Loxapine. Available online: https://www.accessdata.fda.gov/scripts/cder/daf/index.cfm?event=overview.process&ApplNo=022549 (accessed on 11 April 2022).
31. EMA Adasuve. Available online: https://www.ema.europa.eu/en/medicines/human/EPAR/adasuve (accessed on 15 April 2022).
32. Résumé des Caractéristiques du Produit-LOXAPAC 100 Mg, Comprimé Pelliculé-Base de Données Publique des Médicaments. Available online: https://base-donnees-publique.medicaments.gouv.fr/affichageDoc.php?specid=69893582&typedoc=R (accessed on 11 April 2022).

33. Solmi, M.; Murru, A.; Pacchiarotti, I.; Undurraga, J.; Veronese, N.; Fornaro, M.; Stubbs, B.; Monaco, F.; Vieta, E.; Seeman, M.V.; et al. Safety, tolerability, and risks associated with first- and second-generation antipsychotics: A state-of-the-art clinical review. *Ther. Clin. Risk Manag.* **2017**, *13*, 757–777. [CrossRef] [PubMed]
34. Drici, M.-D.; Priori, S. Cardiovascular risks of atypical antipsychotic drug treatment. *Pharmacoepidemiol. Drug Saf.* **2007**, *16*, 882–890. [CrossRef] [PubMed]
35. Sohn, M.; Moga, D.; Blumenschein, K.; Talbert, J. National trends in off-label use of atypical antipsychotics in children and adolescents in the United States. *Medicine* **2016**, *95*, e3784. [CrossRef] [PubMed]
36. Schulz, C.; Haight, R.J. Safety of olanzapine use in adolescents. *Expert Opin. Drug Saf.* **2013**, *12*, 777–782. [CrossRef]
37. Selim, S.; Riesenberg, R.; Cassella, J.; Kunta, J.; Hellriegel, E.; Smith, M.A.; Vinks, A.A.; Rabinovich-Guilatt, L. Pharmacokinetics and Safety of Single-Dose Inhaled Loxapine in Children and Adolescents. *J. Clin. Pharmacol.* **2017**, *57*, 1244–1257. [CrossRef]
38. Roses, A.D. Pharmacogenetics and the practice of medicine. *Nature* **2000**, *405*, 857–865. [CrossRef]
39. Chaplin, M.H. Improving the Reporting of Pharmacogenetic Studies to Facilitate Evidence Synthesis: Anti-Tuberculosis Drug-Related Toxicity as an Example. Ph.D. Thesis, University of Liverpool, Liverpool, UK, 2021; p. 361.
40. Alkelai, A.; Greenbaum, L.; Docherty, A.R.; Shabalin, A.A.; Povysil, G.; Malakar, A.; Hughes, D.; Delaney, S.L.; Peabody, E.P.; McNamara, J.; et al. The benefit of diagnostic whole genome sequencing in schizophrenia and other psychotic disorders. *Mol. Psychiatry* **2021**, *27*, 1435–1447. [CrossRef]
41. Sanders, S.J.; Neale, B.M.; Huang, H.; Werling, D.M.; An, J.-Y.; Dong, S.; Abecasis, G.; Arguello, P.A.; Blangero, J.; Boehnke, M.; et al. Whole genome sequencing in psychiatric disorders: The WGSPD consortium. *Nat. Neurosci.* **2017**, *20*, 1661–1668. [CrossRef]
42. Samer, C.F.; Lorenzini, K.I.; Rollason, V.; Daali, Y.; Desmeules, J.A. Applications of CYP450 Testing in the Clinical Setting. *Mol. Diagn. Ther.* **2013**, *17*, 165–184. [CrossRef] [PubMed]
43. Page, M.J.; McKenzie, J.E.; Bossuyt, P.M.; Boutron, I.; Hoffmann, T.C.; Mulrow, C.D.; Shamseer, L.; Tetzlaff, J.M.; Akl, E.A.; Brennan, S.E.; et al. The PRISMA 2020 statement: An updated guideline for reporting systematic reviews. *BMJ* **2021**, *372*, n71. [CrossRef] [PubMed]
44. Farid-Kapadia, M.; Askie, L.; Hartling, L.; Contopoulos-Ioannidis, D.; Bhutta, Z.A.; Soll, R.; Moher, D.; Offringa, M. Do systematic reviews on pediatric topics need special methodological considerations? *BMC Pediatr.* **2017**, *17*, 57. [CrossRef] [PubMed]
45. Nations, U. Youth. Available online: https://www.un.org/en/global-issues/youth (accessed on 6 April 2022).
46. Newton, L. LibGuides: Original Research: Home. Available online: https://libguides.unf.edu/originalresearch/home (accessed on 18 March 2022).
47. Scherer, R.W.; Saldanha, I.J. How should systematic reviewers handle conference abstracts? A view from the trenches. *Syst. Rev.* **2019**, *8*, 264. [CrossRef] [PubMed]
48. Von Elm, E.; Altman, D.G.; Egger, M.; Pocock, S.J.; Gøtzsche, P.C.; Vandenbroucke, J.P.; STROBE Initiative. The Strengthening the Reporting of Observational Studies in Epidemiology (STROBE) Statement: Guidelines for Reporting Observational Studies. *Ann. Intern. Med.* **2007**, *147*, 573–577. [CrossRef]
49. Ross, S.; Anand, S.S.; Joseph, P.; Paré, G. Promises and challenges of pharmacogenetics: An overview of study design, methodological and statistical issues. *JRSM Cardiovasc. Dis.* **2012**, *1*, 1–13. [CrossRef]
50. Jorgensen, A.L.; Williamson, P.R. Methodological quality of pharmacogenetic studies: Issues of concern. *Stat. Med.* **2008**, *27*, 6547–6569. [CrossRef]
51. Nussbaum, L.A.; Dumitraşcu, V.; Tudor, A.; Grădinaru, R.; Andreescu, N.; Puiu, M. Molecular Study of Weight Gain Related to Atypical Antipsychotics: Clinical Implications of the CYP2D6 Genotype. *Rom. J. Morphol. Embryol.* **2014**, *55*, 877–884.
52. Nussbaum, L.; Grădinaru, R.; Andreescu, N.; Dumitraşcu, V.; Tudor, A.; Suciu, L.; Ştefănescu, R.; Puiu, M. The Response to Atypical Antipsychotic Drugs in Correlation with the Cyp2d6 Genotype: Clinical Implications and Perspectives. *Farmacia* **2014**, *62*, 1191–1201.
53. Le Hellard, S.; Theisen, F.M.; Haberhausen, M.; Raeder, M.B.; Fernø, J.; Gebhardt, S.; Hinney, A.; Remschmidt, H.; Krieg, J.C.; Mehler-Wex, C.; et al. Association between the insulin-induced gene 2 (INSIG2) and weight gain in a German sample of antipsychotic-treated schizophrenic patients: Perturbation of SREBP-controlled lipogenesis in drug-related metabolic adverse effects? *Mol. Psychiatry* **2009**, *14*, 308–317. [CrossRef]
54. Jassim, G.; Fernø, J.; Theisen, F.M.; Haberhausen, M.; Christoforou, A.; Håvik, B.; Gebhardt, S.; Remschmidt, H.; Mehler-Wex, C.; Hebebrand, J.; et al. Association Study of Energy Homeostasis Genes and Antipsychotic-Induced Weight Gain in Patients with Schizophrenia. *Pharmacopsychiatry* **2011**, *44*, 15–20. [CrossRef] [PubMed]
55. Theisen, F.M.; Hinney, A.; Brömel, T.; Heinzel-Gutenbrunner, M.; Martin, M.; Krieg, J.-C.; Remschmidt, H.; Hebebrand, J. Lack of association between the −759C/T polymorphism of the 5-HT2C receptor gene and clozapine-induced weight gain among German schizophrenic individuals. *Psychiatr. Genet.* **2004**, *14*, 139–142. [CrossRef] [PubMed]
56. Gagliano, S.A.; Tiwari, A.K.; Freeman, N.; Lieberman, J.A.; Meltzer, H.Y.; Kennedy, J.L.; Knight, J.; Müller, D.J. Protein kinase cAMP-dependent regulatory type II beta (*PRKAR2B*) gene variants in antipsychotic-induced weight gain. *Hum. Psychopharmacol.* **2014**, *29*, 330–335. [CrossRef] [PubMed]
57. Tiwari, A.K.; Zai, C.C.; Likhodi, O.; Lisker, A.; Singh, D.; Souza, R.P.; Batra, P.; Zaidi, S.H.E.; Chen, S.; Liu, F.; et al. A Common Polymorphism in the Cannabinoid Receptor 1 (CNR1) Gene is Associated with Antipsychotic-Induced Weight Gain in Schizophrenia. *Neuropsychopharmacology* **2010**, *35*, 1315–1324. [CrossRef] [PubMed]

58. Quteineh, L.; Vandenberghe, F.; Morgui, N.S.; Delacrétaz, A.; Choong, E.; Gholam-Rezaee, M.; Magistretti, P.; Bondolfi, G.; Von Gunten, A.; Preisig, M.; et al. Impact of HSD11B1 polymorphisms on BMI and components of the metabolic syndrome in patients receiving psychotropic treatments. *Pharm. Genom.* **2015**, *25*, 246–258. [CrossRef] [PubMed]
59. Saigi-Morgui, N.; Vandenberghe, F.; Delacrétaz, A.; Quteineh, L.; Gholamrezaee, M.; Aubry, J.-M.; von Gunten, A.; Kutalik, Z.; Conus, P.; Eap, C.B. Association of genetic risk scores with body mass index in Swiss psychiatric cohorts. *Pharm. Genom.* **2016**, *26*, 208–217. [CrossRef]
60. Choong, E.; Quteineh, L.; Cardinaux, J.-R.; Gholam-Rezaee, M.; Vandenberghe, F.; Dobrinas, M.; Bondolfi, G.; Etter, M.; Holzer, L.; Magistretti, P.; et al. Influence of *CRTC1* Polymorphisms on Body Mass Index and Fat Mass in Psychiatric Patients and the General Adult Population. *JAMA Psychiatry* **2013**, *70*, 1011–1019. [CrossRef]
61. Menus, Á.; Kiss, Á.; Tóth, K.; Sirok, D.; Déri, M.; Fekete, F.; Csukly, G.; Monostory, K. Association of clozapine-related metabolic disturbances with CYP3A4 expression in patients with schizophrenia. *Sci. Rep.* **2020**, *10*, 21283. [CrossRef]
62. Godlewska, B.R.; Olajossy-Hilkesberger, L.; Ciwoniuk, M.; Olajossy, M.; Marmurowska-Michałowska, H.; Limon, J.; Landowski, J.; Marmurowska-Micha, H. Olanzapine-induced weight gain is associated with the −759C/T and −697G/C polymorphisms of the HTR2C gene. *Pharm. J.* **2009**, *9*, 234–241. [CrossRef]
63. Hong, C.-J.; Lin, C.-H.; Yu, Y.W.-Y.; Chang, S.-C.; Wang, S.-Y.; Tsai, S.-J. Genetic variant of the histamine-1 receptor (glu349asp) and body weight change during clozapine treatment. *Psychiatr. Genet.* **2002**, *12*, 169–171. [CrossRef]
64. Lencz, T.; Robinson, D.G.; Napolitano, B.; Sevy, S.; Kane, J.M.; Goldman, D.; Malhotra, A.K. DRD2 promoter region variation predicts antipsychotic-induced weight gain in first episode schizophrenia. *Pharm. Genom.* **2010**, *20*, 569–572. [CrossRef] [PubMed]
65. Cote, A.T.; Panagiotopoulos, C.; Devlin, A.M. Interaction between the Val158Met catechol-O-methyltransferase gene variant and second-generation antipsychotic treatment on blood pressure in children. *Pharm. J.* **2015**, *15*, 95–100. [CrossRef] [PubMed]
66. Devlin, A.M.; Ngai, Y.F.; Ronsley, R.; Panagiotopoulos, C. Cardiometabolic risk and the MTHFR C677T variant in children treated with second-generation antipsychotics. *Transl. Psychiatry* **2012**, *2*, e71. [CrossRef] [PubMed]
67. Dong, L.; Yan, H.; Huang, X.; Hu, X.; Yang, Y.; Ma, C.; Du, B.; Lu, T.; Jin, C.; Wang, L.; et al. A2BP1 gene polymorphisms association with olanzapine-induced weight gain. *Pharmacol. Res.* **2015**, *99*, 155–161. [CrossRef] [PubMed]
68. Pouget, J.G.; Gonçalves, V.F.; Nurmi, E.L.; Laughlin, C.P.; Mallya, K.S.; McCracken, J.T.; Aman, M.G.; McDougle, C.J.; Scahill, L.; Misener, V.L.; et al. Investigation of TSPO variants in schizophrenia and antipsychotic treatment outcomes. *Pharmacogenomics* **2015**, *16*, 5–22. [CrossRef]
69. Baumann, P.; Barbe, R.; Vabre-Bogdalova, A.; Garran, E.; Crettol, S.; Eap, C.B. Epileptiform Seizure after Sertraline Treatment in an Adolescent Experiencing Obsessive-Compulsive Disorder and Presenting a Rare Pharmacogenetic Status. *J. Clin. Psychopharmacol.* **2006**, *26*, 679–681. [CrossRef]
70. Prows, C.A.; Nick, T.G.; Saldaña, S.N.; Pathak, S.; Liu, C.; Zhang, K.; Daniels, Z.S.; Vinks, A.A.; Glauser, T.A. Drug-Metabolizing Enzyme Genotypes and Aggressive Behavior Treatment Response in Hospitalized Pediatric Psychiatric Patients. *J. Child Adolesc. Psychopharmacol.* **2009**, *19*, 385–394. [CrossRef]
71. Vandel, P.; Haffen, E.; Vandel, S.; Bonin, B.; Nezelof, S.; Sechter, D.; Broly, F.; Bizouard, P.; Dalery, J. Drug extrapyramidal side effects. CYP2D6 genotypes and phenotypes. *Eur. J. Clin. Pharmacol.* **1999**, *55*, 659–665. [CrossRef]
72. Kohlrausch, F.B.; Salatino-Oliveira, A.; Gama, C.S.; Lobato, M.I.; Belmonte-de-Abreu, P.; Hutz, M.H. G-protein gene 825C>T polymorphism is associated with response to clozapine in Brazilian schizophrenics. *Pharmacogenomics* **2008**, *9*, 1429–1436. [CrossRef]
73. Ivashchenko, D.V.; Khoang, S.Z.; Makhmudova, B.V.; Buromskaya, N.I.; Shimanov, P.V.; Deitch, R.V.; Akmalova, K.A.; Shuev, G.N.; Dorina, I.V.; Nastovich, M.I.; et al. Pharmacogenetics of antipsychotics in adolescents with acute psychotic episode during first 14 days after admission: Effectiveness and safety evaluation. *Drug Metab. Pers. Ther.* **2020**, *35*, 20200102. [CrossRef]
74. Nicotera, A.G.; Di Rosa, G.; Turriziani, L.; Costanzo, M.C.; Stracuzzi, E.; Vitello, G.A.; Rando, R.G.; Musumeci, A.; Vinci, M.; Musumeci, S.A.; et al. Role of COMT V158M Polymorphism in the Development of Dystonia after Administration of Antipsychotic Drugs. *Brain Sci.* **2021**, *11*, 1293. [CrossRef] [PubMed]
75. Kohlrausch, F.B.; Salatino-Oliveira, A.; Gama, C.S.; Lobato, M.I.; Belmonte-de-Abreu, P.; Hutz, M.H. Influence of serotonin transporter gene polymorphisms on clozapine response in Brazilian schizophrenics. *J. Psychiatr. Res.* **2010**, *44*, 1158–1162. [CrossRef] [PubMed]
76. Butwicka, A.; Krystyna, S.; Retka, W.; Wolańczyk, T. Neuroleptic malignant syndrome in an adolescent with CYP2D6 deficiency. *Eur. J. Pediatr.* **2014**, *173*, 1639–1642. [CrossRef] [PubMed]
77. Grădinaru, R.; Andreescu, N.; Nussbaum, L.; Suciu, L.; Puiu, M. Impact of the CYP2D6 phenotype on hyperprolactinemia development as an adverse event of treatment with atypical antipsychotic agents in pediatric patients. *Ir. J. Med. Sci.* **2019**, *188*, 1417–1422. [CrossRef]
78. Mosyagin, I.; Dettling, M.; Roots, I.; Mueller-Oerlinghausen, B.; Cascorbi, I. Impact of Myeloperoxidase and NADPH-Oxidase Polymorphisms in Drug-Induced Agranulocytosis. *J. Clin. Psychopharmacol.* **2004**, *24*, 613–617. [CrossRef]
79. Ocete-Hita, E.; Salmerón-Fernández, M.; Urrutia-Maldonado, E.; Muñoz-De-Rueda, P.; Salmerón-Ruiz, M.; Martinez-Padilla, M.; Ruiz-Extremera, O.A. Analysis of Immunogenetic Factors in Idiosyncratic Drug-induced Liver Injury in the Pediatric Population. *J. Pediatr. Gastroenterol. Nutr.* **2017**, *64*, 742–747. [CrossRef]

80. Nelson, C.L.M.; Amsbaugh, H.M.; Reilly, J.L.; Rosen, C.; Marvin, R.W.; Ragozzino, M.E.; Bishop, J.R.; Sweeney, J.A.; Hill, S.K. Beneficial and adverse effects of antipsychotic medication on cognitive flexibility are related to COMT genotype in first episode psychosis. *Schizophr. Res.* **2018**, *202*, 212–216. [CrossRef]
81. Lott, S.A.; Burghardt, P.R.; Burghardt, K.J.; Bly, M.J.; Grove, T.B.; Ellingrod, V.L. The influence of metabolic syndrome, physical activity and genotype on catechol-O-methyl transferase promoter-region methylation in schizophrenia. *Pharm. J.* **2013**, *13*, 264–271. [CrossRef]
82. Houston, J.P.; Kohler, J.; Bishop, J.R.; Ellingrod, V.L.; Ostbye, K.M.; Zhao, F.; Conley, R.R.; Hoffmann, V.P.; Fijal, B.A. Pharmacogenomic Associations with Weight Gain in Olanzapine Treatment of Patients without Schizophrenia. *J. Clin. Psychiatry* **2012**, *73*, 1077–1086. [CrossRef]
83. Konte, B.; Walters, J.T.R.; Rujescu, D.; Legge, S.E.; Pardiñas, A.F.; Cohen, D.; Pirmohamed, M.; Tiihonen, J.; Hartmann, A.M.; Bogers, J.P.; et al. HLA-DQB1 6672G>C (rs113332494) is associated with clozapine-induced neutropenia and agranulocytosis in individuals of European ancestry. *Transl. Psychiatry* **2021**, *11*, 214. [CrossRef]
84. Papazisis, G.; Goulas, A.; Sarrigiannidis, A.; Bargiota, S.; Antoniadis, D.; Raikos, N.; Basgiouraki, E.; Bozikas, V.P.; Garyfallos, G. ABCB1 and CYP2D6 polymorphisms and treatment response of psychotic patients in a naturalistic setting. *Hum. Psychopharmacol. Clin. Exp.* **2018**, *33*, e2644. [CrossRef] [PubMed]
85. Crescenti, A.; Mas, S.; Gassó, P.; Parellada, E.; Bernardo, M.; Lafuente, A. Cyp2d6*3, *4, *5 and *6 Polymorphisms and Antipsychotic-Induced Extrapyramidal Side-Effects in Patients Receiving Antipsychotic Therapy. *Clin. Exp. Pharmacol. Physiol.* **2008**, *35*, 807–811. [CrossRef] [PubMed]
86. Wannasuphoprasit, Y.; Andersen, S.E.; Arranz, M.J.; Catalan, R.; Jurgens, G.; Kloosterboer, S.M.; Rasmussen, H.B.; Bhat, A.; Irizar, H.; Koller, D.; et al. CYP2D6 Genetic Variation and Antipsychotic-Induced Weight Gain: A Systematic Review and Meta-Analysis. *Front. Psychol.* **2021**, *12*, 768748. [CrossRef] [PubMed]
87. Calafato, M.S.; Austin-Zimmerman, I.; Thygesen, J.H.; Sairam, M.; Metastasio, A.; Marston, L.; Abad-Santos, F.; Bhat, A.; Harju-Seppänen, J.; Irizar, H.; et al. The effect of CYP2D6 variation on antipsychotic-induced hyperprolactinaemia: A systematic review and meta-analysis. *Pharm. J.* **2020**, *20*, 629–637. [CrossRef]
88. Prior, T.I.; Baker, G.B. Interactions between the cytochrome P450 system and the second-generation antipsychotics. *J. Psychiatry Neurosci.* **2003**, *28*, 99–112.
89. Olanzapine. Available online: https://www.pharmgkb.org/chemical/PA450688 (accessed on 26 April 2022).
90. Clozapine Pathway, Pharmacokinetics. Available online: https://www.pharmgkb.org/pathway/PA166163661 (accessed on 26 April 2022).
91. Ivanova, S.A.; Filipenko, M.L.; Vyalova, N.M.; Voronina, E.N.; Pozhidaev, I.V.; Osmanova, D.Z.; Ivanov, M.V.; Fedorenko, O.Y.; Semke, A.V.; Bokhan, N. CYP1A2 and CYP2D6 Gene Polymorphisms in Schizophrenic Patients with Neuroleptic Drug-Induced Side Effects. *Bull. Exp. Biol. Med.* **2016**, *160*, 687–690. [CrossRef]
92. Fu, Y.; Fan, C.-H.; Deng, H.-H.; Hu, S.-H.; Lv, D.-P.; Li, L.-H.; Wang, J.-J.; Lu, X.-Q. Association of CYP2D6 and CYP1A2 gene polymorphism with tardive dyskinesia in Chinese schizophrenic patients. *Acta Pharmacol. Sin.* **2006**, *27*, 328–332. [CrossRef]
93. Melkersson, K.I.; Scordo, M.G.; Gunes, A.; Dahl, M.-L. Impact of CYP1A2 and CYP2D6 polymorphisms on drug metabolism and on insulin and lipid elevations and insulin resistance in clozapine-treated patients. *J. Clin. Psychiatry* **2007**, *68*, 697–704. [CrossRef]
94. What Is GRADE? | BMJ Best Practice.
95. Corponi, F.; Fabbri, C.; Serretti, A. Pharmacogenetics in Psychiatry. *Adv. Pharmacol.* **2018**, *83*, 297–331. [CrossRef]
96. Milosavljevic, F.; Bukvic, N.; Pavlovic, Z.; Miljevic, C.; Pešic, V.; Molden, E.; Ingelman-Sundberg, M.; Leucht, S.; Jukic, M.M. Association of CYP2C19 and CYP2D6 Poor and Intermediate Metabolizer Status with Antidepressant and Antipsychotic Exposure: A Systematic Review and Meta-Analysis. *JAMA Psychiatry* **2021**, *78*, 270. [CrossRef]

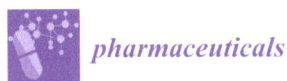

Review

The Potential Application of Extracellular Vesicles from Liquid Biopsies for Determination of Pharmacogene Expression

Henok D. Habtemariam and Henk-Jan Guchelaar *

Department of Clinical Pharmacy and Toxicology, Leiden University Medical Center, 2333 ZA Leiden, The Netherlands; h.d.habtemariam@lumc.nl
* Correspondence: h.j.guchelaar@lumc.nl

Abstract: Pharmacogenomics (PGx) entails the study of heritability of drug response. This may include both variability in genes related to pharmacokinetics (drug absorption, distribution, metabolism and excretion) and pharmacodynamics (e.g., drug receptors or signaling pathways). Individualizing drug therapy taking into account the genetic profile of the patient has the potential to make drug therapy safer and more effective. Currently, this approach relies on the determination of genetic variants in pharmacogenes by genotyping. However, it is widely acknowledged that large variability in gene expression is attributed to non-structural genetic variants. Therefore, at least from a theoretical viewpoint individualizing drug therapy based upon expression of pharmacogenes rather than on genotype may be advantageous but has been difficult to implement in the clinical setting. Extracellular vesicles (EVs) are lipid encapsulated structures that contain cargo such as lipids, nucleic acids and proteins. Since their cargo is tissue- and cell-specific they can be used to determine the expression of pharmacogenes in the liver. In this review, we describe methods of EV isolation and the potential of EVs isolated from liquid biopsies as a tool to determine the expression of pharmacogenes for use in personalized medicine.

Keywords: extracellular vesicles; pharmacogenomics; personalized medicine; exosomes; microvesicles; cytochrome P450; pharmacogene expression

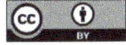

1. Introduction

Pharmacogenomics (PGx) is the study of genetic variation underlying variability in drug response [1]. Specifically, variation in genes that encode for drug metabolizing enzymes, drug transporters, drug receptors or proteins involved in signaling pathways contribute to interindividual variability of drug response. It is now widely acknowledged that variability in pharmacogenes can explain why an individual may experience an adverse drug reaction to a specific medication or could experience inefficient treatment [2]. PGx therefore holds the promise that taking into account an individual's genotype makes drug therapy safer and more effective.

By genotyping, underlying genetic variation such as single nucleotide polymorphisms (SNP) and copy number variations (CNV) can be determined and the drug dose can be adjusted accordingly [2,3]. Common PGx variants have been described with specific therapeutic recommendations for carriers of certain genotypes and have been presented as a PGx passport, representing close to 50 actionable drug-gene interactions [4]. Alternatively, one may use the phenotype of a pharmacogene to apply personalized medicine. In this approach the so called endophenotype [5], such as drug concentration in plasma or urine following administration of a drug probe, is determined as an indirect measure of drug metabolic enzyme activity. Obviously, determining the endophenotype is more invasive and laborious compared to genotyping and it can only be assessed after administering a (probe) drug.

Moreover, the genotype does not always match the phenotype when it comes to drug response. There are several non-genetic factors and epigenetic factors contributing to the expression of pharmacogenes. Examples of non-genetic influences on pharmacogene expression are gender, weight, age and environmental factors [2]. In addition, there are epigenetic modifications known to alter the transcription of pharmacogenes for example through DNA methylation, histone modifications or miRNAs which are known to be involved in the regulation of the drug metabolism gene family cytochrome P450(CYP450) and drug transporter genes [6]. Therefore, at least from a theoretical viewpoint individualizing drug therapy based upon expression of pharmacogenes rather than on genotype may be advantageous but has been difficult to implement in the clinical setting.

To this end, the use of extracellular vesicles (EVs) isolated from liquid biopsies are of great interest. EVs are structures which are secreted by nearly every cell type and are composed of proteins, lipids and nucleic acids that are representative for their cell of origin. Thereby, the cargo of EVs is protected from degradation by their lipid bilayer [7]. Since EVs are involved in cell-cell interaction, they move through the whole body and are able to influence distant cells and tissues [8]. Liquid biopsies, thus, contain EVs from various cell types making them ideal for biomarker research and phenotyping [9]. In this review, background of EVs and methods for isolation and characterization of EVs from liquid biopsies and their application to determine the RNA and protein expression of pharmacogenes in the liver will be discussed and presented as an innovative method for future application in personalized medicine.

2. Extracellular Vesicles

EVs are lipid encapsulated structures that have been conserved through evolution and are found in plants, bacteria and animals [10]. These vesicles were first visualized in the 1950s and were initially considered to be involved in the clearance of cellular debris [11,12]. However, more recent research has shown the involvement of EVs, also, in intercellular communication and development. Through these functions they fulfill a role in determining tissue organization, repair and homeostasis [10,13].

EVs can be categorized as exosomes (30–100 nm) or microvesicles (50–1000 nm), and contain cargo such as proteins, lipids and nucleic acids. The cargo is specific to their donor cell although there are various general EV protein markers that are often used as verification of their presence in the sample. These markers are membrane organizers (tetraspanins: CD9, CD81, CD63, TSPAN6, TSPAN8, CD151, CD37, CD53, Flotilin 1 and 2 for exosomes and CD9, CD81 and CD82 for microvesicles), biogenesis factors (Alix, TSG101), adhesion molecules such as integrins and intercellular adhesion molecules (ICAMs) and intracellular trafficking molecules (RAB, GTPases and annexins) [9,13]. Lipids that are identified to be in the EV layer are sphingomyelin, cholesterol, phosphatidylserine, phosphatidylethanolamine and ceramide [9,14]. The nucleic acids that can be found are mRNA, microRNA, siRNA, circRNA, long non-coding RNA and (mitochondrial) DNA [14–17]. Besides size and cargo, exosomes and microvesicles also vary in the manner that they are formed. Exosomes are formed by inward budding of the cell membrane forming a multi-vesicular body (MVB) in which intra luminal vesicles are formed. After release of these intraluminal vesicles (ILV) they are called exosomes. In contrast, microvesicles are formed by outward budding of the cell membrane [18] (Figure 1). Recent research has revealed variation in morphology between EVs. Electron microscopy has shown much previously unknown variation within Evs showing that Evs can be single, double, double membrane, multilayered or be electron dense [19]. Interestingly, Evs are able to alter the phenotype of their recipient cell by releasing their cargo. In specific EV-cell interaction, vesicles attach to their recipient cells by reciprocated binding to surface receptors. Subsequently, Evs can evoke signaling pathways or be internalized (endocytosis) by the recipient cell. During non-specific interaction the cell membrane simply takes up the Evs through micropinocytosis, phagocytosis or fusion with the membrane [9,14]. Direct fusion of Evs with the membrane results in the release of the cargo directly in the lumen of the recipient cell, while EVs that undergo micropinocytosis or phagocytosis first will come together in the early endosome. The early endosome will be taken up by multi-vesicular body after which the content of the EV will be released or degraded. The EV content can influence both local or distant cells and tissues by autocrine or paracrine communication [20].

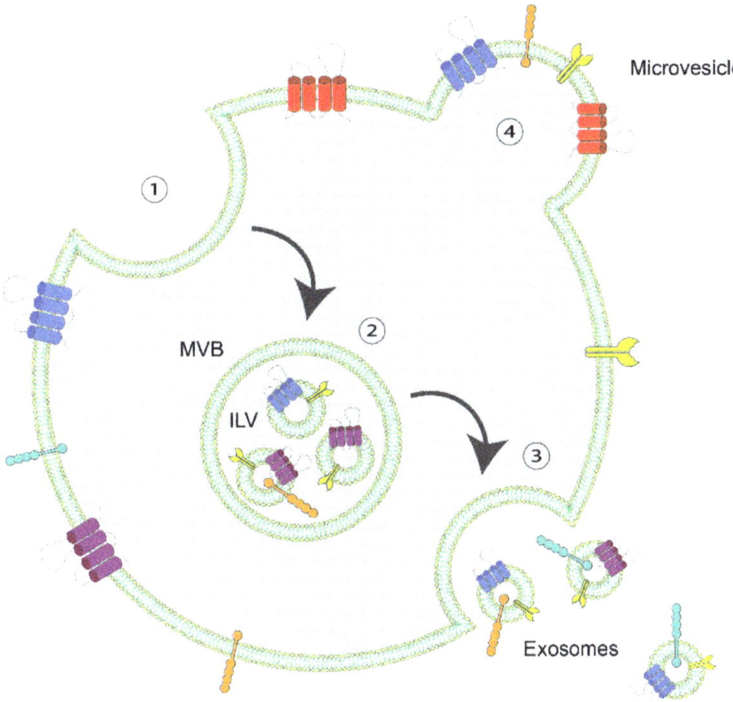

Figure 1. Formation of microvesicles and exosomes. The formation of exosomes by (1) inward budding of the cellular membrane results in the formation of a multivesicular body (MVB) (2) containing intra-luminal vesicles (ILV). After the release of these intra-luminal vesicles the exosomes are formed (3). Microvesicles are formed by outward budding of the cell membrane (4).

Furthermore, EVs are known to be involved in the progression of several pathologies, e.g., the creation of a pre-metastatic niche for cancers and the transport of proteins that are involved in aggregation in neurodegenerative diseases [21]. Moreover, EVs are known to carry pharmacogenomic proteins such as transporters and metabolizing enzymes as well as RNA from pharmacogenes.

2.1. Techniques for EV Isolation and Visualization

EVs can be isolated, visualized and characterized through several methods and from various types of samples. EVs can be isolated from cell culture medium, blood, urine, cerebral spinal fluid and breast milk. The isolation and characterization methods are often chosen in line with the specific sample and goal. The most important factors in choosing the method of isolation are yield and purity [22].

Isolation of EVs can be performed based on size, weight or their composition. Common methods for EV isolation are ultracentrifugation (UC), size-exclusion chromatography (SEC), precipitation, immunoaffinity and filtration methods which can be used in combination (Figure 2) [22].

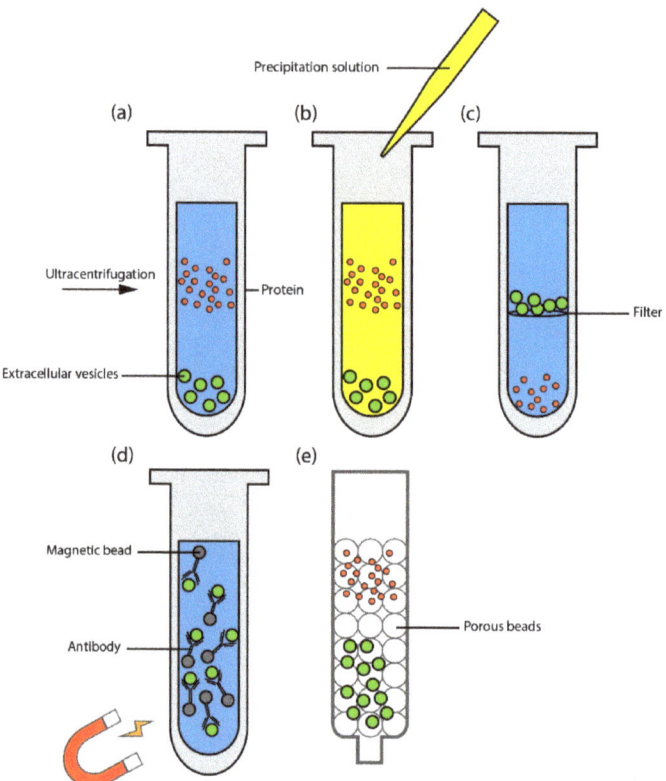

Figure 2. Common EV isolation methods. (**a**). Differential ultracentrifugation is performed at speeds of 100,000× g or higher and leads to heavier particles (extracellular vesicles) descending to the bottom to form a pellet while lighter particles (protein) remain in the supernatant. (**b**). Precipitation techniques employ a solution that makes EVs insoluble. (**c**). Ultrafiltration separated particles in a solution based on size. Filters contain a molecular weight cut-off size specific for EV isolation. (**d**). Immunoaffinity methods require an antibody (for example for CD9, CD81 or CD63) conjugated with beads which are upon binding with EVs separated magnetically. (**e**). Size-exclusion chromatography is a technique in which the sample is separated by running through a gel containing porous beads. The sample is separated in fractions with EVs being in earlier fractions and protein in later fractions.

Ultracentrifugation (UC) is an isolation method that revolves around the weight of the EVs, and is the most commonly used. This method employs centrifugation at high speeds (100,000× g) leading to an EV pellet which is subsequently resuspended in a buffer (Figure 2a) [23]. Size-exclusion chromatography (SEC) is a column-based method which can be used manually by kit or by machine and separates EVs based on size (Figure 2e). Precipitation methods aim to make EVs insoluble by using a substance that initiates hydrophobic reactions (Figure 2b) [24]. Precipitation is significantly simpler and requires less time than the UC or SEC methods. Immunoaffinity methods use antibodies that bind to specific EV surface markers making this method highly specific (Figure 2d). The antibodies used for these methods are directed to tetraspanins such as CD9, CD63 or CD81 which are common EV markers. Moreover, several studies have managed to isolate tissue specific EVs by using tissue specific antibodies. Filtration methods employ membrane filters with pores that have a molecular weight cut-off of 10–100 kDa, a size appropriate for EVs [25] (Figure 2c). Prior to performing these methods of isolation, the sample is often filtered or centrifuged at lower speed to remove excess cell debris [26].

Various studies have been performed comparing several common isolation methods based on various parameters. Alvarez et al. [27] compared the yield, purity and RNA levels of several (modified) EV isolation methods such as UC, filtration and precipitation (ExoQuick) using urine samples. The modified ExoQuick method in which they centrifugated at a higher speed showed the highest yield of urine EVs while filtration and UC combined with filtration showed the lowest yield of EVs. The filtration method did show the highest yield in EV protein although the highest yield in miRNA and mRNA levels were seen in de modified precipitation method [27].

Another isolation method comparison was made on EV isolation from serum samples by SEC, ExoQuick (plus), UC and various other methods. This comparison showed the highest yield in the ExoQuick method in particle sizes 0–1000 nm and 0–60 nm which was followed by SEC and UC respectively. Particles 61–150 nm were also most abundant in the ExoQuick method, though UC showed a slightly higher yield than SEC. Furthermore, serum EV protein levels were investigated in which again the ExoQuick came on top, followed by UC and SEC. The particles per μg of protein was highest in SEC followed by ExoQuick and UC [28].

Several EV isolation methods were also compared by Yang et al. [22] who isolated EVs from plasma using SEC, UC, a filtration method (ExoEasy) and a precipitation (ExoQuick) method. The EVs were isolated from plasma with added fluorescent liposomes to determine fluorescent intensity. The study has shown the most fluorescent intensity in the SEC method as well as the lowest protein contamination. The EV size varied between the methods as the ExoQuick contained EVs larger than 100 nm, while in the other methods, the EVs were smaller than 100 nm. Overall, the ExoQuick method showed the highest yield of EVs, however the SEC method showed the highest purity with lowest free protein levels. RNA isolation proved the ExoEasy to have the highest yield of total miRNA compared to the other methods although SEC showed the highest yield of EV-specific miRNA. The highest percentage of mRNA reads was found in SEC after RNA-seq while the ExoQuick presented the highest percentage of long non-coding-RNA. After assessment of RNA-seq data for long chain RNAs, it was revealed that the ExoQuick and SEC method contained mostly exon reads while the other methods contained mostly intergenic reads [22]. Another study compared several precipitation methods in clinical osteosarcoma plasma samples which interestingly showed besides variation in yield, protein concentration and size distribution between the precipitation kits also variation in group specific yield. This means that some methods showed the highest yield in metastatic osteosarcoma condition while with other methods this was similar to control plasma [24].

Overall, the ExoQuick showed to be the best choice if the goal is to have a high yield of EVs in liquid biopsy samples. There were variations in the size and purity between the methods that varied depending on the type of sample.

After isolation EVs are often subjected to a method for EV visualization such as nanoparticle tracking analysis (NTA) and electron microscopy (EM). NTA is most commonly used and utilizes lasers, microscopy and a camera to visualize the size distribution and concentration of EVs [29]. For more specific visualization of EVs the most common method is EM which can show morphological variation in EVs as well as size on a single EV level [19]. Isolation and visualization of EVs is often followed by downstream applications such as methods to research their composition e.g., biomarkers or EVs are modified to use as carriers for biomolecules.

2.2. Pharmacogenomic Phenotyping Using EVs

The presence of mRNA and proteins/enzymes encoded by pharmacogenes in EVs from liquid biopsies has been studied and proved in various studies. Initially, a study researching expression in plasma derived EVs, found several CYP enzymes and mRNAs coding for drug metabolizing enzymes such as CYP1B1, CYP2A6, CYP2E1 and CYP3A4. In addition, the study revealed that CYP2E1 and CYP3A4 enzymes from EVs were indeed metabolically active [30]. The presence of metabolic enzymes in EVs has also been proven in vitro. Proteomic analysis showed that rat hepatocyte derived EVs contain several CYP enzymes (2A1,2B3,2C11,2D1,2D3,2D10, 2D18 and 2D26) and UDP-glucuronosyltransferases (UGT) (2B2, 2B3 and 2B5) [31].

The fact that EVs contain pharmacogenomic cargo makes them ideal as a non-invasive method for characterizing an individual's PGx profile. EVs from liquid biopsies, specifically their cargo, have been researched and utilized in the context of cancer for prognosis and diagnostics but also neurodegenerative diseases, immunological diseases and cardiovascular disease [32]. For instance, in high-grade prostate cancer diagnostics the use of EVs from liquid biopsy, specifically urine, has been validated and uses one cut point making this a binary predictor [33]. In PGx a single cut point would not suffice since we strive to place individuals in a metabolic category thus very specifically predict the appropriate dose of a medication.

Several studies have found creative and innovative ways to solve challenges in developing a PGx expression assay using EVs from liquid biopsies. The first study on the clinical applications of plasma derived EVs in PGx was performed by Rowland et al. [34] who studied the expression of CYP450 and UGT in plasma EVs with the aim to characterize CYP3A4, which is responsible for the metabolism of more than 30% of all drugs, and its induction by rifampicin. They extracted human liver microsomes from tissue samples by centrifugation as well as EVs from plasma samples. The study subjects were selected based on the genotypes CYP3A4*1/*1 (normal activity) and CYP3A5*3/*3 (no activity) [35] eliminating the possibility of drug clearance by CYP3A5. The participants were exposed to an oral dose of midazolam on the first day and the inducer rifampicin daily (until day 8). qRT-PCR confirmed the presence of CYP1A2, CYP2C8, CYP2C9, CYP2D6, CYP2E1 and CYP3A4 and UGT1A1 UGT1A9, UGT2B4, UGT2B7 and UGT2B10 mRNA in the plasma derived EVs. Mass spectrometry revealed the presence of the enzymes CYP 1A2, 2B6, 2C8, 2C9, 2D6, 2E1, 2J2, 3A4 and 3A5 and UGT 1A1, 1A3, 1A4, 1A6, 1A9, 2B4, 2B7, 2B10 and 2B15 in plasma EVs. Additionally, an ex vivo metabolism assay was performed with plasma EVs involving 4-methylumbelliferone (4-MU) glucuronidation and midazolam hydroxylation by UGT1A1 and CYP3A4, respectively. The study showed a great increase in drug metabolism after activation of EVs by alamethicin on ice versus non-activated EVs which was 150 ± 7.6 pmol/min/mg against 6.5 ± 0.4 pmol/min/mg for 4-MU glucuronidation and 14.3 ± 0.7 pmol/min/mg and 0.35 ± 0.7 pmol/min/mg for midazolam hydroxylation. The activity of CYP3A4 ex vivo highly correlated with EV CYP3A4 protein expression ($R^2 = 0.928$). Most importantly, a correlation was found between the midazolam clearance and plasma EV CYP3A4 mRNA ($R^2 = 0.79$) and protein ($R^2 = 0.90$) expression in vivo [34]. Contrary to Rowland et al. [34], Achour et al. [36] used matching plasma EVs and liver tissue to develop a phenotypic assay for use in PGx. They extracted blood plasma and tissue biopsies from liver cancer patients that underwent surgical cancer removal. From the tissue biopsy they isolated healthy tissue which was subjected to mass-spectrometry to estimate the protein composition while mRNA was extracted from plasma EVs and subsequently sequenced. To prove the representability of plasma EV pharmacogene expression, they compared the RNA expression of EVs to protein expression in liver biopsies and found a correlation between EV expression and liver biopsy expression which improved vastly after normalization for individual shedding using a novel shedding factor. The shedding factor was implemented by dividing the EV expression of a gene of interest by the average EV expression of 12 liver specific markers that are highly expressed and consistently detectable in plasma EVs. The correlation prior to adjustment ranged between $R^2 = 0.00$–0.53 for CYP450 enzymes, $R^2 = 0.00$–0.52 for glucuronosyltransferases (UGT) and $R^2 = 0.04$–0.21 for transporters which after adjustment were $R^2 = 0.50$–$0.75 (p < 0.001)$ for CYP450, $R^2 = 0.36$–0.65 ($p < 0.05$) for glucuronosyltransferases and $R^2 = 0.43$–0.54 ($p < 0.01$) for transporters. A receiver operator characteristic (ROC) analysis, thereby, showed that both the bottom and the top quartile of metabolizers can indeed be predicted with varying accuracies (top quartile AUC ≥ 0.64; bottom quartile AUC ≥ 0.77). Furthermore, an in silico drug trial was performed based on liquid biopsy EV expression using the CYP3A4 metabolized drugs alprazolam, midazolam and ibrutinib. As prior, the categories that were used were the bottom quartile (slow metabolizers), a middle group and top quartile (fast metabolizers). The groups were subjected to three methods of oral administration of medication in the model: a uniform dose, a stratified dose and an individualized dose. After comparison to the uniform dose they showed a 1.7 reduction in variation of drug concentration over time in the stratified condition for all three drugs and in the condition with the individualized dose they showed a 2-fold decrease in variability for alprazolam and midazolam, and a 2.5-fold decrease for ibrutinib. The in silico study confirmed that EV expression based adjustment of drug dose decreases variation in drug plasma levels and could therefore be utilized as a predictor for drug reaction [36].

A novel method for highly specific isolation of liver EVs from a heterogeneous serum sample was introduced by Rodrigues et al. [37,38]. This technique was employed in two of their studies where they studied inducibility of EV pharmacogene expression and drug interactions. They isolated liver EVs from serum by SEC and subsequently an immunoaffinity protocol involving an antibody for the liver enriched marker anti-asiaglycoprotein receptor 1 (ASGR1). In their first research they derived EVs from subjects exposed to oral doses of both midazolam and dextromethorphan (DEX) (day 1) and were daily treated with 300 mg for 8 days or 600 mg for 14 days. The EV samples were assessed prior (day 1) and after rifampicin (day 8 or 15). Midazolam metabolism was found induced as shown by a 72% decrease in midazolam area under the plasma concentration time curve (AUC) after one week of daily 300 mg of the CYP3A4 inducer rifampicin while a two week 600 mg rifampicin use showed a 83% decrease in AUC. Moreover, liver EV CYP3A4 protein expression was significantly increased by rifampicin at both 300 mg ($p = 0.0005$) and 600 mg ($p = 0.0004$). No significant increase was found of liver EV CYP2D6 protein expression as a result of rifampicin treatment. Though, the metabolism of substrate DEX was slightly visible at the 600 mg rifampicin dose, consistent with the fact that CYP2D6 is not or only minimally influenced by rifampicin [39]. They managed to estimate the contribution of CYP2D6 to DEX metabolism by using parameters from previous studies and found a strong correlation between CYP2D6 activity and CYP2D6 liver EV protein expression ($r = 0.917$, $p = 0.0001$). Lastly, proteomic analysis revealed besides CYP3A4 and CYP2D6 also the presence of CYP3A5, OATP1B1 and OATP1B3 proteins in the liver EVs.

Non-hepatic PGx expression was also studied and compared to hepatic EV PGx expression. They determined the CYP3A4 protein concentration in non-liver EVs which showed an average 2- to 3-fold lower CYP3A4 protein expression than in liver EVs. Though, it is important to note that a higher concentration of CYP3A4 in non-liver EVs than in liver EVs was found in half of the samples. Like the protein CYP3A4 expression in liver and non-liver EVs, there was also variation found in the expression at different doses over time liver EVs showed a mean fold increase of 3.5 at 300 mg rifampicin and 3.7 at 600 mg rifampicin. While in non-liver EVs this was shown to be 2.3 at 300 mg rifampicin and 4.4 at 600 mg rifampicin. These findings suggest that there is individual variability in the dominance of the liver with regards to CYP3A4 expression. Moreover, that the level of CYP3A4 inducibility by rifampicin varies per organ. Besides CYP3A4, a proteomic study was performed revealing expression of both hepatic and non-hepatic CYP and transporters in EVs [37].

Another study by the same researchers was performed on the effects of modafinil as a CYP3A4 EV expression inducer. The participants were genotyped for CYP3A5 and were either CYP3A5*1/*3 (expressers) or CYP3A5 *3/*3 (non-expressers). The plasma samples were obtained from subjects that were exposed to a daily oral dose of modafinil for 14 days. The (endo)phenotype was determined by the plasma concentration ratio of 4β-hydroxycholesterol-to-cholesterol day 1 (pre-modafinil), at day 8 and at day 15. The ratio was increased 1.5-fold and 2.1-fold at 8 days and 15 days after daily modafinil administration, respectively. A proteomic analysis revealed that the liver EVs accounted for 78% of the total EV CYP3A4 expression. Moreover, there was a strong correlation between baseline plasma 4βHC/C ratio and liver EV CYP3A4 with ($r = 0.761$, $p = 0.011$), and without inclusion of CYP3A5*1/*3 (r = 0.973, p = 0.001) carriers. Modafinil showed to significantly increase the protein expression of CYP3A4 1.3 fold (1.1–1.5, p = 0.014) in liver EVs, 1.9-fold (1.6–2.2, p = 0.04) in non-liver EVs and 1.4-fold (1.3–1.5, p = 0.014) globally [38].

The studies managed to find correlations between genotype, phenotype and endophenotype. They unfortunately lacked in the amount of study subjects which ranged between n = 5–10 except for the paper by Achour et al. which included 29 participants. Though, in contrary to the other studies Achour et al. did not subject the samples to any genotyping. Overall, these studies demonstrated great potential of using EVs from liquid biopsies for phenotyping the major drug metabolizing liver enzymes.

3. Discussion

The use of EVs isolated from liquid biopsies to determine drug metabolizing phenotypes is a novel, innovative and challenging though promising development. Several techniques are being used to isolate these vesicles, with varying results, though UC is regarded the most popular. Comparative studies have studied variation in yield and purity and showed a difference between isolation methods likely also highly dependent on the type of liquid biopsy (urine, serum or plasma). However, studies also showed disconcordances, e.g., a study on isolation methods of EVs from serum found that the particles had a size between 61 nm and 150 nm for several methods (UC, ExoQuick, SEC) but another study on plasma revealed that the ExoQuick gave EVs of 100 nm or above while the other methods (SEC, UC and ExoEasy) gave smaller vesicles (<100 nm). Therefore, it is important to realize that results could vary if research is reproduced using a different EV isolation methodology or kit and thus standardization of isolation methods is required. This is particularly important in the context of PGx, and clinical research in general, as based on the results a clinical decision in the treatment of a patient may be taken.

Currently, the use of PGx has started to be implemented in clinical practice to individualize drug therapy with genotyping techniques being the main method to profile the individual predicted metabolizer phenotype of patients. However, personalizing therapy based upon metabolizer phenotypes as assessed by mRNA expression of pharmacogenes may prove advantageous. Determining the metabolizer status by drug level measurements after administering a drug or probe could be performed but is invasive, costly and laborious. While a few recent studies have clearly shown that phenotyping of pharmacogenes in EVs from liquid biopsies can performed reliably, there have been (besides standardization of isolation methods) several challenges regarding individual normalization and generalization. Achour et al. [36] approached this problem by introducing a shedding factor through which they managed to normalize the pharmacogene expression in EVs by taking into account expression of other common liver markers [36]. A different method was used by Rodrigues et al. [37,38] who specifically isolated liver EVs from serum samples using an antibody for the liver specific marker ASGR1. The advantage of the latter method is the ability to distinguish hepatic and extrahepatic EV enzymes leading to the discovery of the presence of 78% of CYP3A4 in liver EVs and 22% in non-liver EVs. Indeed, effects of both liver and extrahepatic drug metabolism can be investigated in this setting [37,38].

Both the methods of Achour and Rodrigues include a validation procedure as to determine if expression in EVs is a proxy for drug metabolic capacity. In the study of Achour, expression was compared in EVs and matched liver tissue samples. Unfortunately, the study did not provide the genotype of the patients and only a limited distribution of phenotypes was included. Instead, Rodrigues chose to validate by measuring protein concentration of metabolic enzymes in EVs which is obviously a good representation, but does not represent the place in a human being where actual drug metabolism takes place, and thus lacks correlation with liver activity of involved enzymes [40]. Interestingly, they incorporated genotyping and drug concentration ratio measurements in vivo in their studies. While these studies together clearly proved the potential of using EVs in PGx, a more comprehensive validation is needed before clinical application can takes place.

When validated, the method has great potential in PGx. A main characteristic is that longitudinal measurements can easily be performed using liquid biopsies. This enables to study environmental factors and day-to-day variation in drug metabolism. Indeed, variation in drug response or mRNA expression within a specific genotype are often due to phenoconversion, a mismatch between the genotype and predicted phenotype [40]. This mismatch is a result of non-genetic factors such as weight, gender, age and alcohol consumption but could also be disease related for instance infections that lead to the release of cytokines suppressing expression and/or activity of CYP enzymes [40,41].

In addition, the method makes it possible to assess the in vivo functionality of genetic variants of unknown significance. These variants will be determined more frequently in the near future as the result of using sequencing techniques in PGx. In this way, genotype-phenotype translations can be explored more easily and reliably as compared to current methods [42] mainly dependent on bioinformatics predictions. Moreover, the use of EVs in PGx may open novel possibilities to study drug-drug interaction, especially in pharmacokinetic interactions where drugs inhibit or induce metabolic enzymes.

In conclusion, EVs from liquid biopsy can be used to assess drug metabolizing phenotypes, and has, after careful validation, great potential for use in personalized medicine.

Author Contributions: Conceptualization, H.D.H. and H.-J.G.; writing—original draft preparation, H.D.H.; writing—review and editing, H.D.H. and H.-J.G.; visualization, H.D.H.; supervision, H.-J.G.; All authors have read and agreed to the published version of the manuscript.

Funding: This research received no external funding.

Institutional Review Board Statement: Not applicable.

Informed Consent Statement: Not applicable.

Data Availability Statement: Not applicable.

Acknowledgments: We are grateful for the assistance for the search terms given by Jan Schoones of the Walaeus library (LUMC).

Conflicts of Interest: The authors declare no conflict of interest.

References

1. Roden, D.M.; McLeod, H.L.; Relling, M.V.; Williams, M.S.; Mensah, G.A.; Peterson, J.F.; van Driest, S.L. Pharmacogenomics. *Lancet* **2019**, *394*, 521–532. [CrossRef]
2. Katara, P.; Yadav, A. Pharmacogenes (PGx-genes): Current understanding and future directions. *Gene* **2019**, *718*, 144050. [CrossRef] [PubMed]
3. Katara, P. Single nucleotide polymorphism and its dynamics for pharmacogenomics. *Interdisc. Sci. Comput. Life Sci.* **2014**, *6*, 85–92. [CrossRef]
4. Van der Wouden, C.H.; van Rhenen, M.H.; Jama, W.O.M.; Ingelman-Sundberg, M.; Lauschke, V.M.; Konta, L.; Schwab, M.; Swen, J.J.; Guchelaar, H.-J. Development of the PGx-Passport: A Panel of Actionable Germline Genetic Variants for Pre-Emptive Pharmacogenetic Testing. *Clin. Pharm. Ther.* **2019**, *106*, 866–873. [CrossRef]
5. Lenzenweger, M.F. Endophenotype, intermediate phenotype, biomarker: Definitions, concept comparisons, clarifications. *Depress. Anxiety* **2013**, *30*, 185–189. [CrossRef] [PubMed]
6. Kim, I.-W.; Han, N.; Burckart, G.J.; Oh, J.M. Epigenetic Changes in Gene Expression for Drug-Metabolizing Enzymes and Transporters. *Pharmacother. J. Hum. Pharmacol. Drug Ther.* **2013**, *34*, 140–150. [CrossRef] [PubMed]
7. Szabo, G.; Momen-Heravi, F. Extracellular vesicles in liver disease and potential as biomarkers and therapeutic targets. *Nat. Rev. Gastroenterol. Hepatol.* **2017**, *14*, 455–466. [CrossRef] [PubMed]
8. Patras, L.; Banciu, M. Intercellular Crosstalk Via Extracellular Vesicles in Tumor Milieu as Emerging Therapies for Cancer Progression. *Curr. Pharm. Des.* **2019**, *25*, 1980–2006. [CrossRef]
9. Van Niel, G.; D'Angelo, G.; Raposo, G. Shedding light on the cell biology of extracellular vesicles. *Nat. Rev. Mol. Cell Biol.* **2018**, *19*, 213–228. [CrossRef]
10. Yáñez-Mó, M.; Siljander, P.R.-M.; Andreu, Z.; Zavec, A.B.; Borràs, F.E.; Buzas, E.I.; Buzas, K.; Casal, E.; Cappello, F.; Carvalho, J.; et al. Biological properties of extracellular vesicles and their physiological functions. *J. Extracell. Vesicles* **2015**, *4*, 27066. [CrossRef]
11. Fowler, C.D. NeuroEVs: Characterizing Extracellular Vesicles Generated in the Neural Domain. *J. Neurosci.* **2019**, *39*, 9262–9268. [CrossRef]

12. Maxwell, D.S.; Pease, D.C. The electron microscopy of the choroid plexus. *J. Biophys. Biochem. Cytol.* **1956**, *2*, 467–474. [CrossRef]
13. Azam, Z.; Quillien, V.; Wang, G.; To, S.-S.T. The potential diagnostic and prognostic role of extracellular vesicles in glioma: Current status and future perspectives. *Acta Oncol.* **2019**, *58*, 353–362. [CrossRef] [PubMed]
14. Veerman, R.E.; Akpinar, G.G.; Eldh, M.; Gabrielsson, S. Immune Cell-Derived Extracellular Vesicles—Functions and Therapeutic Applications. *Trends Mol. Med.* **2019**, *25*, 382–394. [CrossRef] [PubMed]
15. Wang, Y.; Zhang, H.; Wang, J.; Li, B.; Wang, X. Circular RNA expression profile of lung squamous cell carcinoma: Identification of potential biomarkers and therapeutic targets. *Biosci. Rep.* **2020**, *40*. [CrossRef]
16. Cai, J.; Han, Y.; Ren, H.; Chen, C.; He, D.; Zhou, L.; Eisner, G.M.; Asico, L.D.; Jose, P.A.; Zeng, C. Extracellular vesicle-mediated transfer of donor genomic DNA to recipient cells is a novel mechanism for genetic influence between cells. *J. Mol. Cell Biol.* **2013**, *5*, 227–238. [CrossRef] [PubMed]
17. Gusachenko, O.N.; Zenkova, M.A.; Vlassov, V. Nucleic acids in exosomes: Disease markers and intercellular communication molecules. *Biochemistry* **2013**, *78*, 1–7. [CrossRef]
18. Yoon, Y.J.; Kim, O.Y.; Gho, Y.S. Extracellular vesicles as emerging intercellular communicasomes. *BMB Rep.* **2014**, *47*, 531–539. [CrossRef]
19. Emelyanov, A.; Shtam, T.; Kamyshinsky, R.; Garaeva, L.; Verlov, N.; Miliukhina, I.; Kudrevatykh, A.; Gavrilov, G.; Zabrodskaya, Y.; Pchelina, S.; et al. Cryo-electron microscopy of extracellular vesicles from cerebrospinal fluid. *PLoS ONE* **2020**, *15*, e0227949. [CrossRef]
20. Pretti, M.A.M.; Bernardes, S.S.; Da Cruz, J.G.V.; Boroni, M.; Possik, P.A. Extracellular vesicle-mediated crosstalk between melanoma and the immune system: Impact on tumor progression and therapy response. *J. Leukoc. Biol.* **2020**, *108*, 1101–1115. [CrossRef] [PubMed]
21. Candelario, K.M.; Steindler, D.A. The role of extracellular vesicles in the progression of neurodegenerative disease and cancer. *Trends Mol. Med.* **2014**, *20*, 368–374. [CrossRef]
22. Yang, Y.; Wang, Y.; Wei, S.; Zhou, C.; Yu, J.; Wang, G.; Wang, W.; Zhao, L. Extracellular vesicles isolated by size-exclusion chromatography present suitability for RNomics analysis in plasma. *J. Transl. Med.* **2021**, *19*, 1–12. [CrossRef] [PubMed]
23. Lapitz, A.; Arbelaiz, A.; O'Rourke, C.J.; Lavin, J.L.; La Casta, A.; Ibarra, C.; Jimeno, J.P.; Santos-Laso, A.; Izquierdo-Sanchez, L.; Krawczyk, M.; et al. Patients with Cholangiocarcinoma Present Specific RNA Profiles in Serum and Urine Extracellular Vesicles Mirroring the Tumor Expression: Novel Liquid Biopsy Biomarkers for Disease Diagnosis. *Cells* **2020**, *9*, 721. [CrossRef] [PubMed]
24. Peng, C.; Wang, J.; Bao, Q.; Wang, J.; Liu, Z.; Wen, J.; Zhang, W.; Shen, Y. Isolation of extracellular vesicle with different precipitation-based methods exerts a tremendous impact on the biomarker analysis for clinical plasma samples. *Cancer Biomark.* **2020**, *29*, 373–385. [CrossRef] [PubMed]
25. Liangsupree, T.; Multia, E.; Riekkola, M.-L. Modern isolation and separation techniques for extracellular vesicles. *J. Chromatogr. A* **2020**, *1636*, 461773. [CrossRef]
26. Pang, B.; Zhu, Y.; Ni, J.; Thompson, J.; Malouf, D.; Bucci, J.; Graham, P.; Li, Y. Extracellular vesicles: The next generation of biomarkers for liquid biopsy-based prostate cancer diagnosis. *Theranostics* **2020**, *10*, 2309–2326. [CrossRef] [PubMed]
27. Alvarez, M.L.; Khosroheidari, M.; Ravi, R.K.; DiStefano, J.K. Comparison of protein, microRNA, and mRNA yields using different methods of urinary exosome isolation for the discovery of kidney disease biomarkers. *Kidney Int.* **2012**, *82*, 1024–1032. [CrossRef] [PubMed]
28. Brennan, K.; Martin, K.; Fitzgerald, S.P.; O'Sullivan, J.; Wu, Y.; Blanco, A.; Richardson, C.; Mc Gee, M.M. A comparison of methods for the isolation and separation of extracellular vesicles from protein and lipid particles in human serum. *Sci. Rep.* **2020**, *10*, 1039. [CrossRef]
29. Chandran, V.I.; Welinder, C.; Månsson, A.-S.; Offer, S.; Freyhult, E.; Pernemalm, M.; Lund, S.M.; Pedersen, S.; Lehtiö, J.; Marko-Varga, G.; et al. Ultrasensitive Immunoprofiling of Plasma Extracellular Vesicles Identifies Syndecan-1 as a Potential Tool for Minimally Invasive Diagnosis of Glioma. *Clin. Cancer Res.* **2019**, *25*, 3115–3127. [CrossRef]
30. Kumar, S.; Sinha, N.; Gerth, K.A.; Rahman, M.A.; Yallapu, M.M.; Midde, N.M. Specific packaging and circulation of cytochromes P450, especially 2E1 isozyme, in human plasma exosomes and their implications in cellular communications. *Biochem. Biophys. Res. Commun.* **2017**, *491*, 675–680. [CrossRef]
31. Conde-Vancells, J.; Rodriguez-Suarez, E.; Embade, N.; Gil, D.; Matthiesen, R.; Valle, M.; Elortza, F.; Lu, S.C.; Mato, J.M.; Falcon-Perez, J.M. Characterization and Comprehensive Proteome Profiling of Exosomes Secreted by Hepatocytes. *J. Proteome Res.* **2008**, *7*, 5157–5166. [CrossRef]
32. Yu, W.; Hurley, J.; Roberts, D.; Chakrabortty, S.; Enderle, D.; Noerholm, M.; Breakefield, X.; Skog, J. Exosome-based liquid biopsies in cancer: Opportunities and challenges. *Ann. Oncol.* **2021**, *32*, 466–477. [CrossRef] [PubMed]
33. McKiernan, J.; Donovan, M.J.; O'Neill, V.; Bentink, S.; Noerholm, M.; Belzer, S.; Skog, J.; Kattan, M.W.; Partin, A.; Andriole, G.; et al. A Novel Urine Exosome Gene Expression Assay to Predict High-grade Prostate Cancer at Initial Biopsy. *JAMA Oncol.* **2016**, *2*, 882–889. [CrossRef]
34. Rowland, A.; Ruanglertboon, W.; Van Dyk, M.; Wijayakumara, D.; Wood, L.S.; Meech, R.; Mackenzie, P.I.; Rodrigues, A.D.; Marshall, J.; Sorich, M. Plasma extracellular nanovesicle (exosome)-derived biomarkers for drug metabolism pathways: A novel approach to characterize variability in drug exposure. *Br. J. Clin. Pharmacol.* **2018**, *85*, 216–226. [CrossRef] [PubMed]

35. Saiz-Rodríguez, M.; Almenara, S.; Navares-Gómez, M.; Ochoa, D.; Román, M.; Zubiaur, P.; Koller, D.; Santos, M.; Mejía, G.; Borobia, A.M.; et al. Effect of the Most Relevant CYP3A4 and CYP3A5 Polymorphisms on the Pharmacokinetic Parameters of 10 CYP3A Substrates. *Biomedicines* **2020**, *8*, 94. [CrossRef]
36. Achour, B.; Al-Majdoub, Z.M.; Grybos-Gajniak, A.; Lea, K.; Kilford, P.; Zhang, M.; Knight, D.; Barber, J.; Schageman, J.; Rostami-Hodjegan, A. Liquid Biopsy Enables Quantification of the Abundance and Interindividual Variability of Hepatic Enzymes and Transporters. *Clin. Pharmacol. Ther.* **2020**, *109*, 222–232. [CrossRef] [PubMed]
37. Rodrigues, A.D.; van Dyk, M.; Sorich, M.J.; Fahmy, A.; Useckaite, Z.; Newman, L.A.; Kapetas, A.J.; Mounzer, R.; Wood, L.S.; Johnson, J.G.; et al. Exploring the Use of Serum-Derived Small Extracellular Vesicles as Liquid Biopsy to Study the Induction of Hepatic Cytochromes P450 and Organic Anion Transporting Polypeptides. *Clin. Pharmacol. Ther.* **2021**, *110*, 248–258. [CrossRef]
38. Rodrigues, A.D.; Wood, L.S.; Vourvahis, M.; Rowland, A. Leveraging Human Plasma-Derived Small Extracellular Vesicles as Liquid Biopsy to Study the Induction of Cytochrome P450 3A4 by Modafinil. *Clin. Pharmacol. Ther.* **2022**, *111*, 425–434. [CrossRef]
39. Berger, B.; Bachmann, F.; Duthaler, U.; Krähenbühl, S.; Haschke, M. Cytochrome P450 Enzymes Involved in Metoprolol Metabolism and Use of Metoprolol as a CYP2D6 Phenotyping Probe Drug. *Front. Pharmacol.* **2018**, *9*, 774. [CrossRef]
40. Klomp, S.D.; Manson, M.L.; Guchelaar, H.-J.; Swen, J.J. Phenoconversion of Cytochrome P450 Metabolism: A Systematic Review. *J. Clin. Med.* **2020**, *9*, 2890. [CrossRef]
41. Crake, R.L.I.; Strother, M.R.; Phillips, E.; Doogue, M.P.; Zhang, M.; Frampton, C.M.A.; Robinson, B.A.; Currie, M.J. Influence of serum inflammatory cytokines on cytochrome P450 drug metabolising activity during breast cancer chemotherapy: A patient feasibility study. *Sci. Rep.* **2021**, *11*, 5648. [CrossRef] [PubMed]
42. Tafazoli, A.; Guchelaar, H.-J.; Miltyk, W.; Kretowski, A.J.; Swen, J.J. Applying Next-Generation Sequencing Platforms for Pharmacogenomic Testing in Clinical Practice. *Front. Pharmacol.* **2021**, *12*, 693453. [CrossRef] [PubMed]

pharmaceuticals

Article

Simple and Robust Detection of *CYP2D6* Gene Deletions and Duplications Using *CYP2D8P* as Reference

Jens Borggaard Larsen [1],* and Steffen Jørgensen [2]

1. Laboratory Unit, The Danish Epilepsy Centre, Filadelfia, Kolonivej 11, DK-4293 Dianalund, Denmark
2. Centre for Engineering and Science, University College Absalon, Parkvej 190, DK-4700 Næstved, Denmark; stjo@pha.dk
* Correspondence: jens.borggaard.larsen@rsyd.dk; Tel.: +45-2987-1237

Abstract: Genotyping of the *CYP2D6* gene is the most commonly applied pharmacogenetic test globally. Significant economic interests have led to the development of a plurality of assays, available for almost any genotyping platform or DNA detection chemistry. Of all the genetic variants, copy number variations are particular difficult to detect by polymerase chain reaction. Here, we present two simple novel approaches for the identification of samples carrying either deletions or duplications of the *CYP2D6* gene; by relative quantification using a singleplex 5′nuclease real-time PCR assay, and by high-resolution melting of PCR products. These methods make use of universal primers, targeting both the *CYP2D6* and the reference gene *CYP2D8P*, which is necessary for the analysis. The assays were validated against a reference method using a large set of samples. The singleplex nature of the 5′nuclease real-time PCR ensures that the primers anneal with equal affinity to both the sequence of the *CYP2D6* and the reference gene. This facilitates robust identification of gene deletions and duplications based on the cycle threshold value. In contrast, the high-resolution melting assay is an end-point PCR, where the identification relies on variations between the amount of product generated from each of the two genes.

Keywords: *CYP2D6*; *CYP2D7P*; *CYP2D8P*; copy number variation; CNV; genotyping; 5′nuclease assay; HRM; high resolution melting; drug metabolization; pharmacogenetics

Citation: Larsen, J.B.; Jørgensen, S. Simple and Robust Detection of *CYP2D6* Gene Deletions and Duplications Using *CYP2D8P* as Reference. *Pharmaceuticals* **2022**, *15*, 166. https://doi.org/10.3390/ph15020166

Academic Editor: Gary J. Stephens

Received: 11 December 2021
Accepted: 27 January 2022
Published: 28 January 2022

Publisher's Note: MDPI stays neutral with regard to jurisdictional claims in published maps and institutional affiliations.

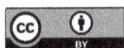

Copyright: © 2022 by the authors. Licensee MDPI, Basel, Switzerland. This article is an open access article distributed under the terms and conditions of the Creative Commons Attribution (CC BY) license (https:// creativecommons.org/licenses/by/ 4.0/).

1. Introduction

The cytochrome p450 monooxidases are a superfamily of enzymes, primarily transcribed in the liver. While many of these enzymes have an essential function in biosynthesis and metabolization of endogenous compounds, others are part of the phase I modification/defense system against xenobiotics [1,2]. This last group constitute pharmacological important enzymes, capable of influencing the treatment of patients prescribed substrate drugs [3]. Alterations in their activity can lead to changes in the metabolic pattern, diminishing the effect of the treatment and/or causing adverse drug reactions [4]. Evolutionary, this group of cytochrome P450 enzymes are believed to have arisen to protect their host against environmental and food produced toxins [5]. As a result, these genes are less stable, allowing faster adaptation, and variants in the forms of deletions or duplications occur at a higher frequency than for other members of the superfamily [4].

One cytochrome P450 gene where copy number variations (CNV) are of particular interest is *CYP2D6*. In humans, the subfamily 2D consists of *CYP2D6* and the two pseudogenes *CYP2D7P* and *CYP2D8P*, located together in a 45 kb region on chromosome 22 [6,7]. Although the evolutionary history of this subfamily dates back to before the divergence between amniotes and amphibians, more than 340 million years ago, its present day organization in hominids is more recent [8,9]. Phylogenetic analysis dates the duplication event and separation between *CYP2D6* and *CYP2D8P* back to the divergence between the new world monkeys and Catarrhini, some 18–5 million years ago [7,9]. In contrast, the

CYP2D7P gene has been acquired more recently by a duplication of *CYP2D6* in the lineage of the great apes. *CYP2D8P* is pseudorized in humans, chimpanzee, and orangutan, by a number of different mutations. In *CYP2D7P*, this is caused by a single frameshift mutation, present in humans and orangutan, but not chimpanzee [7].

The polymorphic nature of the *CYP2D6* gene and its impact on the metabolization of certain drugs had been recognized even before the enzyme was isolated and its gene sequenced [10,11]. Although the enzyme only makes up an estimated 2% of the total content of cytochrome P450 mono-oxidase protein in the liver, it participates in the metabolization of more than 20% of all prescribed drugs [12]. In Caucasians, an estimated 30% of the population has variations in the *CYP2D6* gene, causing changes in metabolic activity [13]. Genotyping of the *CYP2D6* gene is, therefore, a useful tool for predicting the metabolic phenotype and personalizing the treatment of prescribed drugs metabolized by this enzyme. Based on test results, patients are divided into four different groups: poor, intermediate, extensive, and ultrafast metabolizers [10,14]. Ultrafast metabolizers are carriers of one or more fully functional duplication of the gene, while poor metabolizers have two nonfunctional alleles. Abolishment of the enzyme function in an allele can be caused either by single point mutations, or complete or partial deletions of the gene.

Most genotyping methods for copy number variation detection, rely partly or in whole on amplification of the target by PCR [15–22]. Modern real-time PCR techniques are extremely versatile. However, while sensitivity is one of the biggest strengths of this method, it also holds its greatest weakness. Bias can be introduced during amplification that is not only caused by the specificity/annealing temperature of the primers or probes to the target, but may arise due to variations in primer/probe concentrations, the amount of template DNA, or its purity, as well as the concentration of salts or presence of contaminants [23]. This is especially true for assays relying on the multiplexing of primers and probes, or assays that use standard curves or reference samples for relative quantification [24].

The most frequently applied method for routine testing for CNV in the *CYP2D6* gene is by relative quantification, using real-time PCR [15,17,19,25]. By this method, primers amplifying a target sequence from the gene of interest are multiplexed with another primer pair targeting a reference gene. The reference gene is commonly a household gene such as *ALB*, *GAPDH*, or *RNase P*, known not to harbor CNV [16,17,19,26]. During amplification, the products of each primer pair are detected in real-time by monitoring the fluorescence generated from different fluorophores. The relative difference between the two cycle thresholds is then compared to that of a reference wildtype reaction, allowing estimation of copy numbers in the sample.

Although relative quantification by real-time PCR is fast and does not demand additional instrumentation, the use of multiplex PCR makes it less robust. Large fluctuations in the amplification efficiency between identical reactions are common, and routine use necessitates multiple duplicates of each sample, in order to obtain a robust result [23,24,27,28]. One way of optimizing these assays is to design multiplex primer pairs with equal amplification efficiency and with a low level of primer dimer formation. Here, we present a novel approach to this problem, using a singleplex real-time PCR reaction for detection of gene deletions and duplications by relative quantification. Furthermore, by using a single universal primer targeting *CYP2D6* and the reference gene *2D8P*, we developed a high-resolution melting (HRM) end-point PCR method that detects these genotypes based on a melt curve analysis. Both methods allow simple and robust detection of deletions and duplications in the *CYP2D6* gene, and thus are of high clinical relevance in relation to pharmacogenetic testing.

2. Materials and Methods

2.1. Sequence Analysis

The sequences of *CYP2D6*, *CYP2D7P*, and *CYP2D8P* from the latest human genome assembly GHCh38.p13 were downloaded from the National Center for Biotechnology Information (www.ncbi.nlm.nih.gov accession date 11 November 2020) and aligned using

Clustal Omega (www.ebi.ac.uk, 11 November 2020). The webtool boxshade (www.expasy.org—discontinued, 11 November 2020) was used to identify similarities between the three sequences in the alignment. Regions with homology between *CYP2D6* and *CYP2D8P*, and containing heterologous bases to *CYP2D7P*, were then identified by visual inspection of the alignment (Table 1).

Table 1. Alignment of the primed region in exon 9 from *CYP2D6* and the two pseudogenes, *2D7P* and *2D8P*. The alignment is oriented 5′-3′ to the gene. Start and end position of the sequences in the GRCh38.p13 assembly are shown. Letters with gray background mark the location of the *CYP2D6:2D8* universal primers, while the locations of the two gene specific probes/primers are shown in black reversed letters. '*' Indicates conserved bases in the alignment. (A) shows the location of the primers and probes for the 5′nuclease singleplex assay. (B) shows the location of the primers designed for high-resolution melting. Background color shows the location of primers and probes.

Alignment of Target Region from *CYP2D6, 2D7P,* and *2D8P*			
(A) Relative Quantification			
Gene		Alignment Exon 9	
CYP2D6	42126676	CAGCTTCTCGGTGCCCACTGGACAGCCCCGGCCCAGCCACCATGGTGT	
CYP2D7P	42140380	.........C...G..G.C......................TC.C....	
CYP2D8P	42149988	.................C........................TC.C....	
Consensus		********.***.**.*.*****************...*.****	
CYP2D6		CTTTGCTTTCCTGGTGACCCCATCCCCCTATGAGCTTTGTGCTGTGC	42126582
CYP2D7P		.G.CAGC..T....................C................	42140286
CYP2D8P		.G.C.GC..T.........G............................	42149894
Consensus		*.*....**.********.***********.**************	
(B) High Resolution Melting			
Gene		Alignment Exon 9	
CYP2D6	42126676	CAGCTTCTCGGTGCCCACTGGACAGCCCCGGCCCAGCCACCATGGTGT	
CYP2D7P	42140380	.........C...G..G.C......................TC.C....	
CYP2D8P	42149988	.................C........................TC.C....	
Consensus		********.***.**.*.*****************...*.****	
CYP2D6		CTTTGCTTTCCTGGTGACCC	42126609
CYP2D7P		.G.CAGC..T..........	42140313
CYP2D8P		.G.C.GC..T........G.	42149921
Consensus		*.*....**.********.*	

2.2. Design of Primers and Probes for the 5′Nuclease Singleplex PCR

Based on the generated alignment, a universal primer set for *CYP2D6* and *CYP2D8P*, but not *CYP2D7P*, was designed targeting exon 9. A general set of rules for the primer design was used, which included a theoretical annealing temperature of 57–63 °C, primer size of 18–25 nt, and 3′ destabilization, by minimizing the number of C′ and G′ in the last five bases. Bases heterologous to the sequence of *CYP2D7P* were placed in the 3′ end of the primers, if possible, and the amplicon size was minimized.

Two gene specific 5′nuclease probes were designed; one targeting the amplified sequence of *CYP2D6*, and one the sequence of *CYP2D8P*. The probes were designed to have an annealing temperature as close to each other as possible, and a theoretical annealing temperature 6–10 °C higher than that of the primers. A guanine base immediately adjacent to the 5′ labelling was avoided.

Before ordering, each primer and probe sequence was validated in silico using the online software tool Netprimer (Premier Biosoft, http://www.premierbiosoft.com/netprimer/, 11 November 2020), and their specificity to their intended targets was confirmed by performing a Primer-Blast search against the GHCh38.p13 assembly (National Center of Biotechnology Information —www.ncbi.nlm.nih.gov/tools/primer-blast/, 11

November 2020). *CYP2D6* probes were labelled 5′ with FAM, while that of *CYP2D8P* was labelled with CalFluor 560. For quenching of the fluorochrome signal in the intact probe, the 3′ end was labelled with black hole quencher-1 (BHQ-1). All primers and probes were ordered from LGC-Biosearch (Aarhus, Denmark).

2.3. Design of Primers for Use in the High Resolution Melting PCR Assay

To facilitate detection of deletions and duplications using melt curve analysis, a single universal primer was developed capable of amplifying from both the sequence of *CYP2D6* and *CYP2D8P*. As complementary primers, a gene-specific primer was designed for each of the two intended targets. These gene-specific primers generate amplicons variating in size and melt temperature, thereby facilitating separation during analysis. To predict the difference in melt temperatures during the design of the primers, the online tool 'Oligo Calc' (http://biotools.nubic.northwestern.edu, 11 November 2020) was used. The design followed the same rules as for the relative quantification, and the primers were validated *in silico* accordingly.

2.4. Reference Samples and DNA Extraction

Material submitted to the Laboratory of the Danish Epilepsy Centre and tested using a previously published method was used as reference for validation of the assays. Patient samples were anonymized upon retrieval and DNA extraction was performed using a MagNA Pure Compact Nucleic Acid Isolation Kit I (Roche Diagnostic, Basel, Switzerland) applying 200 µL of full blood and a 100 µL elution volume. Following the extraction, samples were quantified using a NanoDrop One spectrophotometer (Thermo Fischer, Waltham, MA, USA), and the DNA concentration was normalized to 20 ng/µL.

2.5. Assay Validation

In total, 48 samples were selected for the validation, based on the genotyping results obtained by the reference method. These samples consisted of 18 tested as wildtype, 20 identified as carriers of a *CYP2D6* deletion variant (*5), and 10 containing one or more duplications of the *CYP2D6* gene.

The applied routine method for CNV genotyping of the reference samples (in the following referred to as *CYP2D6:RNase P*) is accredited by the Danish Accreditation Fund (DANAK) according to the ISO 15189:2013 standard. It relies on relative quantification real-time PCR by amplification of a target sequence in exon 9 of the *CYP2D6* gene. The method is modified from Schaeffler et al. (2003), in that it is multiplexed with a commercial CNV reference kit targeting the *RNase P* gene, instead of the albumin gene described in the original publication [17]. For this study, the assay was performed on duplicates of each sample, in a 20 µL reaction volume containing 10 µL Bio-Rad ITaq Universal Probes Supermix (Bio-Rad Laboratories Inc., Hercules, CA, USA—cat# 1725131), 250 nM of each of the primers of the CYP2D6 assay [17], 150 nM of the probe, 1× RNase P primer/probe mix (Thermo Fischer, Waltham, MA, USA cat# 4403326), and 4 µL of template DNA (20 ng/µL). Temperature cycling was performed in a Bio-Rad CFX Connect real-time PCR instrument, running a program consisting of 3 min at 95 °C, followed by 35 cycles of sequential denaturation for 15 s at 95 °C, and 1 min of elongation at 60 °C. Results were calculated using the $2^{-\Delta\Delta Ct}$ method in the CFX manger v3.1 software (Bio-Rad Laboratories Inc.), by averaging the values from a set of six wildtype samples, used as calibrators and included in each run.

2.6. Detection of CYP2D6 Deletions and Duplications by the 5′ Nuclease Singleplex PCR Assay

The singleplex assay *CYP2D6:2D8P* was performed in 20 µL reaction volumes, containing 10 µL of 2× ITaq Universal Probes Supermix, 250 nM of each of the two primers, 200 nM of each of the probes, together with 4 µL of Template DNA (20 ng/µL). Temperature cycling was performed, applying the same instrument, program, and software setup as for the reference multiplex PCR assay described above. The only exception was that four calibrators instead of six were used per setup.

The PCR efficiency of the *CYP2D6:2D8P*, and the *CYP2D6:RNase P* assay used as reference, was evaluated using standard curve regression. A ten-time dilution series of a wildtype sample, going from 4 ng/μL to 0.004 ng/μL DNA, was generated, and PCR was performed in duplicates using the same reaction concentrations and cycle conditions as above. Using the software CFX Manager v3.1, the PCR efficiency of both probes in each of the two assays was calculated by plotting the logarithmic concentration of the added template DNA against the cycle threshold Cq.

2.7. Detection of CYP2D6 Deletions and Duplications by High-Resolution Melting

For detection of deletions and duplications using HRM, the concentration of the universal forward primer was first optimized against a standard concentration of 250 nM for each of the gene specific primers. The optimization established a concentration at which both of the two amplicons, deferring in size, gave a comparable intensity during melt curve analysis. The optimal concentration of the universal primer was 200 nM for the assay. PCR was performed in 20 μL reaction volumes with 10 μL of Precision Melt Supermix (Bio-Rad cat#1725110) and 2 μL of Template DNA (20 ng/μL), using a Bio-Rad CFX Connect instrument. PCR amplification consisted of an initial denaturation at 95 °C for 3 min, followed by 40 cycles of denaturation at 95 °C for 15 s, annealing of the primers at 60 °C for 30 s, and elongation for 30 s at 72 °C. A melt curve analysis was then performed by first incubating the samples for 3 min at 60 °C, and measuring fluorescence at 0.2 °C/s steps from 70–95 °C. The software package Precision Melt Analysis v1.2 (Bio-Rad Laboratories) was used for normalization of the fluorescence peaks between the samples, and for grouping of the samples according to their melt curve pattern.

2.8. CYP2D6 and CYP2D8P Sequencing

The target region of the singleplex and the HRM assays, were selectively amplified from the *CYP2D6* and *CYP2D8P* gene, using the gene specific primers listed in Table 2, C. PCR was performed in 25 μL reaction volumes with 12.5 μL of CloneAmp HiFi PCR premix (TakaraBio, cat#639298), 250 nM of each primer, and 100 ng genomic DNA. PCR amplification was performed with a Bio-Rad CFX96, using the following conditions: 35 cycles of 98 °C for 10 s, 60 °C for 10 s, and 72 °C for 30 s. The PCR products were gel purified using a 1 % agarose gel. Bands, corresponding to 676 bp for the *CYP2D6* fragment and 670 bp for the *CYP2D8P*, were sequenced by Eurofins Genomics, using the same gene-specific primers as for the PCR amplification.

Table 2. Primers and probes designed and used in this study. 'Size' is the size of the amplicons produced by the primers. (A) Primers and probes designed for the 5′nuclease singleplex *CYP2D6:2D8P* PCR assay for use with relative quantification. Probe labelling: FAM = Fluorescein, CF560 = Calfluor 560, BHQ-1 = Black Hole Quencher 1. (B) Primers designed for detection by high-resolution melting. (C) Gene specific primers designed for sequencing of the *CYP2D6* and *CYP2D8P* target regions of the singleplex and high-resolution melting analysis.

Primers and Probes Designed for this Study		
(A) Primers and probes for relative quantification		
Name	Sequence	Size
CYP2D6:2D8 exon 9 Fwd	5′ CAGCTTCTCGGTGCCCAC 3′	95 bp
CYP2D6:2D8 exon 9 Rev	5′ GCACAGCACAAAGCTCATAGG 3′	
CYP2D6 exon 9 probe	5′ FAM-ACCAGGAAAGCAAAGACACCATGGT-BHQ1 3′	
CYP2D8 exon 9 probe	5′ CF560-TCACCAGAAAGCCGACGACACGAGA-BHQ1 3′	
(B) Primers for high-resolution melting		
Name	Sequence	Size
CYP2D6:2D8 exon 9 Fwd	5′ CAGCTTCTCGGTGCCCAC 3′	
CYP2D6 exon 9 Rev	5′ AGGAAAGCAAAGACACCATGGT 3′	60 bp
CYP2D8 exon 9 Rev	5′ GCGTCACCAGAAAGCCGA 3′	68 bp
(C) Primers for sequencing		
Name	Sequence	Size
CYP2D6 Seq Fwd	5′ GTCTAGTGGGGAGACAAACCA 3′	676 bp
CYP2D8 Seq Fwd	5′ CTAGTGGGGAAGGCAGACCA 3′	670 bp
CYP2D6:2D8 Rev	5′ GCACAGCACAAAGCTCATAGG 3′	

3. Results

3.1. Design and Validation of the 5′Nuclease Singleplex PCR Assay

Sequence alignment identified a common region suitable for designing universal primers, facilitation specific amplification from the *CYP2D6* and *CYP2D8P* genes, but not from *CYP2D7P*. The targets of the primers are located in exon 9, starting at position 42126676 of the *CYP2D6* sequence and position 42149988 of *2D8P* (Table 1). This region is the same as that covered by the assay designed by Schaeffler et al. (2003). The primer pair flank a sequence with heterogeneity between the *CYP2D6* and *CYP2D8P*, thereby facilitating design of specific probes against each of the two genes (Table 2).

The equal affinity of the primers for both gene targets, and the efficiency of the PCR assay, was investigated by comparing a standard curve to that from the reference assay (Figure 1). The obtained slope values for the *CYP2D6:2D8P* assay where -3.39 for the *CYP2D6* probe and -3.37 for the *CYP2D8P*, resulting in a calculated PCR efficiency of 97.3% and 97.9% (Figure 1A). The same analysis for the reference *CYP2D6:RNase P* assay gave a slope of -3.18 and -3.40, respectively, and a calculated efficiency of 105.4% and 96.9% (Figure 1B).

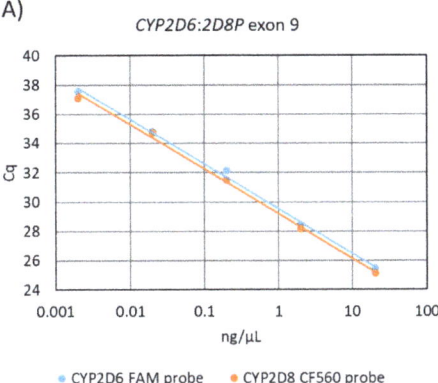

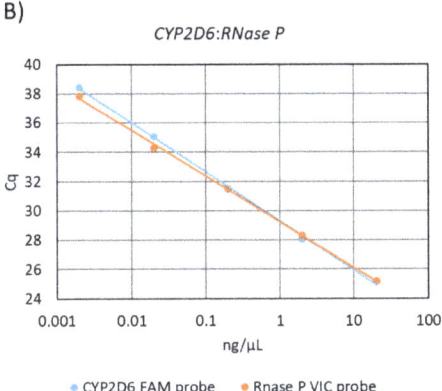

Figure 1. Analysis of primer amplification efficiency by use of the standard curve method, performed by dilution of a wildtype samples. (**A**) Standard curve generated by the 5′nuclease sing-leplex *CYP2D6:2D8P* assay. Slope of the *CYP2D6* probe −3.39 efficiency 97.3%, *CYP2D8P* probe slope −3.37 efficiency 97.9% (**B**) Standard curve generated using the CYP2D6:RNase P reference assay. CYP2D6 probe slope −3.18 and 105.4% efficiency, RNase P probe slope −3.40 calculated efficiency 96.9%.

The *CYP2D6:2D8P* assay was validated against a large set of reference samples ($n = 48$). As a method for comparing the result from the *CYP2D6:2D8P* to that of the reference, the relative quantification (RQ) values obtained by each of the assays were plotted against each other (Figure 2A). This plot clearly separated the samples into the three genotypes (deletion *5, wildtype, duplication xN) and showed 100% consistent results between the two assays. The two assays where further compared by calculating the mean RQ for each of the three genotype groups (Figure 2B). The RQ mean for the reference samples analyzed by the *CYP2D6:2D8P* assay was 0.45 for the deletion *5 allele, 0.94 for the wildtype, and 1.90 for the duplication. In comparison, the values for the *CYP2D6:RNase P* were 0.41, 0.80, and 1.43 for the same set of samples.

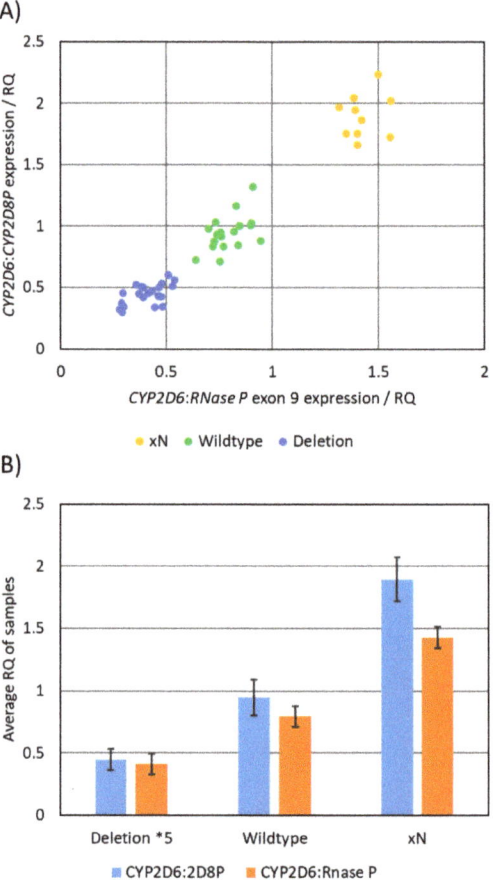

Figure 2. Comparison between the *CYP2D6:2D8P* singleplex, and the *CYP2D6:RNase P* reference assay. (**A**) Graphical representation of results obtained by parallel testing, where the calculated RQ values obtained from the two assays are plotted against each other. The plot separated the samples into three groups based on the copy number of the sample. (**B**) Calculated average RQ value for the samples carrying deletion *5 ($n = 20$), wildtype ($n = 18$), and duplications ($n = 10$).

As both *CYP2D6* and *CYP2D8P* are competing for the same set of primers in the assay, the separation between the genotypes would be expected to increase throughout the PCR reaction. This was verified at the end-point of the PCR for the *CYP2D6:2D8P* assay, by plotting the relative fluorescence from the probes against each other (Figure 3).

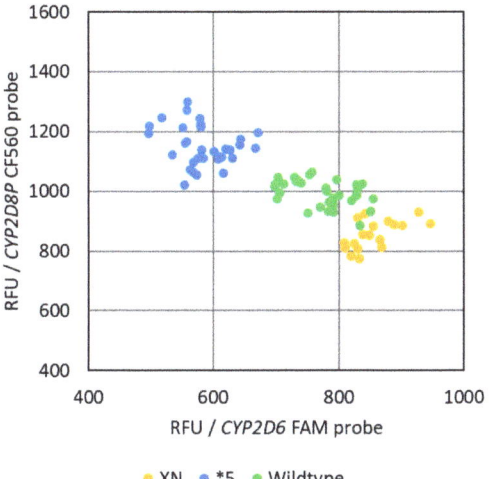

Figure 3. Common end-point PCR allele discrimination plot of the reference samples obtained by the singleplex *CYP2D6:2D8P* assay. The plot shows the differentiation into the three genotype groups, deletions *5, wildtype, and samples with one or more duplicates of the CYP2D6 gene (xN).

3.2. Design and Validation of the High Resolution Melting Assay

The developed genotyping technique using high-resolution melting, relies on a single primer targeting a sequence conserved between the target gene *CYP2D6*, and the reference gene *CYP2D8P*. The single universal primer is multiplexed in the PCR reaction with two gene specific primers, designed to generate amplicons differing in length/melt temperature of the double stranded DNA. This allows separation of the peaks generated by the *CYP2D6* and *CYP2D8P* gene on the melt curve plot (Figure 4). As the universal primer is added at a lower concentration, making it the rate-limiting factor of the PCR, any difference in the starting template amounts between the two gene targets is expected to increase throughout the PCR amplification. Detection of deletions and duplications was thus performed by comparing the melt curves to controls, and looking at the differences in fluorescence, caused by the proportional shift between the amplicons of *CYP2D6* and *2D8P* (Figure 4A).

The proposed method was tested by designing an assay targeting the same region in *CYP2D6* exon 9 and applying the same universal forward primer as for the assay developed for relative quantification in this study (Table 1). Gene specific primers were designed located immediately downstream, resulting in a fragment size of 60 bp for the *CYP2D6* gene, and 68 bp for *CYP2D8P* (Table 2). Optimization was performed on a wildtype sample, to ensure comparable peak heights for both amplicons in the melt curve analysis for this genotype (Figure 4A). This was done by lowering the concentration of the universal primer alone. When tested on samples carrying a deletion or duplications, this resulted in a change in the melt curve pattern, allowing easy discrimination between the three genotypes (Figure 4).

The assay was further validated on the same set of reference samples as used for the relative quantification. The reference samples carrying deletions *5, and homozygote wildtypes, gave a result 100% consistent with the previous findings (Figure 4B). Four of the duplicate samples showed a slightly deviating melt curve pattern. In order to identify the reasons for these discrepancies, this region from both the *CYP2D6* and the *CYP2D8P* gene was sequenced. One of the samples carried a C > T transition within the assay region (Table 1B—*CYP2D8P*—location 42150006), possibly explaining the different melt curve pattern. The discrepancy for the three other samples could not be resolved.

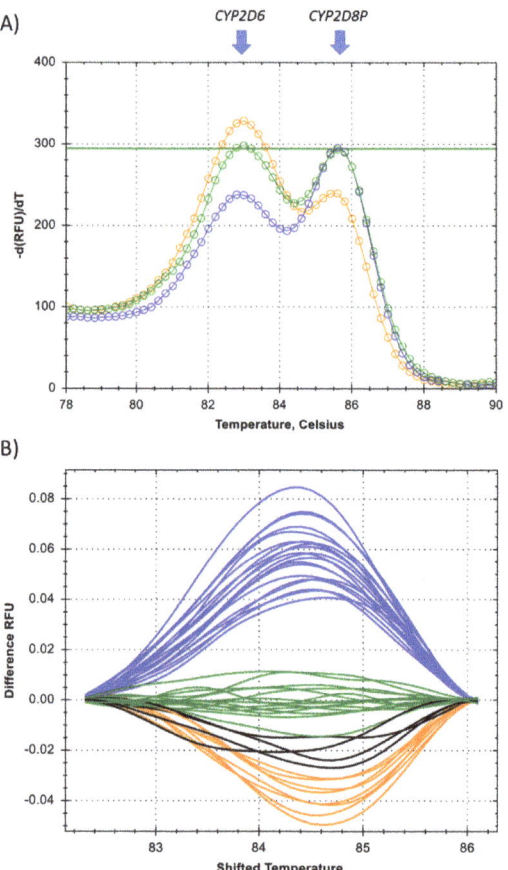

Figure 4. Detection of *CYP2D6* deletions or duplications by high-resolution melting PCR. (**A**) Melt curve showing the proportional change between the two amplicons generated from the *CYP2D6* and the *CYP2D8P* gene, identified by the two arrows. (**B**) Temperature shifted view of the melt curves from all of the reference samples (n = 48) used for the validation of the assay. Clustering was done by automatic calling, using the Precision Melt software from Bio-Rad. Blue = deletions *5, green = wildtype, orange = duplications, and black = unresolved duplicate samples.

4. Discussion

The purpose of the present study was to develop a simple and robust assay for routine pharmacogenetic detection of copy number variations in the *CYP2D6* gene. Previously, the use of *CYP2D8P* as a reference gene for CNV detection of *CYP2D6* was reported in two other studies. While Söderbäck et al. first described a method for genotyping *CYP2D6* by pyrosequencing, Nakamura et al. developed a method combining loop mediated isothermal amplification (LAMP-PCR) and electrochemical detection [21,29]. Both of these studies applied proprietary techniques that require additional instrumentation as well as reagents. In contrast, the methods reported in the current study rely on simple real-time PCR technology. The novelty of this, therefore, relies on two factors:

1. The equal affinity and efficiency of the universal primers when amplifying the two targets located in the *CYP2D6* and *2D8P* gene.
2. The competition of the two targets for the same pool of universal primers, in the later phase of the PCR amplification.

The first is important when performing relative quantification using real-time PCR, as the method relies on cycle threshold values (Cq) obtained during the exponential phase of the reaction. During this phase, the primers and other reagents are not the rate-limiting factor, but rather the efficiency of the primers and the concentration of template DNA. By reducing the number of primers and by having primers with a 100% similar annealing temperature to the two targets, an equal amplification efficiency is obtained for *CYP2D6* and *CYP2D8P* (Figure 1).

The second benefit is a prerequisite for developing an end-point PCR method for identifying deletions and duplications. While a regular multiplex PCR has two (or more) different pools of primers and the depletion of one pool will tend to have no direct effect on the amplification performed by the other, this is not the case using universal primers. Here, following the exponential phase, the two targets will begin to compete for the same pool of free universal primers in the PCR reaction. As this pool becomes depleted, the most abundant template will have a continually increased chance of a primer annealing and initiating amplification. When applied to a sample carrying deletions or duplications in the *CYP2D6* gene, this results in a continuously greater difference between the signal of the target and the reference gene. This principle is applied in the HRM assay, where the identification is based on the difference in fluorescence obtained during melting of the two amplicons (Figure 4). However, it may also be used to develop similar end-point PCR assays based on other chemistries, such as 5′nuclease/Taqman (Figure 3). This has the potential to reduce the overall cost of PCR-based genotyping of the *CYP2D6* gene, by allowing the same workflow and setup for identification of both gene deletions/duplications and single nucleotide polymorphisme (SNP) [30,31]. However, in order for this to work in a 5′nuclease assay, an additional separation between the signal strength of the two probes is required. This is particularly true in order to be able to differentiate between the wildtype and samples harboring duplications of the *CYP2D6* gene (Figure 3). One possible solution could be to use double quenched probes.

Since the clinical relevance of exact copy number calls of duplications is very limited, both assays in their present form are qualitative. This is especially true for the HRM assay, as it is an end-point PCR. In contrast the 5′nuclease singleplex assay relies on the real-time Cq values obtained during the exponential phase of the PCR. With further development, the method, therefore, ought to be useful for exact quantification of duplicates in the *CYP2D6* gene, should that be warranted. This would, however, necessitate a more stringent and elaborate setup than is generally feasible for routine pharmacogenetic testing.

A complicating factor when genotyping the *CYP2D6* gene is the possible presence of partial deletions/duplications or hybrids between the *CYP2D6* and the *2D7P* gene. The location of the two assays presented here allows the discrimination of one common hybrid allele *36 found in tandem CNV. This is a non-functional hybrid allele containing a conversion to *CYP2D7P* within or upstream of exon 9. Therefore, if the target sequence of the assay is upstream from the conversion site, it will be genotyped as a wildtype. In contrast, an assay targeting a region downstream would identify it as a deletion and thereby, correctly, as a non-functional allele [16].

Although the design of an assay applying two universal primers adds restrictions, by lowering the number of possible target sequences in the *CYP2D6* gene, the initial sequence analysis identified other possible locations. One is around the same area in exon 6 targeted by Söderbäck et al. [29]. Other regions of the *CYP2D6* gene may, however, be made accessible by incorporation of single degenerate or modified bases, such as inosine or locked nucleic acids, into the primer sequence.

In contrast to the 5′nuclease singleplex assay, the HRM method only relies on a single universal primer. This increases the potential targets for such assays in the *CYP2D6* gene significantly. The method may, therefore, also be used for detecting deletions and duplications in other genes i.e., *SULT1A1* or *UGT2B17* [28,32].

In conclusion, the novel methods presented in this study allow fast and robust identification of deletions and duplications in the *CYP2D6* gene, applying standard real-time

PCR detection techniques. The outlined approach may also be applicable to other PCR chemistries used for genotyping. In addition, if suitable reference sequences can be identified, these methods could help simplify the routine identification of deletions or duplications in genes other than *CYP2D6*.

Author Contributions: Conceptualization, J.B.L.; methodology, J.B.L. and S.J.; validation, J.B.L. and S.J.; formal analysis, J.B.L.; investigation, J.B.L. and S.J.; data curation, J.B.L.; writing—original draft preparation, J.B.L.; writing—review and editing, J.B.L. and S.J. All authors have read and agreed to the published version of the manuscript.

Funding: This research received no external funding.

Institutional Review Board Statement: Not applicable.

Informed Consent Statement: Not applicable.

Data Availability Statement: Data is contained within this article.

Acknowledgments: The authors would like to thank Annette Pia Møller, Yvonne Grønkjær, Camilla Cederholm, and Anja Sjelhøj from the Danish Epilepsy Centre for technical assistance.

Conflicts of Interest: The authors report no conflict of interest in this work.

References

1. Yang, Y.; Botton, M.R.; Scott, E.R.; Scott, S.A. Sequencing the CYP2D6 Gene: From Variant Allele Discovery to Clinical Pharmacogenetic Testing. *Pharmacogenomics* **2017**, *18*, 673–685. [CrossRef] [PubMed]
2. Thomas, J.H. Rapid Birth-Death Evolution Specific to Xenobiotic Cytochrome P450 Genes in Vertebrates. *PLoS Genet.* **2007**, *3*, 720–728. [CrossRef] [PubMed]
3. Denham, M.J. Adverse Drug Reactions. *Br. Med. Bull.* **1990**, *46*, 53–62. [CrossRef] [PubMed]
4. Esteves, F.; Rueff, J.; Kranendonk, M. The Central Role of Cytochrome P450 in Xenobiotic Metabolism—A Brief Review on a Fascinating Enzyme Family. *J. Xenobiotics* **2021**, *11*, 7. [CrossRef] [PubMed]
5. Fuselli, S.; De Filippo, C.; Mona, S.; Sistonen, J.; Fariselli, P.; Destro-Bisol, G.; Barbujani, G.; Bertorelle, G.; Sajantila, A. Evolution of Detoxifying Systems: The Role of Environment and Population History in Shaping Genetic Diversity at Human CYP2D6 Locus. *Pharm. Genom.* **2010**, *20*, 485–499. [CrossRef] [PubMed]
6. Heim, M.H.; Meyer, U.A. Evolution of a Highly Polymorphic Human Cytochrome P450 Gene Cluster: CYP2D6. *Genomics* **1992**, *14*, 49–58. [CrossRef]
7. Yasukochi, Y.; Satta, Y. Molecular Evolution of the CYP2D Subfamily in Primates: Purifying Selection on Substrate Recognition Sites without the Frequent or Long-Tract Gene Conversion. *Genome Biol. Evol.* **2015**, *7*, 1053–1067. [CrossRef] [PubMed]
8. Sezutsu, H.; le Goff, G.; Feyereisen, R. Origins of P450 Diversity. *Philos. Trans. R. Soc. B Biol. Sci.* **2013**, *368*, 1–11. [CrossRef] [PubMed]
9. Yasukochi, Y.; Satta, Y. Evolution of the CYP2D Gene Cluster in Humansand Four Non-Human Primates. *Genes Genet. Syst.* **2011**, *86*, 109–116. [CrossRef] [PubMed]
10. Taylor, C.; Crosby, I.; Yip, V.; Maguire, P.; Pirmohamed, M.; Turner, R.M. A Review of the Important Role of Cyp2d6 in Pharmacogenomics. *Genes* **2020**, *11*, 1295. [CrossRef]
11. Guengerich, F.P. A History of the Roles of Cytochrome P450 Enzymes in the Toxicity of Drugs. *Toxicol. Res.* **2021**, *37*, 1–23. [CrossRef] [PubMed]
12. Jaquenoud Sirot, E.; van der Velden, J.W.; Rentsch, K.; Eap, C.B.; Baumann, P. Therapeutic Drug Monitoring and Pharmacogenetic Tests as Tools in Pharmacovigilance. *Drug Saf.* **2006**, *29*, 735–768. [CrossRef] [PubMed]
13. Zhou, Y.; Ingelman-Sundberg, M.; Lauschke, V.M. Worldwide Distribution of Cytochrome P450 Alleles: A Meta-Analysis of Population-Scale Sequencing Projects. *Clin. Pharmacol. Ther.* **2017**, *102*, 688–700. [CrossRef] [PubMed]
14. Valdes, R.; Payne, D.A.; Linder, M.W. Laboratory Medicine Practice Guideline: Laboratory Analysis and Application of Pharmacogenetics to Clinical Practice. *Natl. Acad. Clin. Biochem.* **2010**, *37*, 180–193.
15. Leandro-García, L.J.; Leskelä, S.; Montero-Conde, C.; Landa, I.; López-Jimenez, E.; Letón, R.; Seeringer, A.; Kirchheiner, J.; Cascón, A.; Robledo, M.; et al. Determination of CYP2D6 Gene Copy Number by Multiplex Polymerase Chain Reaction Analysis. *Anal. Biochem.* **2009**, *389*, 74–76. [CrossRef]
16. Ramamoorthy, A.; Flockhart, D.A.; Hosono, N.; Kubo, M.; Nakamura, Y.; Skaar, T.C. Differential Quantification of CYP2D6 Gene Copy Number by Four Different Quantitative Real-Time PCR Assays. *Pharm. Genom.* **2010**, *20*, 451–454. [CrossRef]
17. Schaeffeler, E.; Schwab, M.; Eichelbaum, M.; Zanger, U.M. CYP2D6 Genotyping Strategy Based on Gene Copy Number Determination by TaqMan Real-Rime PCR. *Hum. Mutat.* **2003**, *22*, 476–485. [CrossRef]
18. Langaee, T.; Hamadeh, I.; Chapman, A.B.; Gums, J.G.; Johnson, J.A. A Novel Simple Method for Determining CYP2D6 Gene Copy Number and Identifying Allele(s) with Duplication/Multiplication. *PLoS ONE* **2015**, *10*, 2–12. [CrossRef]

19. Bodin, L.; Beaune, P.H.; Loriot, M.A. Determination of Cytochrome P450 2D6 (CYP2D6) Gene Copy Number by Real-Time Quantitative PCR. *J. Biomed. Biotechnol.* **2005**, *2005*, 248–253. [CrossRef]
20. Nguyen, D.L.; Staeker, J.; Laika, B.; Steimer, W. TaqMan Real-Time PCR Quantification Strategy of CYP2D6 Gene Copy Number for the LightCycler 2.0. *Clin. Chim. Acta Int. J. Clin. Chem.* **2009**, *403*, 207–211. [CrossRef]
21. Söderbäck, E.; Zackrisson, A.L.; Lindblom, B.; Alderborn, A. Determination of CYP2D6 Gene Copy Number by Pyrosequencing. *Clin. Chem.* **2005**, *51*, 522–531. [CrossRef] [PubMed]
22. Bjerre, D.; Berg Rasmussen, H.; Indices Consortium, T. Novel Approach for CES1 Genotyping: Integrating Single Nucleotide Variants and Structural Variation. *Pharmacogenomics* **2018**, *19*, 349–359. [CrossRef] [PubMed]
23. Sint, D.; Raso, L.; Traugott, M. Advances in Multiplex PCR: Balancing Primer Efficiencies and Improving Detection Success. *Methods Ecol. Evol.* **2012**, *3*, 898–905. [CrossRef] [PubMed]
24. Markoulatos, P.; Siafakas, N.; Moncany, M. Multiplex Polymerase Chain Reaction: A Practical Approach. *J. Clin. Lab. Anal.* **2002**, *16*, 47–51. [CrossRef] [PubMed]
25. Arneth, B.; Shams, M.; Hiemke, C.; Härtter, S. Rapid and Reliable Genotyping Procedure for Detection of Alleles with Mutations, Deletion, or/and Duplication of the CYP2D6 Gene. *Clin. Biochem.* **2009**, *42*, 1282–1290. [CrossRef] [PubMed]
26. Ramírez, B.; Niño-Orrego, M.J.; Cárdenas, D.; Ariza, K.E.; Quintero, K.; Contreras Bravo, N.C.; Tamayo-Agudelo, C.; González, M.A.; Laissue, P.; Fonseca Mendoza, D.J. Copy Number Variation Profiling in Pharmacogenetics CYP-450 and GST Genes in Colombian Population. *BMC Med. Genom.* **2019**, *12*, 110. [CrossRef]
27. He, Y.; Hoskins, J.M.; McLeod, H.L. Copy Number Variants in Pharmacogenetic Genes. *Trends Mol. Med.* **2011**, *17*, 244–251. [CrossRef]
28. Gaedigk, A.; Twist, G.P.; Leeder, J.S. CYP2D6, SULT1A1 and UGT2B17 Copy Number Variation: Quantitative Detection by Multiplex PCR. *Pharmacogenomics* **2012**, *13*, 91–111. [CrossRef]
29. Nakamura, N.; Fukuda, T.; Nonen, S.; Hashimoto, K.; Azuma, J.; Gemma, N. Simple and Accurate Determination of CYP2D6 Gene Copy Number by a Loop-Mediated Isothermal Amplification Method and an Electrochemical DNA Chip. *Clin. Chim. Acta Int. J. Clin. Chem.* **2010**, *411*, 568–573. [CrossRef]
30. Larsen, J.B.; Rasmussen, J.B. Pharmacogenetic Testing Revisited: 5′ Nuclease Real-Time Polymerase Chain Reaction Test Panels for Genotyping CYP2D6 and CYP2C19. *Pharm. Pers. Med.* **2017**, *10*, 115–128. [CrossRef]
31. Lu, H.C.; Chang, Y.S.; Chang, C.C.; Lin, C.H.; Chang, J.G. Developing and Evaluating the HRM Technique for Identifying Cytochrome P450 2D6 Polymorphisms. *J. Clin. Lab. Anal.* **2015**, *29*, 220–225. [CrossRef] [PubMed]
32. Vijzelaar, R.; Botton, M.R.; Stolk, L.; Martis, S.; Desnick, R.J.; Scott, S.A. Multi-Ethnic SULT1A1 Copy Number Profiling with Multiplex Ligation-Dependent Probe Amplification. *Pharmacogenomics* **2018**, *19*, 761–770. [CrossRef] [PubMed]

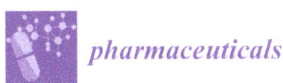

Article

Genotyping for HLA Risk Alleles to Prevent Drug Hypersensitivity Reactions: Impact Analysis

Lisanne E. N. Manson [1,2], Wilbert B. van den Hout [3] and Henk-Jan Guchelaar [1,2,*]

1. Department of Clinical Pharmacy and Toxicology, Leiden University Medical Center, 2333 ZA Leiden, The Netherlands; L.E.N.Manson@lumc.nl
2. Leiden Network for Personalized Therapeutics, 2333 ZA Leiden, The Netherlands
3. Department of Biomedical Data Sciences, Leiden University Medical Center, 2333 ZA Leiden, The Netherlands; W.B.van_den_Hout@lumc.nl
* Correspondence: H.J.Guchelaar@lumc.nl

Abstract: Human Leukocyte Antigen (HLA) variants can be a risk factor for developing potentially fatal drug hypersensitivity reactions. Our aim was to estimate the potential impact of genotyping for the HLA risk alleles incorporated in the Dutch Pharmacogenetics Working Group (DPWG) guidelines in The Netherlands. We estimated the number of hypersensitivity reactions and associated deaths that can be avoided annually by genotyping for these HLA risk alleles. Additionally, the cost-effectiveness was estimated. Nationwide implementation of genotyping HLA risk alleles before initiating drugs with an actionable drug–gene interaction can potentially save the life of seven allopurinol initiators and two flucloxacillin initiators each year in The Netherlands. Besides these deaths, 28 cases of abacavir hypersensitivity, 24 cases of allopurinol induced SCARs, 6 cases of carbamazepine induced DRESS and 22 cases of flucloxacillin induced DILI can be prevented. Genotyping *HLA-B*5701* in abacavir initiators has a number needed to genotype of 31 to prevent one case of abacavir hypersensitivity and is cost-saving. Genotyping *HLA-B*5801* in allopurinol initiators has a number needed to genotype of 1149 to prevent one case of SCAR but is still cost-effective. Genotyping before initiating antiepileptic drugs or flucloxacillin is not cost-effective. Our results confirm the need for mandatory testing of *HLA-B*5701* in abacavir initiators, as indicated in the drug label, and show genotyping of *HLA-B**5801 in allopurinol initiators should be considered.

Keywords: HLA; drug hypersensitivity; pharmacogenomics; abacavir; allopurinol; flucloxacillin; antiepileptic drugs; cost-effectiveness

1. Introduction

Adverse drug reactions (ADRs) are a major cause of morbidity and mortality in modern healthcare. An adverse drug reaction (ADR) is defined by the World Health Organization as "a response to a drug which is noxious and unintended, and which occurs at doses normally used in humans for the prophylaxis, diagnosis, or therapy of disease, or for the modifications of physiological function" [1]. Two types of ADRs are distinguished, type A and type B reactions. Whereas type A reactions can be predicted from the drug's pharmacological mechanism of action, type B reactions, or idiosyncratic reactions, cannot be predicted as such and are often much rarer than type A reactions.

Bouvy et al. performed a review of all epidemiological studies quantifying ADRs in a European setting and found a median percentage of ADR related hospital admissions of 3.5% of all admissions and a fatality rate of approximately 0.15% indicating that ADRs represent a significant burden on European healthcare [2]. Incidence numbers of idiosyncratic ADRs are scarcely available within Caucasian cohorts, but according to Asian studies the incidence of drug hypersensitivity of hospitalized patients is estimated to be 1.8–4.2 per 1000 hospital admissions [3,4]. They are rare but, due to them being unpredictable and often severe with high mortality rates, genetic biomarkers to identify patients at higher

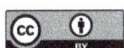

risk of drug hypersensitivity are of utmost importance in preventing these hypersensitivity reactions, hospital admissions and potentially death.

In 2005, the Dutch Pharmacogenetics Working Group (DPWG) was established by the Royal Dutch Pharmacist's Association with the objective to develop pharmacogenetics-based therapeutic (dose) recommendations [5]. Many of its guidelines concern pharmacokinetic and pharmacodynamic gene-drug interactions to prevent type A ADRs. But also guidelines related to risk alleles in the HLA gene and associated idiosyncratic drug reactions are available.

The guidelines include *HLA-B*5701* and abacavir hypersensitivity reaction (ABC-HSR), *HLA-B*5801* and allopurinol associated severe cutaneous adverse drug reactions (SCARs) including Stevens–Johnson syndrome (SJS), toxic epidermal necrolysis (TEN) and drug reaction with eosinophilia and systemic symptoms (DRESS) and *HLA-B*5701* and flucloxacillin induced liver injury (DILI). Additionally there are guidelines about *HLA-B*1502, HLA-B*1511* and *HLA-A*3101* and carbamazepine induced SCARs and *HLA-B*1502* and lamotrigine, oxcarbazepine and phenytoin associated SJS/TEN [6–13].

In many populations, these HLA tests have been proven to be effective in predicting susceptibility for the specific drug hypersensitivity reactions and in a recent paper the diagnostic test criteria including sensitivity and specificity have been described [14]. However, it is yet unclear what the impact of genotyping for these HLA risk alleles would be in a European population.

Genotyping for HLA risk alleles potentially has a high impact for the individual patient and nationwide. Therefore we aim to make a quantitative estimate of the potential impact of genotyping for HLA risk alleles in The Netherlands by estimating the number of drug hypersensitivity reactions that can be avoided annually by switching patients to an alternative drug if they tested positive for the specific HLA risk allele. Additionally we determined how many deaths could be prevented annually by this approach. In addition, we performed a cost-effectiveness study to determine whether testing for HLA risk alleles is cost-effective.

2. Results

2.1. Nationwide Dispensing Data

An overview of first dispensations obtained from the Dutch Foundation for Pharmaceutical Statistics or Stichting Farmaceutische Kerngetallen (SFK) of abacavir, allopurinol, carbamazepine, flucloxacillin, lamotrigine, oxcarbazepine and phenytoin for the period 1 January–31 December 31, 2019 is shown in Table 1 [15]. First dispensations are defined as a dispensation without a previous dispensation within the prior 12 months [16]. Flucloxacillin is the most represented drug of the seven drugs with almost 19,000 first dispensations per million patients followed by allopurinol with around 1700 first dispensations and carbamazepine with nearly 600 dispensations per million patients.

Table 1. An overview of the first dispensations for drugs with an actionable HLA associated DPWG recommendation dispensed in Dutch pharmacies [15].

Name Drug	No. First Dispensations	First Dispensations per Million Patients
FLUCLOXACILLIN	296,467	18,529
ALLOPURINOL	27,585	1724
CARBAMAZEPINE	9520	595
LAMOTRIGINE	6426	402
OXCARBAZEPINE	1219	76
ABACAVIR monotherapy or in combination with other antiviral drugs	873	55
PHENYTOIN	678	42

2.2. Frequencies of HLA Variants

The frequency of HLA variants is derived from Dutch populations from the Allele Frequency Net Database and literature [17,18]. The most common HLA risk alleles in The Netherlands are *HLA-B*5701* and *HLA-A*3101*. *HLA-B*1511* was not found in any of the four Dutch populations while *HLA-B*1502* was only found once. The weighted averages of the allele frequencies and calculated carrier frequencies of the five HLA risk alleles mentioned in the DPWG guidelines are shown in Table 2.

Table 2. Allele frequencies and carrier frequencies of HLA risk alleles in the Dutch population [17,18].

HLA Risk Allele	Allele Frequency	Carrier Frequency
*HLA-A*3101*	0.0338	0.0665
*HLA-B*1502*	0.0007	0.0014
*HLA-B*1511*	0.0000	0.0000
*HLA-B*5701*	0.0336	0.0661
*HLA-B*5801*	0.0069	0.0138

2.3. Positive Predictive Values

The probability that following a positive HLA test result, the individual will develop the specific drug hypersensitivity when exposed to the drug of interest, is the positive predictive value (PPV). The positive predictive values of the HLA-drug hypersensitivity reactions are shown in Table 3. The PPVs were retrieved from literature and existing guidelines. The *HLA-B*5701* test for abacavir hypersensitivity has by far the highest PPV of approximately 48%. The PPV of *HLA-B*5801* for allopurinol-induced SJS/TEN is also relatively high with 5.5%. On the other hand, all other PPVs are below 1%.

Table 3. Positive predictive values of HLA-drug hypersensitivity interactions.

Drug	HLA Variant	Outcome	PPV	Source
Abacavir	*HLA-B*5701*	Abacavir hypersensitivity reaction	48%	DPWG guideline [12]
Allopurinol	*HLA-B*5801*	SJS/TEN	5.5%	Lonjou et al. [19]
		DRESS	0.72%	Gonçalo et al. [20]
Flucloxacillin	*HLA-B*5701*	DILI	0.11%	Daly et al. [21]
Carbamazepine	*HLA-B*1502*	SJS/TEN	0.14%	Amstutz et al. [22]
	*HLA-B*1511*	SJS/TEN	0.5%	DPWG guideline [7]
	*HLA-A*3101*	DRESS	0.89%	Genin et al. [23]
		SJS/TEN	0.02%	DPWG guideline [7]
Oxcarbazepine	*HLA-B*1502*	SJS	0.73%	Chen et al. [24] DPWG guideline [10]
Lamotrigine	*HLA-B*1502*	SJS/TEN	0.4%	DPWG guideline [9]
Phenytoin	*HLA-B*1502*	SJS/TEN	0.65%	Chen et al. [25] DPWG guideline [11]

2.4. Mortality

The mortality rates of abacavir hypersensitivity reaction (ABC-HSR), SJS/TEN, SJS, DRESS and DILI used in our analysis are shown in Table 4. Abacavir hypersensitivity has a mortality of about 0.07%, DRESS of 2%, DILI of 7.6% while SJS and SJS/TEN have a high mortality of 24% and 34%.

Table 4. Mortality rates of hypersensitivity reactions.

Type of Hypersensitivity Reaction	Mortality (Reference)
ABC-HSR	0.07% [26]
DRESS	2% [27]
SJS	24% [28]
SJS/TEN	34% [28]
DILI	7.6% [29]

2.5. Hypersensitivity Reactions and Deaths Prevented by HLA Genotyping

Table 5 summarizes the estimated annual number of actionable genotypes, HLA associated hypersensitivity reactions and deaths caused by these hypersensitivity reactions in The Netherlands. As is shown in Table 5, *HLA-B*5701* testing, which is already mandatory for abacavir prior to start, is estimated to prevent 28 hypersensitivity reactions per year but less than one death each year. This is due to a high allele carrier frequency and positive predictive value but low mortality rate of 0.07%. This low mortality rate can probably be explained by the fact that abacavir hypersensitivity reaction is more severe after a rechallenge and the drug is usually withdrawn after a first reaction.

Table 5. An overview of actionable genotypes amongst drug initiators and the estimated number of hypersensitivity reactions and deaths caused by hypersensitivity reactions that can be prevented by HLA genotyping.

Drug	HLA Allele	Outcome	First Prescriptions	Carrier Frequency	PPV	Mortality	Actionable Genotypes	Hypersensitivity Reactions	Deaths
Abacavir	B*5701	ABC-HSR	873	0.0661	0.48	0.0007	57.71	27.70	0.02
Allopurinol	B*5801	SJS/TEN	27,585	0.0138	0.055	0.34	380.67	20.94	7.12
Allopurinol	B*5801	DRESS	27,585	0.0138	0.007	0.02	380.67	2.74	0.05
Carbamazepine	B*1502	SJS/TEN	9520	0.0014	0.0014	0.34	13.33	0.02	0.01
Carbamazepine	B*1511	SJS/TEN	9520	0	0.005	0.34	0.00	0.00	0.00
Carbamazepine	A*3101	DRESS	9520	0.0665	0.0089	0.02	633.08	5.63	0.11
Carbamazepine	A*3101	SJS/TEN	9520	0.0665	0.0002	0.34	633.08	0.13	0.04
Flucloxacillin	B*5701	DILI	296,467	0.0661	0.0011	0.076	19,596.47	12.56	1.64
Lamotrigine	B*1502	SJS/TEN	6426	0.0014	0.004	0.34	9.00	0.04	0.01
Oxcarbazepine	B*1502	SJS	1219	0.0014	0.0073	0.24	1.71	0.01	0.00
Phenytoin	B*1502	SJS/TEN	678	0.0014	0.0065	0.34	0.95	0.01	0.00

*HLA-B*5801* testing of all allopurinol starters and switching to an alternative drug when tested positive would prevent 21 cases of SJS/TEN and 3 cases of DRESS each year and is estimated to prevent 7 deaths each year.

Our results show that for some drugs-gene interactions, genotyping for HLA in the Dutch population would prevent less than one hypersensitivity reaction per year. This includes *HLA-B*1502* genotyping for lamotrigine, oxcarbazepine and phenytoin starters and *HLA-B*1511* testing for carbamazepine starters. *HLA-A*3101* testing for carbamazepine starters and switching to an alternative drug when tested positive would prevent 6 cases of DRESS per year.

*HLA-B*5701* testing for all flucloxacillin starters is estimated to prevent 22 hypersensitivity reactions and 2 deaths per year, but almost 300,000 people would need to be genotyped for *HLA-B*5701* each year.

2.6. Cost-Effectiveness Model

The net annual costs for the Dutch population for the genotyping strategy versus the standard care was calculated per drug–gene interaction. We considered a cost of 2 million euros per prevented death to be cost-effective [30]. Our results in Table 6 show that *HLA-B*5701* testing for abacavir starters is calculated to be cost saving. Annually, genotyping all 873 abacavir initiators and switching 58 *HLA-B*5701* positive patients to an alternative drug saves €34,000 in net costs in the Netherlands. Although not cost saving like testing for abacavir, genotyping *HLA-B*5801* for allopurinol starters would still be cost-effective. Annually, this would cost about 2 million euros and prevents 24 cases of allopurinol induced SCARS and 7 deaths. Ignoring the prevented ADR, the corresponding cost-effectiveness ratio is €282,000 to prevent one death. This is considered very cost-effective. Genotyping for HLA risk alleles for starters of antiepileptic drugs and flucloxacillin is not cost-effective. *HLA-B*1502*, *HLA-B*1511* and *HLA-A*3101* genotyping for carbamazepine initiators comes closest to being cost-effective with costs of 5 million euros per prevented death.

Table 6. Cost-effectiveness model parameters and results (all in euros).

Drug	HLA Allele	Outcome	Costs HLA Test	Costs Lab	Standard Costs per Day	Alternative Medsper Day	Costs per ADR	Net Costs NL	Net Costs per Patient	Costs per Prevented ADR	Costs per Prevented Death
abacavir	B*5701	ABC-HSR	79		29.62	29.54	3700	−34,000	−39	−1200	−1,770,000
allopurinol	B*5801	SJS/TEN	79		0.20	0.60	9100	2,040,000	74	97,000	287,000
allopurinol	B*5801	DRESS	79		0.20	0.60	6800	2,220,000	80	808,000	40,400,000
cllopurinol total			79		0.20	0.60		2,020,000	73	85,000	282,000
carbamazepine	B*1502	SJS/TEN	79		0.45	0.86	9100	754,000	79	41,400,000	119,000,000
carbamazepine	B*1511	SJS/TEN	79		0.45	0.86	9100	752,000	79	-	-
carbamazepine	A*3101	DRESS	79		0.45	0.86	6800	808,000	83	143,000	7,170,000
carbamazepine	A*3101	SJS/TEN	79		0.45	0.86	9100	846,000	89	6,680,000	19,600,000
carbamazepine total			79		0.45	0.86		808,000	83	143,000	4,990,000
flucloxacillin	B*5701	DILI	79	19	0.62	0.62	13,500	23,500,000	79	1,090,000	14,300,000
lamotrigine	B*1502	SJS/TEN	79		0.36	0.86	9100	509,000	79	14,100,000	41,600,000
oxcarbazepine	B*1502	SJS	79		0.87	0.86	9100	96,000	79	7,700,000	22,700,000
phenytoin	B*1502	SJS/TEN	79		0.21	0.86	9100	54,000	79	8,700,000	25,600,000

3. Discussion

Nationwide implementation of genotyping for specific HLA risk alleles before initiating drugs with an actionable drug–gene interaction and switching when tested positive can potentially save the life of 7 allopurinol initiators and 2 flucloxacillin initiators each year in The Netherlands. Besides these deaths, 28 cases of abacavir hypersensitivity, 24 cases of allopurinol induced SCARs, 6 cases of carbamazepine induced DRESS and 22 cases of flucloxacillin induced DILI can be prevented. Our analysis confirms the importance of mandatory testing of *HLA-B*5701* for abacavir starters since the number needed to genotype is only 31. Indeed, only 873 patients have to be genotyped and of these 58 *HLA-B*5701* positive patients have to switch to an alternative therapy to prevent 28 cases of abacavir hypersensitivity. This approach saves The Netherlands the limited amount of 34,000 euros each year. Promising seems to be *HLA-B*5801* testing for allopurinol starters with a number needed to genotype of 1149 initiators to prevent one case of SJS/TEN or DRESS. Testing of 27,585 allopurinol starters would prevent 21 cases of SJS/TEN, 3 cases of DRESS and 7 deaths each year. Especially patients with chronic renal insufficiency have a high chance of developing SJS/TEN when exposed to allopurinol. In this patient group, the PPV is tenfold higher. Therefore, genotyping for *HLA-B*5801* of this specific patient group would be the most obvious step forward for HLA testing in the Dutch population. HLA genotyping for AEDs and flucloxacillin is not cost-effective.

To our knowledge, this study is the first nationwide impact analysis and cost-effectiveness study of all, according to the CPIC and DPWG guidelines, actionable HLA-drug interactions. The analysis includes abacavir, allopurinol, carbamazepine, oxcarbazepine, lamotrigine, phenytoin and flucloxacillin. Zhou et al. have developed a global cost-effectiveness model to estimate country-specific cost-effectiveness thresholds for pre-emptive genetic testing for abacavir, allopurinol and carbamazepine [31]. However, in this study, The Netherlands was only included in the cost-effectiveness analysis of carbamazepine. Our study shows that testing for *HLA-B*1502* and *HLA-A*3101* is not cost-effective in the Dutch population. This is in disagreement with Zhou at al who estimated that HLA-A*3101 testing for carbamazepine is likely to be cost-effective, although the carrier frequency used in both studies is comparable. However, they assumed the costs of HLA testing would be only USD 40, which we currently consider too low.

Although our study focusses on the impact and cost-effectivity of genotyping for HLA risk alleles in The Netherlands, the results may be generalizable to other Caucasian European populations, if carrier frequencies and healthcare costs in those populations are comparable to the Dutch values.

A limitation of our study is that we used mainly input data of Caucasian populations. This leads to underestimating the usefulness of *HLA-B*1502* and *HLA-B*1511* for patients with Asian ancestry in The Netherlands for which HLA-B*1502 and HLA-B*1511 genotyping may be more useful than for the average Dutch population. However, because only 5.5% of the Dutch population has migrated from Asia, and of this 5.5% the majority comes from Indonesia where HLA studies are relatively scarce, this was considered to be the best approach. In contrast, we may have overestimated the usefulness of *HLA-B*1502* and *HLA-B*1511* for Caucasian lamotrigine, oxcarbazepine and phenytoin initiators. No data for a PPV in Caucasian populations was found for these drug–gene interactions and therefore we used PPVs originating from Asian studies which may have led to an overestimation of the utility of the HLA tests.

For an estimation of the number of patients initiating abacavir, allopurinol, flucloxacillin or one of the four AEDs we used data of first dispensations from the Dutch Foundation for Pharmaceutical Statistics. Conventionally, first dispensations are defined as a pharmacy dispensation without a previous dispensation of the same drug in the prior 12 months in the community pharmacy [16]. This probably leads to an overestimation of actual first starters, especially for flucloxacillin. The other drugs are often used chronically for many years while flucloxacillin can be used for a short duration multiple times in a lifetime but with more than 12 months between consecutive uses.

For the costs of treating the drug hypersensitivity reactions, we used the average of the prices charged by the Dutch academic hospitals. To check whether these are representative, we compared the used to costs found in the literature. The price used for abacavir hypersensitivity reaction was comparable to the costs of treating abacavir hypersensitivity reaction in a UK study and a German study [32,33]. The costs for treating DRESS used in this study (6800 euros) was considerably lower than found in a US study (17,000 USD) [34]. This is consistent with the generally higher price level of US healthcare, as compared to other high-income countries [35]. The average price for Dutch academic hospitals we used for SJS/TEN (9100 euros) was considerably lower than in a Dutch study in a burn center specialized in SJS/TEN [36]. We attribute this to the longer treatment duration and especially ICU stay for the severe cases that are referred to this burn center, as compared to the SJS/TEN in our study. Overall, we can conclude that the prices used in our cost-effectiveness model are comparable to costs in other western countries and can therefore be considered reliable estimates.

In this study we only focused on HLA associated hypersensitivity reactions and we did not take into account any other ADR of the studied drugs or of the drugs that could be used in case of a hypersensitivity reaction. Obviously, if a patient is tested positive for an HLA risk allele and the physician prescribes an alternative drug, this drug may also cause ADRs, or it might be less effective. Febuxostat, for instance, seems to have more cardiovascular adverse drug reactions than allopurinol but can also cause cutaneous hypersensitivity reactions, though these are rarer than with allopurinol and not associated with an HLA risk allele or other predictive biomarker [37–39].

We performed a cost-effectiveness analysis where we calculated genotyping for abacavir to be cost-saving, and genotyping for allopurinol to be cost-saving while for the other drugs genotyping is not cost-effective. We used a threshold of 2 million euros per prevented death, although the literature is not very clear what the threshold should be [30]. In many countries economic thresholds in terms of costs-per-QALY are used [40]. However, we felt using QALYs for our calculations would require making many uncertain assumptions and exploratory calculations suggested it would not change our conclusion.

Currently, the implementation of HLA testing in patients starting drugs with a known gene-drug interaction in The Netherlands remains low, despite available guidelines and actionability. Only for abacavir initiators, genotyping for *HLA-B*5701* is mandatory and routinely done and our study confirms this approach is cost-saving. The other HLA alleles are rarely tested before initiating drug therapy. Our study shows genotyping *HLA-B*5801* for allopurinol starters is cost-effective and can reduce morbidity and mortality and therefore it should be considered in pharmacogenetic implementation programs. Also genotyping carbamazepine starters with Asian ancestry should be considered, because of the high prevalence of *HLA-B*1502* in this population. However, genotyping all carbamazepine starters, regardless of ethnicity, is not cost-effective. Also genotyping for flucloxacillin, oxcarbazepine, lamotrigine and phenytoin is not cost-effective in the Dutch population.

4. Materials and Methods

4.1. Selection of Drug Gene Interactions

Gene-drug interactions with an actionable therapeutic recommendation for carriers of HLA risk alleles were selected from the DPWG guidelines. These include abacavir-*HLA-B*5701*, allopurinol-*HLA-B*5801*, carbamazepine-*HLA-B*1502*, *A*3101* and *B*1502*, flucloxacillin-*HLA-B*5701*, lamotrigine-*HLA-B*1502*, oxcarbazepine-*HLA-B*1502* and phenytoin-*HLA-B*1502*. The drug hypersensitivity reactions in this article are the drug hypersensitivity reactions as described in the DPWG guidelines [7–13].

4.2. Source of Nationwide Dispensing Data

Dutch dispensing data from "first dispensations" of the 7 selected drugs were collected for the period 1 January–31 December 2019 from the Dutch Foundation for Pharmaceutical Statistics or Stichting Farmaceutische Kengetallen (SFK). SFK is the Dutch Foundation for Pharmaceutical Statistics and collects exhaustive data about the use of dispensed drugs in the Netherlands. It contains data from more than 98% of the approximately 2000 community pharmacies in the Netherlands. These pharmacies combined serve about 15.8 million people from the population in The Netherlands [15]. Conventionally, first dispensations are defined as a dispensation without a previous dispensation within the prior 12 months in the community pharmacy [16].

4.3. Frequencies of HLA Variants

The allele frequencies of the HLA variants in the Dutch population were collected from the Allele Frequency Net Database and from a PubMed search. In the Allele Frequency Net Database all populations concerning the country The Netherlands were included. A PubMed search was performed using the search terms "(hla [ti]) AND (dutch [ti]) OR Netherlands [ti])" and relevant articles which include allele frequencies of the HLA variants of interest were included.

Three Dutch cohorts were found in the Allele Frequency Net Database and one cohort was retrieved using the PubMed search [17,18]. A weighted average of the allele frequencies of the 4 populations was calculated by performing a meta-analysis in R. Because of low heterogeneity, a fixed effects model was used.

The carrier frequency was subsequently calculated as follows:

$$\text{Carrier frequency} = 1 - (1 - \text{allele frequency})^2.$$

4.4. Positive Predictive Values

The PPVs for the actionable drug–gene interactions were retrieved from studies performed in Caucasian populations or from the DPWG guideline. If available, numbers for Caucasian populations were used, otherwise PPVs derived from other populations were used.

4.5. Morbidity and Mortality of Outcomes

The hypersensitivity reactions included in this article are abacavir hypersensitivity, allopurinol induced SCARs including DRESS and SJS/TEN, carbamazepine induced SCAR, lamotrigine and phenytoin induced SJS/TEN and oxcarbazepine induced SJS. Finally flucloxacillin induced DILI was also included. Estimates of the mortality of the included drug hypersensitivity reactions were collected from literature [26–29]. If possible, mortality estimates from European or other mainly Caucasian countries were used.

4.6. Estimation of Hypersensitivity Reactions and Deaths Prevented by Pre-Emptively Genotyping

The number of actionable drug–gene interactions is calculated by multiplying the number of first prescriptions by the allele carrier frequency of the associated HLA risk allele. Subsequently the estimated annual number of drug hypersensitivity reactions is calculated by multiplying the number of actionable drug–gene interactions by the positive predictive value of the HLA test for the outcome. Thus the annual number of drug hypersensitivity reactions is calculated by:

$$N_{ADR} = DISP \times CF \times PPV \quad (1)$$

N_{ADR} = number HLA associated hypersensitivity reactions prevented, DISP = number of first dispensations, CF = carrier frequency of HLA risk allele, PPV = positive predictive value of HLA test.

The annual number of deaths caused by HLA associated hypersensitivity reactions is calculated by multiplying the estimated number of drug hypersensitivity reactions by the mortality of the outcome:

$$N_{death} = N_{ADR} \times MORT \quad (2)$$

N_{death} = number of HLA associated deaths prevented, N_{ADR} = number HLA associated hypersensitivity reactions prevented, MORT = mortality.

4.7. Healthcare Costs

We compared the cost of two treatment strategies; no genetic test and initiation of the HLA allele associated drug, and testing for the HLA risk allele and switching to an alternative drug not associated with the same HLA risk allele when a patient tests positive for the HLA risk allele.

Costs are calculated with a one-year time-horizon, and reported in Euros at price level 2021. The costs of single-variant HLA tests were based on single-gene prices for genotyping (DNA amplification, manually) and a fixed price per lab-order for handling and administration set in the four hospitals who test for *HLA-B*5701* separately. The cost of drugs for the relevant reference drugs and the alternatives was based on the most common indication for the drug. The costs of the reference and alternative drugs were collected from the national drug price registry by selecting the most suitable dose and formulation [41]. The alternative drugs were chosen from existing guidelines for the most common indication of the drugs of interest.

In the case of flucloxacillin, unlike the other drugs of interest, the DPWG guideline does not recommend an alternative drug but instead recommends to monitor liver function. Only with increasing liver values, an alternative drug is recommended [8]. For the costs of the monitoring, the average cost from the Dutch academic hospitals was used for testing ALAT and ASAT and also includes a fixed price per lab-order for handling and administration and blood withdrawal. According to previous research, 0.0097% of all flucloxacillin initiators patients experience increasing liver values [42].

The costs used in the cost-effectiveness model are shown in Table 7.

Table 7. Model inputs for the healthcare costs.

Input	Costs in Euros	Source
HLA-A*3101 test	79	Average of 4 Dutch hospitals
HLA-B*1502 test	79	Average of 4 Dutch hospitals
HLA-B*1511 test	79	Average of 4 Dutch hospitals
HLA-B*5701 test	79	Average of 4 Dutch hospitals
HLA-B*5801 test	79	Average of 4 Dutch hospitals
Liver monitoring for HLA-B*5701 positive flucloxacillin users	19	Average of price charged by the Dutch academic hospitals
Triumeq (dolutegravir/abacavir/lamivudine)	29.62 per day	Medicijnkosten.nl [41]
Biktarvy (bictegravir/emtricabine/tenofoviralafenamide)	29.54 per day	Medicijnkosten.nl [41]
Allopurinol	0.20 per day	Medicijnkosten.nl [41]
Febuxostat	0.62 per day	Medicijnkosten.nl [41]
Lamotrigine	0.36 per day	Medicijnkosten.nl [41]
Phenytoin	0.21 per day	Medicijnkosten.nl [41]
Oxcarbazepine	0.87 per day	Medicijnkosten.nl [41]
Carbamazepine	0.45 per day	Medicijnkosten.nl [41]
Levetiracetam	0.86 per day	Medicijnkosten.nl [41]
Flucloxacillin	0.62 per day	Medicijnkosten.nl [41]
Clarithromycin	0.48 per day	Medicijnkosten.nl [41]
Abacavir hypersensitivity reaction	3700	Average of price charged by the Dutch academic hospitals
DRESS	6800	Average of price charged by the Dutch academic hospitals
SJS/TEN	9100	Average of price charged by the Dutch academic hospitals
SJS	9100	Average of price charged by the Dutch academic hospitals
DILI	13,500	Average of price charged by the Dutch academic hospitals

For the costs of treating drug hypersensitivity reactions the average of the prices charged by the seven academic hospitals (Amsterdam University Medical Center, University Medical Center Groningen, Leiden University Medical Center, Maastricht University Medical Center+, Radboud University Medical Center, Erasmus University Medical Center and University Medical Center Utrecht in The Netherlands was used. However, as a check to see whether these costs are representative a literature search was performed to compare the prices from the academic hospitals to the costs in previous clinical studies.

For abacavir hypersensitivity the price for "intensive treatment for allergy" was used (3700 euros). The European RegiSCAR study found a median stay of 17 days for DRESS patients. Because of this, the price for "6 to 28 days of treatment for inflammation of the skin" was used (6800 euros). For SJS, SJS/TEN and TEN the price for "6 to 28 days of treatment for a skin condition with blisters" was used (9100 euros). The costs used for DILI are an average of the prices for patient receiving a liver transplantation after suffering from DILI and patients not needing a liver transplantation. In the DILIN prospective study 3.8% of the patients suffering from DILI needed a liver transplant [29]. The price for "liver transplantation with a living donor with a maximum of 28 days due to severe liver failure" was used for patients needing a liver transplantation while the price for "hospital admission of 6–28 days for a disease of the liver" was used for the remaining 96.2% not needing a liver transplant.

4.8. Cost-Effectiveness Model

The net annual costs for the Dutch population for the genotyping strategy versus the standard care was calculated per drug–gene interaction as following:

$$\text{DISP} \times C_{test} + \text{HLA}^+ \times C_{mon} + (\text{HLA}^+ - \text{ADR}) \times 365 \times (C_{alt} - C_{ref}) - \text{ADR} \times C_{ADR} \quad (3)$$

With DISP as the number of first dispersions, C_{test} as the costs of the HLA test, HLA+ as the number of patients carrying the risk allele, C_{mon} as the costs for monitoring liver values in the case of flucloxacillin, ADR as the number of patients developing drug hypersensitivity, C_{alt} and C_{ref} as the daily drug costs of respectively the alternative and reference drug and C_{ADR} as the estimated costs of an hypersensitivity reaction.

We calculated cost-effectiveness ratios by dividing this impact on costs by the impact on the number of ADRs and deaths.

5. Conclusions

This study confirms the need for mandatory testing of *HLA-B*5701* in abacavir initiators, as indicated in the drug label, since it only has a number needed to genotype of 31 and implementation of this test is calculated to be cost-saving. Genotyping all carbamazepine, oxcarbazepine, lamotrigine, phenytoin and flucloxacillin initiators is not cost-effective in the overall Dutch population. However, our study shows genotyping *HLA-B*5801* for allopurinol starters is cost-effective and can reduce morbidity and mortality and therefore it should be considered in pharmacogenetic implementation programs.

Author Contributions: Conceptualization, L.E.N.M. and H.-J.G.; methodology, L.E.N.M., H.-J.G. and W.B.v.d.H.; formal analysis, L.E.N.M. and W.B.v.d.H.; data curation, L.E.N.M. and W.B.v.d.H.; writing—original draft preparation, L.E.N.M.; writing—review and editing, L.E.N.M., H.-J.G. and W.B.v.d.H.; visualization, L.E.N.M.; supervision, L.E.N.M., H.-J.G. and W.B.v.d.H.; funding acquisition, none. All authors have read and agreed to the published version of the manuscript.

Funding: The research leading to these results has received funding from the European Community's Horizon 2020 Programme under grant agreement No. 668353 (U-PGx).

Institutional Review Board Statement: Ethical review and approval were waived for this study, due to using only publically available data and retrospective data as provided by the SFK.

Informed Consent Statement: Not applicable.

Data Availability Statement: Data is contained within the article.

Conflicts of Interest: The authors declare no conflict of interest.

References

1. World Health Organization. *International Drug Monitoring: The Role of National Centres*; WHO Technical Report Series No. 498; World Health Organization: Geneva, Switzerland, 1972.
2. Bouvy, J.C.; De Bruin, M.L.; Koopmanschap, M.A. Epidemiology of adverse drug reactions in Europe: A review of recent observational studies. *Drug Saf.* **2015**, *38*, 437–453. [CrossRef] [PubMed]
3. Park, C.S.; Kim, T.B.; Kim, S.L.; Kim, J.Y.; Yang, K.A.; Bae, Y.J.; Cho, Y.S.; Moon, H.B. The use of an electronic medical record system for mandatory reporting of drug hypersensitivity reactions has been shown to improve the management of patients in the university hospital in Korea. *Pharmacoepidemiol. Drug. Saf.* **2008**, *17*, 919–925. [CrossRef] [PubMed]
4. Thong, B.Y.; Leong, K.P.; Tang, C.Y.; Chng, H.H. Drug allergy in a general hospital: Results of a novel prospective inpatient reporting system. *Ann. Allergy Asthma Immunol.* **2003**, *90*, 342–347. [CrossRef]
5. Swen, J.J.; Huizinga, T.W.; Gelderblom, H.; de Vries, E.G.; Assendelft, W.J.; Kirchheiner, J.; Guchelaar, H.J. Translating pharmacogenomics: Challenges on the road to the clinic. *PLoS Med.* **2007**, *4*, e209. [CrossRef]

6. Cheung, Y.K.; Cheng, S.H.; Chan, E.J.; Lo, S.V.; Ng, M.H.; Kwan, P. HLA-B alleles associated with severe cutaneous reactions to antiepileptic drugs in Han Chinese. *Epilepsia* 2013, *54*, 1307–1314. [CrossRef] [PubMed]
7. Koninklijke Nederlandse Maatschappij ter bevordering der Pharmacie. CARBAMAZEPINE HLA -B*1502–A*3101–B*1511. Available online: https://kennisbank.knmp.nl/article/farmacogenetica/6237-6238-6239.html (accessed on 31 October 2016).
8. Koninklijke Nederlandse Maatschappij ter bevordering der Pharmacie. FLUCLOXACILLINE HLA -B*5701. Available online: https://kennisbank.knmp.nl/article/farmacogenetica/4652.html (accessed on 20 November 2017).
9. Koninklijke Nederlandse Maatschappij ter bevordering der Pharmacie. LAMOTRIGINE HLA -B*1502. Available online: https://kennisbank.knmp.nl/article/farmacogenetica/6932.html (accessed on 14 May 2018).
10. Koninklijke Nederlandse Maatschappij ter bevordering der Pharmacie. OXCARBAZEPINE HLA -B*1502. Available online: https://kennisbank.knmp.nl/article/farmacogenetica/6931.html (accessed on 14 May 2018).
11. Koninklijke Nederlandse Maatschappij ter bevordering der Pharmacie. FENYTOINE HLA -B*1502. Available online: https://kennisbank.knmp.nl/article/farmacogenetica/6927.html (accessed on 14 May 2018).
12. Koninklijke Nederlandse Maatschappij ter bevordering der Pharmacie. ABACAVIR HLA -B*5701. Available online: https://kennisbank.knmp.nl/article/farmacogenetica/2356.html (accessed on 14 May 2018).
13. Koninklijke Nederlandse Maatschappij ter bevordering der Pharmacie. ALLOPURINOL HLA -B*5801. Available online: https://kennisbank.knmp.nl/article/farmacogenetica/6391.html (accessed on 14 May 2018).
14. Manson, L.E.N.; Swen, J.J.; Guchelaar, H.J. Diagnostic Test Criteria for HLA Genotyping to Prevent Drug Hypersensitivity Reactions: A Systematic Review of Actionable HLA Recommendations in CPIC and DPWG Guidelines. *Front. Pharmacol.* 2020, *11*, 567048. [CrossRef]
15. The Dutch Foundation for Pharmaceutical Statistics (SFK). SFK. 2019, Database. Available online: https://www.sfk.nl/publicaties/data-en-feiten/data-en-feiten-2019 (accessed on 20 November 2017).
16. Sodihardjo-Yuen, F.; van Dijk, L.; Wensing, M.; De Smet, P.A.; Teichert, M. Use of pharmacy dispensing data to measure adherence and identify nonadherence with oral hypoglycemic agents. *Eur. J. Clin. Pharmacol.* 2017, *73*, 205–213. [CrossRef]
17. Gonzalez-Galarza, F.F.; McCabe, A.; Santos, E.J.M.D.; Jones, J.; Takeshita, L.; Ortega-Rivera, N.D.; Cid-Pavon, G.M.D.; Ramsbottom, K.; Ghattaoraya, G.; Alfirevic, A.; et al. Allele frequency net database (AFND) 2020 update: Gold-standard data classification, open access genotype data and new query tools. *Nucleic Acid Res.* 2020, *48*, D783–D788. [CrossRef]
18. Hou, L.; Enriquez, E.; Persaud, M.; Steiner, N.; Oudshoorn, M.; Hurley, C.K. Next generation sequencing characterizes HLA diversity in a registry population from the Netherlands. *Hla* 2019, *93*, 474–483. [CrossRef]
19. Lonjou, C.; Borot, N.; Sekula, P.; Ledger, N.; Thomas, L.; Halevy, S.; Naldi, L.; Bouwes-Bavinck, J.N.; Sidoroff, A.; de Toma, C.; et al. A European study of HLA-B in Stevens-Johnson syndrome and toxic epidermal necrolysis related to five high-risk drugs. *Pharm. Genom.* 2008, *18*, 99–107. [CrossRef]
20. Goncalo, M.; Coutinho, I.; Teixeira, V.; Gameiro, A.R.; Brites, M.M.; Nunes, R.; Martinho, A. HLA-B*58:01 is a risk factor for allopurinol-induced DRESS and Stevens-Johnson syndrome/toxic epidermal necrolysis in a Portuguese population. *Br. J. Dermatol.* 2013, *169*, 660–665. [CrossRef]
21. Daly, A.K.; Donaldson, P.T.; Bhatnagar, P.; Shen, Y.; Pe'er, I.; Floratos, A.; Daly, M.J.; Goldstein, D.B.; John, S.; Nelson, M.R.; et al. HLA-B*5701 genotype is a major determinant of drug-induced liver injury due to flucloxacillin. *Nat. Genet.* 2009, *41*, 816–819. [CrossRef] [PubMed]
22. Amstutz, U.; Ross, C.J.; Castro-Pastrana, L.I.; Rieder, M.J.; Shear, N.H.; Hayden, M.R.; Carleton, B.C. HLA-A 31:01 and HLA-B 15:02 as genetic markers for carbamazepine hypersensitivity in children. *Clin. Pharmacol. Ther.* 2013, *94*, 142–149. [CrossRef]
23. Genin, E.; Chen, D.P.; Hung, S.I.; Sekula, P.; Schumacher, M.; Chang, P.Y.; Tsai, S.H.; Wu, T.L.; Bellon, T.; Tamouza, R.; et al. HLA-A*31:01 and different types of carbamazepine-induced severe cutaneous adverse reactions: An international study and meta-analysis. *Pharmacogenomics J* 2014, *14*, 281–288. [CrossRef] [PubMed]
24. Chen, C.B.; Hsiao, Y.H.; Wu, T.; Hsih, M.S.; Tassaneeyakul, W.; Jorns, T.P.; Sukasem, C.; Hsu, C.N.; Su, S.C.; Chang, W.C.; et al. Risk and association of HLA with oxcarbazepine-induced cutaneous adverse reactions in Asians. *Neurology* 2017, *88*, 78–86. [CrossRef]
25. Chen, Z.; Liew, D.; Kwan, P. Real-world cost-effectiveness of pharmacogenetic screening for epilepsy treatment. *Neurology* 2016, *86*, 1086–1094. [CrossRef] [PubMed]
26. Mounzer, K.; Hsu, R.; Fusco, J.S.; Brunet, L.; Henegar, C.E.; Vannappagari, V.; Stainsby, C.M.; Shaefer, M.S.; Ragone, L.; Fusco, G.P. HLA-B*57:01 screening and hypersensitivity reaction to abacavir between 1999 and 2016 in the OPERA((R)) observational database: A cohort study. *AIDS Res. Ther.* 2019, *16*, 1. [CrossRef]
27. Kardaun, S.H.; Sekula, P.; Valeyrie-Allanore, L.; Liss, Y.; Chu, C.Y.; Creamer, D.; Sidoroff, A.; Naldi, L.; Mockenhaupt, M.; Roujeau, J.C.; et al. Drug reaction with eosinophilia and systemic symptoms (DRESS): An original multisystem adverse drug reaction. Results from the prospective RegiSCAR study. *Br. J. Dermatol.* 2013, *169*, 1071–1080. [CrossRef]
28. Sekula, P.; Dunant, A.; Mockenhaupt, M.; Naldi, L.; Bouwes Bavinck, J.N.; Halevy, S.; Kardaun, S.; Sidoroff, A.; Liss, Y.; Schumacher, M.; et al. Comprehensive survival analysis of a cohort of patients with Stevens-Johnson syndrome and toxic epidermal necrolysis. *J. Invest. Dermatol.* 2013, *133*, 1197–1204. [CrossRef]
29. Hayashi, P.H.; Rockey, D.C.; Fontana, R.J.; Tillmann, H.L.; Kaplowitz, N.; Barnhart, H.X.; Gu, J.; Chalasani, N.P.; Reddy, K.R.; Sherker, A.H.; et al. Death and liver transplantation within 2 years of onset of drug-induced liver injury. *Hepatology* 2017, *66*, 1275–1285. [CrossRef]

30. Lindhjem, H.; Navrud, S.; Braathen, N.A.; Biausque, V. Valuing mortality risk reductions from environmental, transport, and health policies: A global meta-analysis of stated preference studies. *Risk Anal.* **2011**, *31*, 1381–1407. [CrossRef] [PubMed]
31. Zhou, Y.; Krebs, K.; Milani, L.; Lauschke, V.M. Global Frequencies of Clinically Important HLA Alleles and Their Implications For the Cost-Effectiveness of Preemptive Pharmacogenetic Testing. *Clin. Pharmacol. Ther.* **2021**, *109*, 160–174. [CrossRef]
32. Hughes, D.A.; Vilar, F.J.; Ward, C.C.; Alfirevic, A.; Park, B.K.; Pirmohamed, M. Cost-effectiveness analysis of HLA B*5701 genotyping in preventing abacavir hypersensitivity. *Pharmacogenetics* **2004**, *14*, 335–342. [CrossRef] [PubMed]
33. Wolf, E.; Blankenburg, M.; Bogner, J.R.; Becker, W.; Gorriahn, D.; Mueller, M.C.; Jaeger, H.; Welte, R.; Baudewig, M.; Walli, R.; et al. Cost impact of prospective HLA-B*5701-screening prior to abacavir/lamivudine fixed dose combination use in Germany. *Eur. J. Med. Res.* **2010**, *15*, 145–151. [CrossRef] [PubMed]
34. Wolfson, A.R.; Zhou, L.; Li, Y.; Phadke, N.A.; Chow, O.A.; Blumenthal, K.G. Drug Reaction with Eosinophilia and Systemic Symptoms (DRESS) Syndrome Identified in the Electronic Health Record Allergy Module. *J. Allergy Clin. Immunol. Pract.* **2019**, *7*, 633–640. [CrossRef]
35. Papanicolas, I.; Woskie, L.R.; Jha, A.K. Health Care Spending in the United States and Other High-Income Countries. *JAMA* **2018**, *319*, 1024–1039. [CrossRef] [PubMed]
36. Oen, I.M.; van der Vlies, C.H.; Roeleveld, Y.W.; Dokter, J.; Hop, M.J.; van Baar, M.E. Epidemiology and costs of patients with toxic epidermal necrolysis: A 27-year retrospective study. *J. Eur. Acad. Dermatol. Venereol.* **2015**, *29*, 2444–2450. [CrossRef]
37. Lin, C.W.; Huang, W.I.; Chao, P.H.; Chen, W.W.; Hsiao, F.Y. Risk of cutaneous adverse reactions associated with allopurinol or febuxostat in real-world patients: A nationwide study. *Int. J. Clin. Pract.* **2019**, *73*, e13316. [CrossRef] [PubMed]
38. Park, H.W.; Kim, D.K.; Kim, S.H.; Kim, S.; Chae, D.W.; Yang, M.S.; Oh, Y.K.; Lee, J.P.; Jung, J.W.; Shin, J.; et al. Efficacy of the HLA-B(*)58:01 Screening Test in Preventing Allopurinol-Induced Severe Cutaneous Adverse Reactions in Patients with Chronic Renal Insufficiency-A Prospective Study. *J. Allergy Clin. Immunol. Pract.* **2019**, *7*, 1271–1276. [CrossRef]
39. White, W.B.; Saag, K.G.; Becker, M.A.; Borer, J.S.; Gorelick, P.B.; Whelton, A.; Hunt, B.; Castillo, M.; Gunawardhana, L. Cardiovascular Safety of Febuxostat or Allopurinol in Patients with Gout. *N. Engl. J. Med.* **2018**, *378*, 1200–1210. [CrossRef] [PubMed]
40. Cameron, D.; Ubels, J.; Norström, F. On what basis are medical cost-effectiveness thresholds set? Clashing opinions and an absence of data: A systematic review. *Glob. Health Action* **2018**, *11*, 1447828. [CrossRef] [PubMed]
41. Zorginstituut Nederland. Available online: https://www.medicijnkosten.nl/ (accessed on 20 November 2017).
42. Wing, K.; Bhaskaran, K.; Pealing, L.; Root, A.; Smeeth, L.; van Staa, T.P.; Klungel, O.H.; Reynolds, R.F.; Douglas, I. Quantification of the risk of liver injury associated with flucloxacillin: A UK population-based cohort study. *J. Antimicrob. Chemother.* **2017**, *72*, 2636–2646. [CrossRef] [PubMed]

MDPI
St. Alban-Anlage 66
4052 Basel
Switzerland
Tel. +41 61 683 77 34
Fax +41 61 302 89 18
www.mdpi.com

Pharmaceuticals Editorial Office
E-mail: pharmaceuticals@mdpi.com
www.mdpi.com/journal/pharmaceuticals

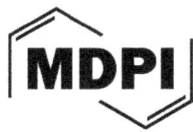

www.ingramcontent.com/pod-product-compliance
Lightning Source LLC
LaVergne TN
LVHW070407100526
838202LV00014B/1404